OFFICE
EMERGENCIES

OFFICE
EMERGENCIES

Marjorie A. Bowman, M.D., MPA
Chair, Department of Family Practice
University of Pennsylvania Hospital
Philadelphia, Pennsylvania

William G. Baxt, M.D.
Professor and Chair
Department of Emergency Medicine
University of Pennsylvania Hospital
Philadelphia, Pennsylvania

SAUNDERS
An Imprint of Elsevier Science

OFFICE EMERGENCIES   ISBN 0–7216–7779–7
Copyright 2003, Elsevier Science (USA). All rights reserved.

Notice

Medicine is an ever-changing field. Standard safety precautions must be followed but as new research and clinical experience broaden our knowledge, changes in treatment and drug therapy may become necessary or appropriate. Readers are advised to check the most current product information provided by the manufacturer of each drug to be administered to verify the recommended dose, the method and duration of administration, and contraindications. It is the responsibility of the treating physician, relying on experience and knowledge of the patient, to determine dosages and the best treatment for each individual patient. Neither the Publisher nor the authors assume any liability for any injury and/or damage to persons or property arising from this publication.

The Publisher

Library of Congress Cataloging-in-Publication Data

Office emergencies/edited by Marjorie A. Bowman, William G. Baxt.
   p. cm.
   ISBN 0–7216–7779–7
   1. Medical emergencies. 2. Ambulatory medical care. 3. Family medicine. I. Bowman, Marjorie A.
   II. Baxt, William G.
RC86.7.O35 2003
616′.025–dc21   2002075760

Acquisitions Editor: Steven Merahn, MD
Developmental Editor: Joanie Milnes
Senior Project Manager: Natalie Ware

RT/MVY
Printed in the United States of America.

Last digit is the print number: 9 8 7 6 5 4 3 2 1

Contributors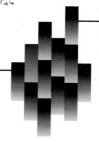

Louise Acheson, M.D., M.S.
Associate Professor of Family Medicine and
   Assistant Professor of Reproductive Biology, Case
   Western Reserve University and University
   Hospitals of Cleveland, Ohio
   Precipitous Delivery

Amy J. Behrman, M.D.
Associate Professor, Emergency Medicine,
   University of Pennsylvania School of Medicine;
   Director, Occupational Medicine, University of
   Pennsylvania, Philadelphia, Pennsylvania
   Environmental Emergencies

Ian M. Bennett, M.D., Ph.D.
Clinical Instructor, Department of Family Practice
   and Community Medicine, University of
   Pennsylvania, Philadelphia, Pennsylvania
   Infectious Emergencies

Marjorie A. Bowman, M.D., MPA
Professor and Chair, Department of Family Practice
   and Community Medicine, University of
   Pennsylvania, Philadelphia
   Hyperglycemia and Hypoglycemia

Victor Caraballo, M.D.
Medical Director, Independence Blue Cross,
   Philadelphia, Pennsylvania
   Coma and Altered Mental Status

Kevin M. Curtis, M.D., FACEP
Assistant Professor, Section of Emergency Medicine,
   Dartmouth-Hitchcock Medical Center, Lebanon,
   New Hampshire
   Head and Neck Emergencies

Elizabeth M. Datner, M.D.
Assistant Professor, Department of Emergency
   Medicine, Hospital of the University of
   Pennsylvania, Philadelphia, Pennsylvania
   First Trimester Emergencies; Spinal Injury

Francis DeRoos, M.D.

Assistant Professor, University of Pennsylvania
   School of Medicine;
   Residency Director, Department of Emergency
   Medicine, Hospital of the University of
   Pennsylvania, Philadelphia, Pennsylvania
   Acute Poisonings

Marilyn V. Howarth, M.D.

Assistant Professor, Occupational and Emergency
   Medicine, University of Pennsylvania School of
   Medicine; Director, Occupational and
   Environmental Consultation Services, Hospital of
   the University of Pennsylvania, Philadelphia,
   Pennsylvania
   Chemical Terrorism

John M. Howell, M.D., FACEP

Clinical Professor of Emergency Medicine,
   Georgetown University School of Medicine,
   Washington, D.C.; Director of Clinical Affairs,
   Department of Emergency Medicine, INOVA
   Fairfax Hospital, Falls Church, Virginia
   Chest Pain; Hyperglycemia and Hypoglycemia

Andy Jagoda, M.D., FACEP

Professor of Emergency Medicine, Mount Sinai
   School of Medicine, New York, New York
   Seizures

Jay R. Kostman, M.D.

Clinical Associate Professor of Medicine, University
   of Pennsylvania School of Medicine; Head,
   Division of Infectious Diseases, Presbyterian
   Medical Center, Philadelphia, Pennsylvania
   Infectious Emergencies

Steven Larson, M.D.

Assistant Professor of Emergency Medicine,
   University of Pennsylvania School of Medicine;
   Department of Emergency Medicine, Hospital of
   the University of Pennsylvania, Philadelphia,
   Pennsylvania
   Asthma; Orthopedic Urgencies; Anaphylaxis

Raymond H. Lucas, M.D.

Assistant Professor, Department of Emergency
   Medicine, George Washington University School
   of Medicine, Washington, D.C.; Chairman,
   Department of Emergency Medicine, Prince
   Georges Hospital Center, Cheverly, Maryland
   Transport and Transfer of Emergency Patients

Katherine Margo, M.D.
Assistant Professor and Predoctoral Director,
  University of Pennsylvania School of Medicine,
  Philadelphia, Pennsylvania
  Orthopedic Urgencies

C. Crawford Mechem, M.D., M.S.
Assistant Professor, University of Pennsylvania
  School of Medicine; Division Head, Emergency
  Medical Services, Department of Emergency
  Medicine, Hospital of the University of
  Pennsylvania; EMS Medical Director, Philadelphia
  Fire Department, Philadelphia, Pennsylvania
  Bioterrorism

Zachary F. Meisel, M.D., M.P.H.
Chief Resident, Department of Emergency Medicine,
  Hospital of the University of Pennsylvania,
  Philadelphia, Pennsylvania
  Hypertensive Urgencies

Richard A. Neill, M.D.
Assistant Professor, University of Pennsylvania
  School of Medicine, and Residency Program
  Director, Department of Family Practice and
  Community Medicine, Hospital of the University
  of Pennsylvania, Philadelphia, Pennsylvania
  Upper Airway Obstruction

James M. Nicholson, M.D.
Assistant Professor, University of Pennsylvania
  School of Medicine, Philadelphia, Pennsylvania
  Third Trimester Emergencies

David E. Nicklin, M.D.
Assistant Professor, Family Practice and Community
  Medicine, University of Pennyslvania School of
  Medicine, Philadelphia, Pennsylvania
  Chest Pain; Gastrointestinal Bleeding

Eugene Orientale, Jr., M.D.
Associate Professor, Family Medicine, University of
  Connecticut School of Medicine; Director,
  Principles of Clinical Medicine, St. Francis
  Hospital and Medical Center, Hartford,
  Connecticut
  *Electrolyte Disturbances; Transport and Transfer of
  Emergency Patients*

Iris M. Reyes, M.D., FACEP
Assistant Professor of Emergency Medicine,
  University of Pennsylvania School of Medicine;
  Philadelphia, Pennsylvania
  *Cardiac Ischemia; Hypertensive Urgencies; Psychosis;
  Chemical Terrorism*

Matthew H., Rusk, M.D., FACP

Director of Ambulatory Education, Department of
  Medicine, Hospital of the University of
  Pennsylvania; Assistant Professor of Medicine,
  University of Pennsylvania School of Medicine,
  Philadelphia, Pennsylvania
  Coma and Altered Mental Status

Ellen Sakornbut, M.D.

Executive Director, Northeast Iowa Medical
  Education Foundation, Waterloo, Iowa
  Acute Abdominal Pain; First Trimester Emergencies

Suzanne Moore Shephard, M.D., M.S., D.T.M.&H., FACEP

Associate Professor, Director of Education and
  Research, Penn Travel Medicine, Department of
  Emergency Medicine, Hospital of the University of
  Pennsylvania, Philadelphia, Pennsylvania
  Spinal Injury

William H. Shoff, M.D., D.T.M.&H.

Associate Professor and Director, Penn Travel
  Medicine, Department of Emergency Medicine,
  Hospital of the University of Pennsylvania,
  Philadelphia, Pennsylvania
  Spinal Injury

Robert Silbergleit, M.D.

Assistant Professor, Emergency Medicine, University
  of Michigan, Ann Arbor, Michigan
  Vascular Emergencies

John G. Spangler, M.D., M.P.H.

Associate Professor, Department of Family and
  Community Medicine, Wake Forest University
  School of Medicine, Winston-Salem, North
  Carolina
  Vascular Emergencies

Roger J. Zoorob, M.D., M.P.H.

Vice Chair, Residency Program Director, Louisiana
  State University Health Sciences Center School of
  Medicine, Department of Family Practice, Family
  Practice Residency Program, Kenner, Louisiana
  Acute Shortness of Breath

Preface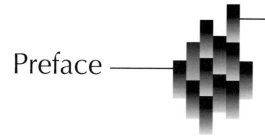

This book is designed to provide quick and accurate information on a broad range of urgent problems and emergencies that present by telephone or in person at a primary care office or urgent care center. Chapters have been kept brief, practical, and highly concise to allow for rapid reference by the busy practitioner who needs fast answers to emergency questions. Tips for recognition of emergencies by both triage staff members and clinicians are provided. Specific steps for staff and clinicians, to prioritize treatment, are given, including the need for equipment in the office and during any required transfer. Office emergencies presenting in the pediatric age group are considered specifically. The authors are academic primary care physicians and emergency medicine physicians, providing authoritative information based on both literature evidence and practical experience. This combines the state-of-the-art in emergency care with the realities of practice in an outpatient office, both near and far from hospital facilities. The book also includes chapters devoted to both chemical and biological terrrorism, which have recently become major concerns for all primary practitioners.

Many physicians and health care providers will find this book useful: family physicians, general internists, emergency physicians practicing urgent care, physician assistants, nurse practitioners, and other office physicians or health care providers in whose practice location emergencies may arise.

Acknowledgements

Our special thanks and gratitude go to Dr. James Scott, who initiated this book, including the conceptualization and format. We greatly appreciate the work of our editors and copy editors. Our sincere appreciation is also extended to the many contributors who have sacrificed their time and given of their talents, even when the co-editors were taskmasters.

Dr. Marjorie A. Bowman
Dr. William G. Baxt

Contents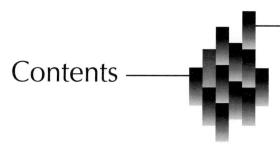

Chapter 1

Upper Airway Obstruction

Richard Neill

CLINICAL RECOGNITION

Early symptoms of upper airway obstruction vary by cause and can include stridor, paroxysmal cough, inability to swallow saliva, prurulent nasal discharge with sneezing, hoarseness, or rhonchorous breathing. If symptoms are severe and remain untreated, patients rapidly become apneic and cyanotic and lose consciousness. Death follows within minutes unless the airway can be restored. Fortunately, most patients presenting to physicians' offices have less severe symptoms, which allows additional time for assessment and tailoring of treatment to specific causes.

The differential diagnosis is less important than the initial management given the life-threatening consequences of untreated airway obstruction. In general, however, the differential diagnosis includes foreign body obstruction, anaphylaxis, infectious causes (e.g., epiglottitis, peritonsillar or hypopharyngeal abscess), tumor, and trauma. Less common causes include blood clots, thyroiditis, and achalasia. See Table 1–1 for a complete list of causes of upper airway obstruction in children and adults.

Patient age and concurrent symptoms assist the clinician in narrowing diagnostic possibilities and guiding initial management plans. A toddler presenting with fever, stridor, and drooling should be presumed to have epiglottitis, although croup can mimic these symptoms. Generalized wheezing implies reactive airway disease, although localized wheezes may indicate a foreign body. Antecedent upper respiratory symptoms and a deviated uvula suggest peritonsillar abscess. Lip or tongue swelling with wheezing raises suspicion of anaphylaxis.

1

Table 1–1. Differential Diagnosis of Upper Airway Obstruction by Location

Location	Causes
Mouth/pharynx	Suppurative parotitis
	Tonsillar hypertrophy/peritonsillar abscess
	Ludwig's angina
	Macroglossia
	Sublingual hematoma
	Lingual cellulitis
	Retropharyngeal abcess
Larynx	Cancer
	Hamartoma
	Laryngeal stenosis
	Laryngeal edema due to anaphylactic reactions/C1 inhibitor
	deficiency/angiotensin-converting enzyme inhibitor use
	Postextubation
	Burns
	Laryngeal tuberculosis
Epiglottis	Epiglottitis
	Redundant epiglottic fold
Vocal cords	Polyps, papillomatosis
	Vocal cord palsy
	Unilateral
	Cancer, recurrent laryngeal nerve injury, vagal nerve injury
	Bilateral
	Laryngeal dystonia due to Parkinson's or Gerhardt's syndrome,
	neuroleptic medications, Shy-Drager syndrome,
	olivopontocerebellar atrophy
	Metabolic disturbances such as hypokalemia, hypocalcemia
	Relapsing polychondritis
	Intracranial tumors
	Odontoid peg subluxation
	Laryngeal dyskinesia
	Rheumatoid arthritis
	Foreign bodies
Trachea	Tracheomalacia
	Tumors
	Compression
	Thyroid goiter/carcinoma
	Esophageal
	Foreign body
	Esophageal achalasia
	Vascular
	Arterial puncture
	Ruptured thoracic aorta
	Superior vena cava obstruction
	Aortic dissection
	Pulmonary vascular sling
	Innominate artery aneurysm
	Fluid extravasation from central catheter
	Bronchogenic cysts
	Hodgkin's with mediastinal involvement
	Tracheal stenosis
	Subglottic
	Laryngotracheobronchitis (croup)
	Wegener's granulomatosis
	Tracheal
	Post-tracheostomy
	Postintubation
	Tracheal narrowing
	Mucous ball from transtracheal catheter
	Tracheitis

Adapted from Aboussouan LS, Stoller JK: Diagnosis and management of upper airway obstruction. Clin Chest Med 15:35–53, 1994.

PHONE TRIAGE ◄——————————————————

When patients are triaged by telephone, a positive response to any of the following questions warrants emergent evaluation:

Is the patient unable to speak?

Is there nasal flaring, or are neck muscles used to breathe?

Is the patient unable to breathe when lying down?

Is there a blue or gray discoloration in the fingernail beds, lips, or ear lobes?

Initial Management

The initial management decision involves an assessment of the severity of obstruction. In severe or abrupt cases, cardiopulmonary resuscitation principles apply. When symptoms are less severe, additional diagnostic studies can help guide treatment.

Frank stridor, hoarseness, inability to speak, and diminished sensorium all indicate more serious obstruction. When any of these is present, the clinician should initiate evaluation of airway, breathing, and circulation (ABCs) immediately (Fig. 1–1). Check the patient for response by asking, "Are you OK?" If the patient does not respond, call for assistance, then position the patient on the back to facilitate resuscitation. Assess respiratory efforts by looking for chest movement, listening for breath sounds at the patient's mouth, and feeling for air movement on your cheek. If the patient is apneic, inspect and clear the airway of any foreign material. Then use a head tilt and chin lift to open the airway, and prepare for artificial ventilation (with attention to the neck if cervical instability is suspected). If the patient remains apneic after positioning and airway clearing have been done, initiation of artificial respiration is called for, preferably with the use of a bag-valve mask. Two short rescue breaths should be attempted with an insufflation time of 1.5 to 2.0 seconds for each. Assess the adequacy of ventilation again by looking, listening, and feeling. Inadequate ventilation should prompt a second attempt to clear the airway, followed by up to five repeated attempts at ventilation. Continued inability to ventilate despite repeated attempts to clear the airway warrants cricothyroidotomy if your office is so equipped. Although many authorities recommend maneuvers to remove impacted food when aspiration is suspected, this more commonly occurs as a witnessed event outside the physician's office.

Less severe obstruction may allow additional diagnostic testing before treatment, but airway obstruction can develop rapidly, even when the initial presentation may be reassuring. For this reason, any suspected

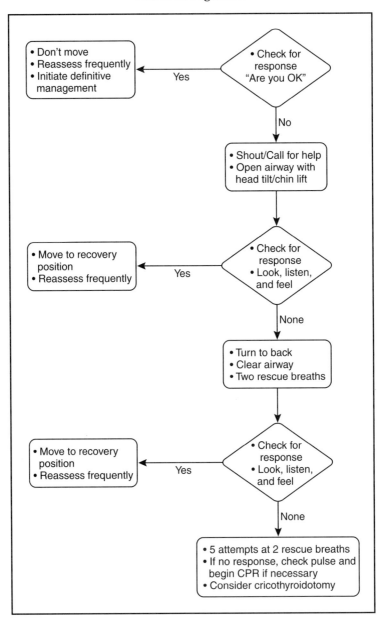

Figure 1–1. Algorithm for initial management of suspected airway obstruction in the office. Adapted from Circulation 95(8):2174–2179, April 15, 1997. CPR, cardiopulmonary resuscitation.

airway obstruction should prompt referral to a setting in which airway emergencies can be managed definitively. This can be important when one is considering diagnoses such as epiglottitis, wherein oral examination might precipitate obstruction, or peritonsillar abscess, for which drainage under controlled conditions is recommended. Anaphylactic shock and foreign body aspiration represent two additional circumstances in which initial findings may rapidly progress to life-threatening emergencies because of airway obstruction.

Plain film or computed tomographic imaging is helpful in locating foreign bodies, differentiating epiglottitis from croup, demarcating tumors or abscesses, and assessing adequacy of endotracheal tube placement.

Stabilization for transport has been established when a stable airway and adequate oxygenation are ensured. Although some patients may be stable for transport without requiring additional ventilatory support, for most patients, rapid access to supplies necessitates ambulance transport with trained personnel. The least invasive measures, such as supplemental oxygen via nasal cannula or mask, can be augmented by bag-valve mask ventilation, or in more urgent circumstances, by laryngeal mask airways, endotracheal intubation, or cricothyroidotomy.

Equipment and Medications

Many companies now sell prepackaged emergency kits for office-based practice that include the majority of supplies needed for management of airway obstruction and other common office emergencies.[1] Physicians can also equip their own kits by paying attention to regular restocking of expired medications (Table 1–2).

Disposition and Transfer

An adequate airway allows ventilation sufficient to maintain oxygenation as measured by physical examination or through direct measurement by pulse oximetry or arterial blood gas determination. Return of pink color, normal vital signs, and disappearance of symptoms of distress all suggest adequate ventilation.

Table 1–2. Supplies for Office Management of Airway Obstruction

Bag-valve masks for infants, children, adolescents, and adults
Endotracheal tubes—sizes 3 mm, 5 mm, 7 mm with stylet
Laryngoscopes with light source—adult and pediatric with curved/straight blade as preferred
Oxygen canister with tubing for attachment to bag-valve mask
Non-rebreather masks
Oropharyngeal airways, various sizes
Suction device with appropriate sterile tubing
Nebulizer
Epinephrine 1:1000
Albuterol solution for inhalation/albuterol inhaler
Ammonia inhaler

Because of the variety of causes underlying upper airway obstruction, it is impossible to recommend a single course for disposition of patients treated in the office. Although some patients may be safely managed and discharged home following office treatment (e.g., nasal foreign body removal), a majority will require ambulance transport to the nearest facility capable of handling life-threatening airway obstruction. Transport personnel should, at a minimum, have Advanced Cardiac Life Support (ACLS) training and be capable of both maintaining airway control and initiating additional measures when airway control is lost.

The nature of the obstruction may also dictate transport to higher-level emergency facilities in some circumstances. Traumatic obstruction with airway involvement warrants referral to trauma centers with appropriate surgical and anesthesia personnel. Air ambulance is warranted to expedite transport of patients with airway obstruction when definitive care is unattainable in the current setting. In these instances, airway management efforts should continue during transport until stabilization is attained and definitive treatment for the underlying cause can ensue.

Epidemiology and Pathophysiology

Many excellent reviews of the broad causes of airway obstruction have been written.[2-8] Fortunately, life-threatening upper airway obstruction rarely presents in office practice. By its nature, onset, and course, airway obstruction more commonly presents either in hospitalized patients or in the community, with transport of patients directly to emergency care settings.

Foreign body aspiration is the most common cause of acute upper airway obstruction.[9] Although this is more common in children, adults with dysphagia or other neurologic impairment of swallowing may also present in this manner. Aspiration usually causes acute onset of wheezing, stridor, and/or hoarseness. In children, these symptoms may occur hours to days after aspiration, when inflammatory changes in the upper airways augment the obstruction, causing a subacute onset of obstructive symptoms, often accompanied by fever that confuses the presentation.

Pediatrics

Upper airway obstruction in children is distinctly different from that in adults owing to congenital deformities not typically seen in adults. Also, children's smaller airways succumb more easily to inflammatory processes that are easily tolerated by adults.[10-12] A good example of this is croup (laryngotracheobronchitis). When croup occurs, an infection, usually parainfluenza virus, causes inflammation of the trachea and larynx, leading to reduced caliber of the supraglottic airway with a resulting characteristic stridorous inspiration followed by a barky cough. Although similar viral infection occurs in older children and adults, the larger caliber of their airways prevents the disturbances in laminar airflow seen in affected children.

Episodes of epiglottitis have diminished dramatically since the introduction of vaccines effective against the most common causative agent, *Haemophilus influenzae* type b. Lateral neck radiographs help to differentiate croup from epiglottitis when they show the characteristic "thumbprint" sign, indicating a swollen, boggy epiglottis. Radiographs should be performed before any invasive examination of the oropharynx in children suspected of having epiglottitis given rare reports of examination-induced laryngospasm that causes acute worsening of obstruction.

Physicians should become familiar with the hospitals in their referral area that are capable of handling pediatric emergencies.

References

1. Statkit. Banyan International Corporation, 2118 E. Interstate 20, P.O. Box 1779, Abilene, Tex 79604–1779. Phone: 800-351-4530. Internet: http://www.StatKit.com.
2. Aboussouan LS, Stoller JK: Diagnosis and management of upper airway obstruction. Clin Chest Med 15:35–53, 1994.
3. Deem S, Bishop MJ: Evaluation and management of the difficult airway. Crit Care Clin 11:1–27, 1995.
4. Josephson GD, Josephson JS, Krespi YP, et al: Airway obstruction. New modalities in treatment. Med Clin North Am 77:539–549, 1993.
5. Eagle CJ: The compromised airway: Recognition and management. Can J Anaesth 39(5 Pt 2):40–52, 1992.
6. Fitzpatrick PC, Guarisco JL: Pediatric airway foreign bodies. J Louisiana State Med Soc 150:138–141, 1998.
7. John SD, Swischuk LE: Stridor and upper airway obstruction in infants and children. Radiographics 12:625–643, 1992.
8. Kharasch M, Graff J: Emergency management of the airway. Crit Care Clin 11:53–66, 1995.
9. Somanath BP, Singhi S: Airway foreign bodies in children. Indian Pediatr 32:890–897, 1995.
10. Shechtman FG: Office evaluation of pediatric upper airway obstruction. Otolaryngol Clin North Am 25:857–865, 1992.
11. Tobias JD: Airway management for pediatric emergencies. Pediatr Ann 25:317–320, 1996.
12. Rencken I, Patton WL, Brasch RC: Airway obstruction in pediatric patients. From croup to BOOP. Radiol Clin North Am 36:175–187, 1998.

Chapter 2
Asthma
Steven Larson

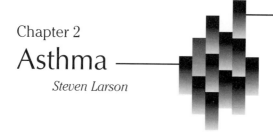

Asthma is a disease of the airways manifested by "increased airway responsiveness to stimuli, resulting in bronchoconstriction, bronchial wall edema, and the development of thick, tenacious secretions."[1] These changes produce increased airway resistance, decreased forced expiratory volume in 1 second (FEV_1), reduced flow rates, lung hyperinflation, increased ventilation-perfusion (V/Q) mismatch, and ultimately, increased labor of breathing.

Asthma affects an estimated 4% to 5% of the U.S. population. Although asthma is a disease found in people of all ages, it predominantly manifests early in life; nearly 50% of patients are diagnosed before age 10, and an additional 30% are diagnosed before age 40. Asthma is typically an episodic disease, with acute exacerbations interspersed between symptom-free periods. The average asthmatic patient spends 5 to 8 days annually in bed, with an additional 15 days of diminished activity each year.[2]

Asthma is a heterogeneous disease that shares as a common denominator increased airway reactivity in response to a variety of initiating stimuli. It is typically classified into two broad groups: allergic and idiosyncratic. Allergic asthma is found in less than 10% of the asthmatic population. It develops early in childhood and is associated with inhaled allergens, a family history of asthma/allergies (e.g., rhinitis, urticaria, eczema), increased levels of immunoglobulin E (IgE), increased eosinophilia, and positive skin testing. Idiosyncratic asthma implies a lack of classification based on the absence of defined immunologic mechanisms. Included in this category is asthma associated with a variety of physical, environmental, or pharmacologic stimuli.

CLINICAL RECOGNITION

Asthma classically presents as a triad of cough, shortness of breath, and wheezing. At the onset of an asthma flare, patients sense a constrictive sensation in the chest. They typically present with heightened levels of anxiety, tachycardia, and tachypnea. Patients with severe attacks find it difficult to complete sentences. They may sit upright in an attempt to maximize their respiratory efforts. On examination,

9

retractions of the sternocleidomastoid muscles, as well as the intercostal muscles, may be noted in patients experiencing moderate to severe asthmatic attacks. Audibly harsh wheezing in both the inspiratory and expiratory phases of respiration may be noted. Diffuse expiratory wheezing with a prolonged expiratory phase may be noted on auscultation. The absence of wheezing on examination does not exclude asthma from the diagnosis. The presence of wheezing is dependent on air velocity and turbulence. The finding of a "silent chest" is ominous in acute asthma, suggesting insufficient air movement and impending respiratory collapse.

Evaluation of the asthmatic patient's respiratory status is crucial on a minute-by-minute basis as rapid deterioration of ventilatory efforts may result in respiratory arrest. Clinicians need to rely on their clinical skills to determine a baseline for their patient's condition, as well as the efficacy of their therapeutic interventions. In addition to auscultation, physicians must pay close attention to mental status changes in their patients, as these may be the earliest clinical indicators of respiratory failure. Mental status changes in asthmatic patients may be subtle, ranging from confusion and somnolence to anxiety and panic, and should raise concern of impending "fatigue" of the accessory muscles of respiration with resultant hypoxia and hypercarbia from inadequate ventilation.

 PHONE TRIAGE ◄————————————————————

The severity of an asthma flare can be difficult to gauge over the phone. Patients who are unable to complete sentences owing to shortness of breath require immediate medical attention. They should be directed at once to either their primary care provider's office or the nearest emergency department.

Additionally, careful attention should be paid to patients' "asthma history": Have they used steroids? Have they ever been intubated? How frequent are their flares? When was their last hospital admission? Are they having fevers, chills, or a change in sputum production? The patient with a history of severe asthmatic attacks (manifested by use of steroids, previous intubations, and multiple hospitalizations) must be considered high risk for a bad outcome, as is the patient with repeated visits for an attack over a short period. The latter group is representative of patients who experience increased morbidity and mortality from status asthmaticus.

Finally, patients often present with asthma flares in the setting of upper respiratory infection, as well as exposure to known stimuli. One must consider infection in any febrile asthmatic patient, and the history should include questions about recent earaches, sore throats, or changes in sputum production.

LABORATORY RECOGNITION

When patients are on the verge of fatigue or are experiencing a severe asthmatic flare, it may be difficult for the clinician to gauge the severity of the attack. Given the broad spectrum of clinical presentations for the acute asthmatic patient, a rapid and objective index for staging the illness and evaluating therapy is useful. Although some clinicians advocate the use of arterial blood gases (ABGs) to stage the severity of illness, neither pretreatment nor post-treatment ABGs are useful in predicting outcome.[3]

The FEV_1 and the peak expiratory flow rate (PEFR) are two tools that can help clinicians gauge the severity of an asthma flare, as well as patient response to therapy. For use in the outpatient or emergency setting, the PEFR (standardized according to the patient's age, sex, and height) is the easier measurement to obtain and serves as a powerful adjunct to the clinician's examination, providing a quantitative baseline measure of respiratory reserve. Additionally, when followed serially, the PEFR is a reliable indicator of therapeutic efficacy. As a reference point, an initial PEFR of less than 100 L/min (less than 20% predicted) is indicative of severe obstruction.[4]

Laboratory testing is generally of little help in management of the asthmatic patient; however, a complete blood count (CBC) may be useful in the infected patient with sepsis or pneumonia. Individuals with fever or a change in sputum may warrant a chest radiograph to evaluate for pneumonia; however, this remains a clinical decision.

Initial Management

The goal in management of an acute asthma flare is the rapid reversal of airway obstruction. Traditionally, this is accomplished through therapeutic interventions aimed at providing immediate relief from smooth muscle bronchospasm as well as reducing the inflammatory response of the airway. As a prelude to pharmacologic intervention, intravenous access is recommended for patients with severe asthma (PEFR < 100). Supplemental

ASTHMA

oxygen should be administered to maintain a pulse oximeter level greater than 90%.

The mainstay of initial treatment involves the use of adrenergic agents that bind to cell receptors to produce α and/or β stimulation. Selective stimulation of β_2 receptors through the use of β_2 agonists results in the synthesis of cyclic adenosine monophosphate (cAMP) and the subsequent relaxation of bronchial smooth muscle. Additionally, β_2 stimulation inhibits mast cell release of histamine, a causative agent of bronchospasm. The effects of β_2 stimulation are rapid in onset. Adrenergic agents are administered either by inhalation or through subcutaneous delivery.

Inhalation of aerosolized medication offers direct delivery to airway mucosa. In the setting of an acute asthma flare, it is the preferred route of delivery for adrenergic agents. Inhalational delivery of medications can be accomplished either by the aerosolized, hand-held nebulizer or via metered-dose inhaler (MDI). Evidence suggests that the MDI is equal to the nebulizer in providing bronchodilatation; however, patient difficulty with appropriate use of the MDI (particularly in the setting of an acute flare) makes the nebulizer the preferred method of delivery in the emergency department.[5]

Albuterol, a β_2-selective, long-acting medication, is the preferred adrenergic agent for use in acute asthma exacerbations. It is administered in 2.5-mg doses (mixed with normal saline solution) via a nebulizer three times over 60 to 90 minutes.[6]

Subcutaneous delivery of epinephrine, an endogenous catecholamine that exerts both α and β smooth muscle effects, has historically been used in the treatment of asthma. Although it is effective in the setting of an acute asthma flare, the resulting tachycardia and hypertension and the increased incidence of cardiac dysrhythmia limit its clinical usefulness. This treatment should be used with caution in the elderly population. Terbutaline is a β_2-specific, longer-acting agent with bronchodilatory effects similar to those of subcutaneous epinephrine. Both agents can be an effective adjunct to nebulizer therapy, particularly in those patients with a markedly depressed PEFR, in whom mechanical ability to use a nebulizer is diminished.

Corticosteroids play a well-defined role in the management of both acute and chronic asthma. Glucocorticoids, powerful regulators of cellular inflammation, decrease cellular inflammation and bronchial hyperresponsiveness. Clinical improvement can be noted within 3 hours of administration; however, significant improvement in pulmonary function typically occurs within 6 to 12 hours. Either methylprednisolone 60 to 125 mg IV or prednisone 60 mg orally is administered.

Anticholinergic agents, particularly atropine-like agents, are potent bronchodilators that override the smooth muscle constrictor and secretory actions of the parasympathetic nervous system. Undesirable side effects limit their use; however, quaternary derivatives, which are poorly absorbed through mucosal surfaces, cause fewer side effects, making them a useful adjunct to β_2-agonist therapy in patients with severe obstruction. Their onset of action is typically 30 minutes and their effects last up to 8 hours. They are administered via the nebulizer simultaneously with albuterol in dosages ranging from .25 to .5 mg for ipratroprium.

Disposition and Transfer

The decision to refer a patient on to an emergency department remains a clinical one. Clearly, patients with impending respiratory compromise (silent chest) and/or those individuals demonstrating an alteration in their sensorium consistent with either hypercarbia or hypoxia give cause for prompt activation of the 911 system. However, in those individuals with moderate to severe asthma flares, as manifested by a peak expiratory flow less than 50% predicted, it is reasonable to attempt to stabilize and potentially reverse their clinical course in the office setting through an aggressive series of treatments using the various bronchodilating agents discussed earlier (Fig. 2–1). Through repeated treatments and periods of observation and reassessment, the progress of the acute asthmatic patient can be followed safely. Patients demonstrating a good response to initial therapy, as manifested by a PEFR greater than 70 predicted and marked improvement in symptoms, may be safely discharged home from

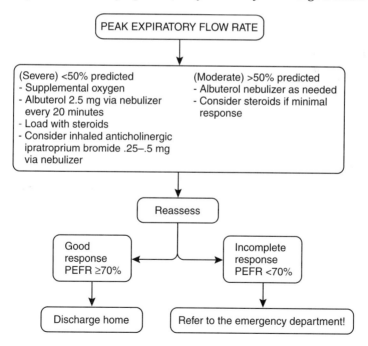

Figure 2–1. Emergent office management of the acute asthmatic patient.

the office on inhalational β-adrenergic therapy and corticosteroids. For those individuals failing to improve symptomatically or who are unable to attain a PEFR greater than 70% predicted, referral to the emergency department for further management is necessary. Additionally, patients with clinical evidence of an underlying respiratory tract infection should be managed cautiously, given the presence of a cause for persistent bronchospasm.

Pediatrics

Children with an asthma flare classically present with wheezing and respiratory distress. As in adults, however, cough, shortness of breath, fatigue, and/or chest pain may be principal symptoms. A rapid initial assessment of the child's respiratory status should include close attention to mental status, the use of accessory muscles, nasal flaring, and the presence of wheezing. When possible, measurement of the patient's PEFR should be attained. Treatment with oxygen, albuterol, steroids, and serial examination follows the algorithm outlined in Figure 2–1.

References

1. Sears ME: The definition and diagnosis of asthma. Allergy 48:12, 1993.
2. Cydulka RA: Asthma. In Harwood-Nuss A (ed): The Clinical Practice of Emergency Medicine, 3rd ed. Philadelphia, Lippincott, 2001, pp 740–745.
3. Nowak RM, Tomlanovich MC, Sarkar DD: Arterial blood gases and pulmonary function testing in acute bronchial asthma: Predicting patient outcomes. JAMA 249:2043, 1983.
4. Nowak RM, Pensler MI, Sarkar DD: Comparison of peak expiratory flow and FEV1, admission criteria for acute bronchial asthma. Ann Emerg Med 11:64, 1982.
5. Idris AH, McDermott MF, Raucci JC, et al: Emergency department treatment of severe asthma. Metered dose inhaler plus holding chamber is equivalent in effectiveness to nebulizer. Chest 103:665, 1993.
6. U.S. Department of Health and Human Services: Management of exacerbations of asthma. In Guidelines for the Diagnosis and Management of Asthma: National Asthma Education Program Expert Panel Report 2 (NIH Publication 97–4051). Bethesda, Md, Department of Health and Human Services, April 1997.

Chapter 3
Cardiac Ischemia

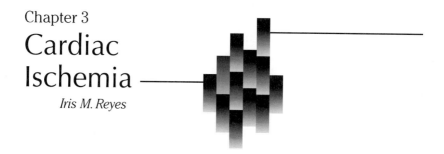

Iris M. Reyes

Chest pain is one of the most common symptoms for which patients seek evaluation in emergency departments. It is also one of the most complex, with diagnoses ranging from non–life-threatening conditions such as muscle strain and indigestion, to those requiring emergent lifesaving intervention such as myocardial ischemia or infarction, thoracic dissection, and pulmonary embolus. Many patients with acute coronary syndromes defined as acute myocardial infarctions or unstable angina have atypical presentations that are difficult to diagnose in the outpatient setting with a history, physical examination, and electrocardiogram (ECG). The ECG may be normal or nondiagnostic up to 55% of the time. If the patient is not admitted for further evaluation, the diagnosis may be missed. Misdiagnosis of an acute coronary syndrome can result in serious morbidity or mortality for the patient. It is also a frequent cause of malpractice suits against emergency physicians.

In the United States, approximately 1.5 million hospitalizations occur annually for acute coronary syndromes. Despite significant innovations over the past 20 years, the percentage of patients admitted to hospitals may actually be increasing. The reasons for this are well known to most emergency physicians. Approximately 2% to 8% of patients with myocardial infarction are mistakenly discharged from emergency departments.[1] Short-term mortality rates as high as 25% have been documented for these patients.[2] This rate is twice that of patients hospitalized for myocardial infarction. The legal costs are enormous as well. It is estimated that 20% of money awarded against emergency physicians is related to the misdiagnosis of acute coronary syndromes.

The attempt by cautious emergency physicians to lower the misdiagnosis rate has led to an increase in the hospitalization rate of patients presenting with symptoms or findings suspicious for an acute coronary syndrome. Of those admitted under these circumstances, approximately 30% are found to have an acute myocardial infarction or unstable angina. In the United States, annual health care costs for these potentially unnecessary hospitalizations can be as high as $5 billion.[3]

Key guidelines for the diagnosis and management of acute myocardial infarction have been published by several agencies, including the American College of Emergency Physicians (www.acep.org), the Agency for Health Care Policy and Research (www.ahcpr.gov), the American College of Cardiology (www.acc.org), the American Heart Association (www.Americanheart.org), and the National Heart Attack Alert Program (www.nhlbi.nih.gov).[4-7] The goal of these guidelines is the timely and appropriate care of patients presenting with an acute myocardial infarction, unstable angina, or other life-threatening conditions such as aortic dissection and pulmonary embolus. In addition to hastening the implementation of therapy for patients with acute coronary syndromes, these guidelines may assist in expediting the evaluation of low-risk patients.

CLINICAL RECOGNITION ◄———————————

Evaluation of patients with acute chest pain for an acute coronary syndrome includes obtaining a history that reviews the character of the symptoms and provides an assessment of significant risk factors. A physical examination should be performed that specifically addresses vital signs, along with a cardiopulmonary evaluation. An assessment for evidence of heart failure should be performed.

Familiarization with the classical signs and symptoms of cardiac ischemia will assist the clinician in diagnosing the vast majority of patients who present with acute coronary syndromes. However, a significant number of

Box 3–1. *Classical Symptoms of Myocardial Ischemia*		
Chest pain:	Described as—	Pressure
		Tightness
		Heaviness
		Radiating to neck, jaw, shoulders, back or one or bothe arms
		Indigestion or "heartburn"
	Associated with—	Nausea and/or vomiting
		Diaphoresis
		Palpitations
		Shortness of breath
		Lightheadedness
		Dizziness
		Loss of consciousness

Box 3–2. *Atypical Symptoms Associated with Myocardial ischemia*

Chest pain: But present with— Dizziness
                                  Nausea and or vomiting
                                  Abdominal discomfort or pain
                                  Shortness of breath
                                  Fatigue
                                  Palpitations
                                  Isolated neck/jaw/back/arm pain
                                  Diaphoresis

---

patients do not present with these classical symptoms. It is essential that the clinician maintain a high degree of suspicion for acute myocardial infarction (AMI), especially in the treatment of those with significant risk factors, as noted in the "Phone Triage" section of this chapter. Note that the lack of known risk factors does not preclude the patient from having an AMI. Atypical symptoms, age younger than 55 years, female gender, ethnic minorities, lack of significant risk factors, few or no electrocardiographic abnormalities, and misinterpretation of the ECG are all important factors in the misdiagnosis of AMI. Box 3–1 lists the typical presenting complaints. Box 3–2 reviews some atypical symptoms that have been associated with myocardial ischemia.

Electrocardiography is the most common diagnostic study performed in emergency departments and outpatient settings to assess for evidence of myocardial ischemia. Although it has become a standard study in the

CARDIAC
ISCHEMIA

Box 3–3. *ECG Changes With Acute Coronary Syndrome*

• Transmural MI	ST-segment elevation
• Ischemia	ST-segment depression
• New left bundle branch block	
• Inferior wall	Abnormalities in leads II, III, aVF
• Anteroseptal wall	Abnormalities in precordial leads V1–V3
• Anterolateral wall	Abnormalities in precordial leads V1–V6
• Lateral wall	Abnormalities in I, aVL, V4–V6
• Posterior wall	Tall R waves and ST-segment depression in V1, V2
• Right ventricular wall	Abnormalities in V4R-V6R
• Nondiagnostic or normal ECG in 50% of AMI	

AMI, acute myocardial infarction; ECG, electrocardiogram; MI, myocardial infarction.

evaluation of patients for myocardial ischemia, the ECG can be normal or nondiagnostic in approximately one half of those with AMI. Box 3–3 lists the typical findings found in patients with diagnostic electrocardiograms. Note that the ECG represents a single point in time in what is a dynamic process. It is easy to miss capture of instability of the ST segments in ongoing ischemia. In the setting of a nondiagnostic ECG in patients with symptoms suspicious for recurrent or ongoing myocardial ischemia, the performance of automated serial 12-lead ECG monitoring (SECG) or repeated ECGs at standard intervals after presentation may be more revealing. Patients with symptoms suspicious for an acute coronary syndrome who have a nondiagnostic ECG must be referred to an emergency department and admitted for further evaluation.

 PHONE TRIAGE ◄————————————

Patients with suspected acute coronary syndrome with symptom duration longer than 20 minutes, symptoms suggestive of hemodynamic instability, and/or recent syncope or presyncope are to be referred to an emergency department or a chest pain center.[8] A medical practitioner should perform the evaluation in a facility equipped to perform a 12-lead ECG. Emergency transport via ambulance is recommended unless waiting for one would impose a long delay.

The American College of Emergency Physicians (ACEP) guidelines recommend that the routine evaluation of patients with nontraumatic chest pain should address the following[9]:
1. History
   a. Character of the pain—onset; severity; quality; location; radiation; frequency; duration; comparison with previous episodes of similar pain; precipitating factors; relationship to exertion, respiration, stress, or movement; response to therapy
   b. Age—should be documented with knowledge that men older than 33 and women older than 40 are at higher risk, but AMI has been documented at younger ages. Young age should not be used as an exclusion criterion in assessment for AMI
   c. Associated symptoms—nausea, vomiting, diaphoresis, shortness of breath, dyspnea on exertion, paroxysmal nocturnal dyspnea, cough, fevers, chills, sweats, dizziness, syncope, palpitations, productive cough, fatigue, weight change
   d. Medical history—past illnesses, especially known coronary artery disease, previous myocardial infarction, percutaneous transluminal coronary angioplasty (PTCA), coronary artery bypass graft (CABG),

hyperlipidemia, diabetes; review medications—assess for presence of cardiac medications, allergies, previous surgery, substance abuse, relevant diagnostic studies, and recent immobilization
2. Risk factors
   a. Known coronary artery disease
   b. Family history of coronary artery disease in a first-degree relative younger than age 55
   c. Diabetes mellitus
   d. Hypertension
   e. Cigarette use
   f. Left ventricular hypertrophy
   g. Elevated cholesterol levels
   h. Recent cocaine use
   i. Age—men older than 33; women older than 40

 LABORATORY RECOGNITION ◄───

Laboratory analyses performed in the evaluation of suspicious chest pain include the serum markers—creatine kinase MB fraction (CK-MB), myoglobin, and troponin. In addition to serum markers, an assessment of possible factors that may precipitate myocardial ischemia should be performed. This includes testing for underlying anemia and electrolyte derangement. Coagulation studies are necessary in the event that heparin or fibrinolytic therapy will be used.

Serum marker analysis in the diagnosis of AMI is standard, but much controversy exists as to which marker is the best measure of myocardial necrosis. The use of CK-MB mass became the gold standard in the 1990s. Currently, cardiac troponin T (cTnT) and troponin I (cTnI) are purported to be as sensitive as CK-MB but more specific for unstable ischemic syndromes. These also remain elevated for days after an AMI. The role of myoglobin in the diagnosis of AMI remains unclear. It is believed to be the earliest marker of myocardial necrosis with a rapid rise and early decrease. Because of this early decrease, myoglobin should never be used as the sole marker for AMI.

The single measurement of serum biochemical markers drawn within 6 hours of the onset of symptoms does not reliably include or exclude the diagnosis of AMI. Also, patients with unstable angina may have negative markers despite ongoing symptoms.

ACEP guidelines for serum marker testing of patients with acute chest pain include baseline CK-MB and troponin C or I on initial evaluation. If the baseline results are negative, testing for these markers should be repeated at 6 to 10 hours from symptom onset. If this timing is unknown, then the time of arrival to the emergency department should be used.

Treatment

- Cardiac monitoring
- Intravenous (IV) access
- Oxygen administration
- Pulse oximetry
- Blood pressure monitoring
- Aspirin administration—80 to 325 mg PO
- If systolic blood pressure is greater than 90 to 100 mm Hg, administer nitroglycerin 0.3 to 0.4 mg sublingually every 5 minutes × 3 doses
- If heart rate is greater than 50 to 60 and no associated hypotension or congestive heart failure (CHF) is noted, administer IV β blocker
- Intravenous heparin should be given for AMI and unstable angina
- Angiotensin-converting enzyme inhibitors may provide a decrease in mortality when given on a short-term basis

The National Heart Attack Alert Program (NHAAP) guidelines specifically recommend that the "GI cocktail" should NOT be used as a diagnostic tool to differentiate between gastrointestinal (GI) and cardiac causes of chest pain. A "GI cocktail" is a commonly used concoction in emergency departments to treat chest pain presumed to be a result of esophageal irritation. It consists of a mixture of viscous lidocaine, an antacid, and an anti spasmodic. This approach frequently leads to erroneous conclusions.

Fibrinolysis

Large randomized trials involving the use of fibrinolytic therapy have shown reduced mortality in some patients presenting with an acute myocardial infarction. Patients who benefited from this treatment were those with a clinical presentation suggestive of an AMI and ECG evidence of myocardial injury (ST elevation) in two or more contiguous leads, or bundle branch block (BBB). Those who were treated within the first 12 hours of symptom onset showed improvement. Patients benefited most from earliest treatment. Use of fibrinolytic therapy in this group demonstrated benefit despite age, gender, history of previous myocardial infarction, diabetes, systolic blood pressure,[9] or heart rate.

Primary Coronary Angioplasty

Primary coronary angioplasty has a clear role in the patient presenting with evidence of an AMI and cardiogenic shock. It is also indicated in those with an AMI who have an absolute contraindication to fibrinolytic use. Its role as the primary intervention in AMI is otherwise controversial. The ACEP clinical policy for the treatment of AMI recommends the use of primary angioplasty when performed by experienced personnel within 90 minutes of diagnosis of AMI. Review of numerous studies indicates that in this setting, it is as effective as fibrinolytic therapy for those patients who meet reperfusion criteria.

Glycoprotein IIb/IIIa Inhibitors

The use of this class of medications is recommended for patients with symptoms of AMI without ST-segment elevation who have refractory ischemia and/or high-risk features. This treatment is contraindicated in patients who have a major contraindication because of the risk of bleeding.

Disposition and Transfer

All patients with symptoms suspicious for an acute coronary syndrome should be referred to the nearest emergency department. Whenever possible, the physician should initiate treatment with an aspirin, oxygen supplementation, intravenous access, and sublingual nitroglycerin. Vital signs should be monitored closely. Transfer of office patients with active chest pain should be provided via an Advanced Cardiac Life Support (ACLS)-equipped ambulance.

Complications

- Sudden death—occurs in 50% of patients with AMI before they reach a hospital
- Congestive heart failure—if at least 25% of the myocardium is impaired
- Cardiogenic shock—common if greater than 40% of the myocardium is affected
- Papillary muscle rupture—occurs as a result of autolysis of the infarcted myocardium
- Hypotension—common in inferior AMI with right ventricular infarction
- Dysrhythmias—including supraventricular bradydysrhythmias and ventricular dysrhythmias
- Conduction disturbances

References

1. Pope JH, Aufderheide TP, Ruthazer R, et al: Missed diagnoses of acute cardiac ischemia in the emergency department. N Engl J Med 342:1163–1170, 2000.

2. Lee TH, Goldman L: Evaluation of the patient with acute chest pain. N Engl J Med 342:1187–1195, 2000.
3. Mehta RH, Eagle KA: Missed diagnoses of acute coronary syndromes in the emergency room—continuing challenges. N Engl J Med 342:1207–1210, 2000.
4. American College of Emergency Physicians. Clinical policy: Critical issues in the evaluation and management of adult patients presenting with suspected acute myocardial infarction or unstable angina. Ann Emerg Med 35:521–544, 2000.
5. Braunwald E, Antman EM, Beasley JW, et al: ACC/AHA guidelines for the management of patients with unstable angina: A report of the American College of Cardiology/American Heart Association Task Force on Practice Guidelines (Committee on the Management of Patients with Unstable Angina). J Am Coll Cardiol 36:970–1062, 2000.
6. Lee TH: Diagnosis and management of acute myocardial infarction: AHA/ACC guidelines summary. In Braunwald E, Zipes DP, Libby P (eds): Heart Disease: A Textbook of Cardiovascular Medicine, 6th ed. Philadelphia, WB Saunders, 2001.
7. U.S. Department of Health and Human Services: National Heart Attack Alert Program Coordinating Committee 60 Minutes to Treatment Working Group: Emergency Department: Rapid Identification and Treatment of Patients with Acute Myocardial Infarction (NIH Publication No. 93-3278). Rockville, Md, National Heart, Lung, and Blood Institute, Public Health Service, U.S. Department of Health and Human Services, September 1993.
8. Storrow AB, Gibler WB: Chest pain centers: Diagnosis of acute coronary syndromes. Ann Emerg Med 35:449–461, 2000.
9. American College of Emergency Physicians: Clinical policy for the initial approach to adults presenting with a chief complaint of chest pain, with no history of trauma. Ann Emerg Med 25:274–299, 1995.

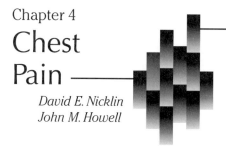

Chapter 4

Chest
Pain

David E. Nicklin
John M. Howell

The patient who complains of chest pain in the primary care office is an urgent challenge. The symptom most commonly is due to benign disease processes, but it can represent an acute, life-threatening crisis. In a recent study of 10,689 patients presenting to emergency departments with chest pain suggestive of acute ischemic events, 1866 (17%) met the criteria for acute cardiac ischemia (8% had myocardial infarction and 9% had unstable angina).[1] Psychosomatic disease, panic attacks, and musculoskeletal pain are other common causes of chest discomfort. A prospective study of 399 episodes of chest pain in patients seen in primary care offices over a 1-year period found that 60% of chest pain diagnoses were not "organic" in origin (i.e., not due to cardiac, gastrointestinal [GI], or pulmonary disease). Musculoskeletal chest pain accounted for 36% of all diagnoses (of which costochondritis accounted for 13%) followed by reflux esophagitis (13%).[2] Stable angina pectoris was responsible for 11% of chest pain episodes, and unstable angina or myocardial infarction occurred in only 1.5%. Esophageal spasm and gastroesophageal reflux disease are also common causes of acute noncardiac chest pain.[3]

The correct diagnosis can generally be made from a detailed history, supported by specific physical findings and an electrocardiogram (ECG) and/or chest radiograph. One study found that physicians, using only the history and physical examination, correctly diagnosed nonorganic (i.e., not due to cardiac, GI, or pulmonary disease) versus organic causes of chest pain in 88% of patients. Twelve percent of patients were misdiagnosed as having chest pain of organic origin; no organic diagnosis was missed.[4]

CLINICAL RECOGNITION

The evaluation of acute chest pain should thus begin with a clinical history, focus on risk factors, a pain history, an examination that emphasizes vital signs, cardiovascular findings, and ECG or chest

23

radiograph, when indicated. Chest pain due to myocardial infarction, pulmonary embolus, aortic dissection, or esophageal rupture may result in sudden death. When initial evaluation suggests any of these diagnoses, emergent stabilization and ambulance transfer to the emergency department are required. Recognition of each of these entities is discussed in this chapter. Tables 4–1 and 4–2 show an overview of the approach to chest pain differential diagnosis.

Table 4–1. Historical Findings in Patients with Chest Pain Disorders

Differential Diagnosis	Character of Discomfort	Factors Worsening Symptoms	Factors Improving Symptoms	Risk Factors
Cardiovascular Disorders				
Acute myocardial infarction	Classically dull, crushing, substernal CP with radiation,* usually longer than 20 min; may be burning, pleuritic, or absent; usually occurs during early morning	Exertion, although may occur at rest	Rest, oxygen, nitrates, and calcium channel blockers	Arteriosclerosis as suggested by DM, HTN, male gender, tobacco use, hyperlipidemia, family history, postmeno-pausal state
Stable angina	Same as AMI with consistent frequency, duration, and severity; inciting stimuli remain relatively constant	Same as AMI	Same as AMI	Same as AMI
Unstable angina	Same as AMI with increased severity, duration, and frequency relative to patient's baseline, although each episode is generally of shorter duration than AMI; may have a stable pattern with less exertion	Same as AMI	Same as AMI	Same as AMI
Prinzmetal's angina	Similar to AMI; typically occurs during early morning	Occurs at rest and with exertion	Nitrates and calcium channel blockers	
Cocaine-related ischemia	May be atypical, but cocaine-related AMI often described as classically dull, crushing, substernal chest pain	Use of cocaine immediately preceding symptoms or hours to days earlier	Rest, oxygen, nitrates, and calcium channel blockers	May have some, all, or no risk factors for arteriosclerosis

Table 4–1. Historical Findings in Patients with Chest Pain Disorders *(Continued)*

Differential Diagnosis	Character of Discomfort	Factors Worsening Symptoms	Factors Improving Symptoms	Risk Factors
Cardiovascular Disorders *Continued*				
Mitral valve prolapse	CP usually atypical for myocardial ischemia but occasionally typical; anxiety, palpitations, depression, and hyperventilation may be present; may present with TIA	Psychological stress	β blockers, anxiolytics	Female gender, family history
Aortic stenosis	Angina associated with exertional dyspnea and syncope, usually during the 5th–7th decades	Same as AMI, and symptoms may be marked with minimal exertion	Same as AMI	Rheumatoid arthritis, advanced age, and congenital condition
Hypertrophic cardio-myopathy	Angina associated with dyspnea, fatigue, and syncope; first manifestation may be sudden death	Same as AMI	Same as AMI	Family history, Friedreich's ataxia
Pericarditis	Substernal pain that may be severe and increased with swallowing and breathing	Supine position	Sitting forward	Viral illness, TB, recent AMI, uremia, mononucleosis, postirradiation, sarcoid, SLE, RA, drugs
Aortic dissection	Severee, tearing pain localized to anterior chest, back, abdomen, or lumbar region; steady nature; may be associated with leg weakness	None	None	Uncontrolled hypertension, Marfan's syndrome, Turner's syndrome, trauma, pregnancy, aortic coarctation, atherosclerosis
Pulmonary Disorders				
Massive pulmonary embolism	Dyspnea with substernal, dull, heavy, or arching chest pain	None	None	Hypercoagulability as suggested by immobilization, cancer, BCP, DVT, post-partum state, prior DVT or

Table continued on following page

CHEST PAIN

Table 4–1. Historical Findings in Patients with Chest Pain Disorders *(Continued)*

Differential Diagnosis	Character of Discomfort	Factors Worsening Symptoms	Factors Improving Symptoms	Risk Factors
Pulmonary Disorders *Continued*				
				PE, chronic disease, other cause of hyperviscosity
Submassive pulmonary embolism	Painless, acute, unexplained dyspnea on exertion on rest	None	None	Same as for massive pulmonary embolism
Pulmonary infarction	Dyspnea with sharp, respirophasic pain, often with cough and hemoptysis	None	None	Same as massive pulmonary embolism and sickle cell disease
Pneumothorax, simple	Unilateral, pleuritic chest pain of acute onset	Trauma; frequently occurs spontaneously	None	Tobacco use; prior history of pneumothorax
Pneumothorax, tension	Same as simple pneumothorax, except dizziness and hypotension also present	Same as simple pneumothorax	None	Same as simple pneumothorax
Pneumonia	Usually localized, pleuritic, and associated with cough and fever; diarrhea or vomiting possible with atypical pneumonia	None	None	Tobacco use, COPD, seizure disorders, chronic disease
Pleurisy	Pleuritic, lower chest pain, typically sharp and may be associated with viral symptoms	None	None	Viral illnesses
Gastrointestinal Disorders				
Esophageal rupture	Usually left-sided, pleuritic CP associated with fever and SOB	Vomiting	None	Alcoholism, trauma, caustic ingestion, instrumentation, foreign body ingestion
Esophageal reflux and spasm	Substantial CP with radiation to arms, back, and neck; may be associated with heartburn and regurgitation; persistent, dull, background ache possible; may	Exertion, tobacco use, and methylxanthines; pain may occur 20–30 min after meals	Nitrates, calcium channel blockers, antacids, and rest; dietary manipulations and elevating the head of the bed	Hiatal hernia, gastric reflux

Table continued on following page

Table 4–1. Historical Findings in Patients with Chest Pain Disorders *(Continued)*

Differential Diagnosis	Character of Discomfort	Factors Worsening Symptoms	Factors Improving Symptoms	Risk Factors
Gastrointestinal Disorders *Continued*				
	have nocturnal cough from recurrent aspiration; may occur with esophageal dysmotility			
Esophageal dysmotility	Occasionally severe retrosternal CP that may radiate to neck, arms, back, and jaw; usually lasts seconds to minutes; may coexist with esophageal reflux	Pain may begin immediately or within minutes of swallowing solids or liquids; anti-cholinergics and stress	Nitrates and calcium channel blockers	Diabetic neuropathy, esophageal irradiation, esophageal foreign body, and various collagen vascular disorders (i.e., PSS)
Gastric ulcer disease	Dull, boring epigastric pain that may penetrate with posterior wall ulcers; perforation manifests with RLQ and/or shoulder pain; RUQ discomfort in 10%; low thoracic chest discomfort may mimic AMI	Postprandial state (delayed exacerbation of pain), frequently within 1–2 hrs of retiring; salicylates, NSAIDs, and various drugs that cause gastric irritation	Meals (immediate relief), antacids, carafate, and and H_2 blockers	Tobacco use, stress, hypercalcemia, CRF, alcoholic cirrhosis, COPD, renal transplantation
Pancreatitis	Dull, boring epigastric and periumbilical pain that penetrates; frequently associated with vomiting; may radiate to low chest	Lying flat, alcohol ingestion	Sitting forward	Alcohol ingestion, GB disease, trauma, renal failure, elevated lipid and calcium levels, viral illnesses, drugs, connective tissue disorders, scorpion envenomations
Cholelithiasis or cholecystitis	May be steady or colicky; classic RUQ radiating to right back or subscapular region; discomfort may be epigastric and LUQ; lower	Fatty meals, meperidine	Anticholinergics, nasogastric suction	Female gender, obesity, pregnancy, Native North Americans, cirrhosis, hemolysis, elevated

Table continued on following page

Table 4–1. Historical Findings in Patients with Chest Pain Disorders *(Continued)*

Differential Diagnosis	Character of Discomfort	Factors Worsening Symptoms	Factors Improving Symptoms	Risk Factors
Gastrointestinal Disorders *Continued*				
	thoracic chest discomfort may mimic AMI; fever and chills in the setting of cholecystitis			cholesterol and estrogen levels, ileal resection, clofibrate, cystic fibrosis
Musculoskeletal and Integumentary Disorders				
Musculo-skeletal causes	Pain usually sharp, lancinating, localized, and increased with breathing or motion; may be dull and substernal	Body movement; nerve root compression may be worse with sneezing or coughing, neck and shoulder movement	May be relieved with rest	Lifting large weights, poor posture, chest wall deformity
Herpes zoster	Sharp, burning, unilateral pain; discomfort may precede exanthem by 4–7 d	Stress, viral illness, immuno-suppression	Slight relief from oral pain medications	Age >50 yr, although it occurs at any age; underlying malignancy

From Emergency Medicine, vol 1, T17–1. Howell JM et al (eds): Philadelphia, WB Saunders, 1998, pp 10–132.

*The text discusses atypical presentations.

AMI, acute myocardial infarction; BCP, birth control pills; COPD, chronic obstructive pulmonary disease; CP, chest pain; CRF, chronic renal failure; DM, diabetes mellitus; DVT, deep venous thrombophlebitis; GB, gallbladder; GI, gastrointestinal; HJR, hepatojugular reflux; HTN, hypertension; LUQ, left upper quadrant; NSAIDs, nonsteroidal anti-inflammatory drugs; PE, pulmonary embolus; PSS, progressive systemic sclerosis; RA, rheumatoid arthritis; RLQ, right lower quadrant; RUQ, right upper quadrant; SLE, systemic lupus erythematosus; SOB, shortness of breath; TB, tuberculosis; TIA, transient ischemic attack

Table 4–2. Physical Findings in Patients with Chest Pain Disorders

Differential Diagnosis	Pertinent Physical Findings
Cardiovascular Disorders	
Acute myocardial infarction*	S_3, S_4, jugular venous distension, hepatojugular reflux, peripheral edema, rales, low-grade temperature, tachycardia, tachypnea, and hypertension or hypotension; irregular pulse
Stable and unstable angina	Similar to myocardial infarction, but JVD, HJR, rales, peripheral edema, and fever are absent or not exacerbated; mild hypertension
Prinzmetal's angina	Mild tachycardia, tachypnea, and hypertension; S_3 and S_4 may be present during episodes of pain
Cocaine-related ischemia	Similar to AMI and angina, with associated sequelae of cocaine intoxication: severe hypertension, tachycardia, euphoria; may occur after cocaine use with no sequelae of intoxication

Table 4–2. Physical Findings in Patients with Chest Pain Disorders *(Continued)*

Differential Diagnosis	Pertinent Physical Findings
Mitral valve prolapse	Mid to late systolic murmur and/or click; findings may move earlier in systole with Valsalva maneuver and amyl nitrite examination; tachycardia and tachypnea possible in anxious individuals
Aortic stenosis	Classic systolic murmur is a crescendo-decrescendo sound heard best at the right upper sternal border and radiating to the carotids; less frequent findings include an opening systolic snap, a delayed, weak carotid pulse, a bifid carotid pulse (bisferious pulse), and a prominent apical impulse
Hypertrophic cardiomyopathy	Systolic crescendo-decrescendo murmur, heard best at the left lower sternal border and increased with maneuvers that decrease preload (e.g., Valsalva); less frequent findings are fourth heart sound, double apical impulse, and rapidly rising carotid pulse
Pericarditis	One-, two-, or three-component pericardial rub (two components in diastole, one in systole); rub is evanescent and usually heard best with the patient sitting forward; low-grade fever; pericardial tampanode may develop with hypotension, muffled heart sounds, and elevated jugular venous pressure
Aortic dissection	Tachycardia and tachypnea; patient initially hypertensive, but falling blood pressure is a harbinger of catastrophe; acute hemiparesis and/or hemianesthesia; blood pressure discrepancy between arms and between arms and legs; lower extremity motor weakness; murmur or aortic regurgitation; Beck's triad of hypotension, muffled heart sounds, and JVD
Pulmonary Disorders	
Pulmonary embolism	Tachycardia, tachypnea, fever, rales, wheezes, pleural friction rub; lower extremity swelling, tenderness, and palpable cord possible; RV gallop, RV heave, loud P_2, and hypotension may be present in severe cases (e.g., massive PE)
Pneumothorax, simple	Diminished breath sound unilaterally, although breath sounds may be normal; mild tachycardia and tachypnea
Pneumothorax, tension	Markedly diminished breath sounds, contralateral tracheal deviation, hypotension (variable), tachycardia, respiratory insufficiency or failure
Pneumonia	Localized rhonchi, rales, or diminished breath sounds on auscultation; fever, tachypnea, and tachycardia possible
Gastrointestinal Disorders	
Esophageal rupture	Fever, tachycardia, tachypnea, hypotension; dullness and diminished breath sounds at the left lung base; subcutaneous emphysema (especially in the supraclavicular regions) and mediastinal emphysema (Hamman's sign or "crunch")
Esophageal reflux	Minimal signs; mild tachycardia and tachypnea possible
Esophageal dysmotility	Tachypnea and tachycardia; difficulty swallowing secretions in severe cases; signs of heart failure absent
Peptic ulcer disease	Epigastric, RUQ, and LUQ tenderness; RLQ tenderness in some cases of gastric perforation; hematochezia and bloody or coffee-ground nasogastric aspirate; hypotension and marked tachycardia in severe cases
Pancreatitis	Epigastric, RUQ, and LUQ tenderness; low-grade fever, tachycardia, and occasionally hypotension; clinical signs of pleural effusion, usually left-sided; jaundice infrequent; blue discoloration about the umbilicus (Cullen's sign) and evidenc of resolving flank hematoma (Turner's sign) are uncommon and late findings

Table continued on following page

Table 4–2. Physical Findings in Patients with Chest Pain Disorders *(Continued)*

Differential Diagnosis	Pertinent Physical Findings
Cholelithiasis or cholecystitis	Tenderness in the RUQ or epigastrium; inspiratory arrest on palpation of the RUQ (Murphy's sign); simple cholangitis characterized by abdominal tenderness, fever, and jaundice (Charcot's triad); presentation of suppurative cholangitis is similar to simple infection with the addition of shock and depression of central nervous system function (Reynold's pentad)
Musculoskeletal and Integumentary Disorders	
Musculoskeletal causes	Chest wall tenderness, with light to moderate pressure, which completely reproduces the patient's discomfort; repeated attempts to elicit tenderness may cause false-positive results; discomfort elicited by Spurling's maneuver, horizontal arm flexion, or Adson's maneuver; Dejerine's sign (increased pain with cough or sneeze) also may be present
Herpes zoster	Pain may precede exanthem by 1–2 wk; exanthem is dermatomal, unilateral, and initially maculopapular; later findings are grouped vesicles on a red base

From Emergency Medicine, vol I, T17–2. Howell JM et al (eds): Philadelphia, WB Saunders, 1998, p. 135
*Although these findings suggest AMI, the patient with AMI more commonly has normal examination findings.
AMI, acute myocardial infarction; HJR, hepatojugular reflux; JVD, jugular venous distention; PE, pulmonary embolus; LUQ, left upper quadrant; RLQ, right lower quadrant; RUQ, right upper quadrant; RV, right ventricular.

The presence of risk factors and the age of the patient population are important determinants of coronary artery disease prevalence. In one retrospective review, only 7% of patients younger than age 35 who had chest pain were diagnosed with ischemic heart disease.[5] In contrast, the incidence of cardiac diagnoses may approach 50% in patients with chest pain after the age of 40.[6] A previous diagnosis of coronary disease greatly increases risk. Other important risk factors include:

- Hyperlipidemia
- Diabetes
- Left ventricular hypertrophy
- Family history of premature coronary artery disease (CAD)
- Hypertension
- Cigarette smoking
- Cocaine use (risk of acute myocardial infarction [AMI] was increased 24-fold in the 60 minutes after cocaine use)[7]

A majority of younger patients with chest pain due to CAD have risk factors other than age. In a retrospective study of 209 patients younger than 40 years of age presenting with an AMI, 98% had one or more of the conventional coronary risk factors, including cigarette smoking (80%), family history (40%), hypertension (26%), hyperlipidemia (20%), and cocaine use (7%).[8] In contrast, a history of symptomatic gastroesophageal reflux, gallstones, panic disorder, asthma, or musculoskeletal pain may reduce the likelihood of an ischemic cause, if the present symptoms are similar to those that occurred with the previous diagnosis.

History

Typical descriptions of ischemic chest discomfort include squeezing, tightness, pressure, "gas," or fullness in the chest, or the patient may demonstrate the symptom by placing his or her fist in the center of the chest. Patients often deny having "pain." Ischemic discomfort is generally diffuse and cannot be localized by the patient. Pain localized to a small area is more commonly of chest wall or pleural origin. Some patients with cardiac ischemia describe a sharp or stabbing discomfort. Such a description is low risk only if the pain has a pleuritic or positional component and is reproducible by palpation, and the patient has no history of angina or myocardial infarction.[9] The pain of myocardial ischemia often radiates to the neck, jaw, upper extremities (right or left), or shoulder.[9] The onset of ischemic pain is often gradual and intensity increases over a period of minutes; the pain caused by pneumothorax or a vascular event such as aortic dissection or acute pulmonary embolism typically has an abrupt onset with full intensity at the beginning. Chest discomfort that lasts only seconds or pain that is constant over weeks is not due to cardiac ischemia. Chest discomfort provoked by exertion is a classical symptom of angina. Cold, emotional stress, meals, or sexual intercourse may also provoke ischemic pain. Pain made worse by swallowing, after meals, and by lying prone is likely of esophageal origin. Body position, movement, or deep breathing may exacerbate chest pain of musculoskeletal origin. Sublingual nitroglycerin relieves myocardial ischemia, as well as esophageal spasm. A "GI cocktail" (i.e., viscous lidocaine, antacid, and an anticholenergic) also may relieve both GI and ischemic chest pain.[10] Nonspecific symptoms often associated with myocardial ischemia include nausea, vomiting, diaphoresis, palpitations, and shortness of breath. One national study found that patients with myocardial ischemia presenting as exertional dyspnea without chest discomfort were 2.7 times more likely to be sent home from the emergency department than those with chest pain; ischemia should be carefully considered in such patients.[1] Women and nonwhite patients were also more frequently discharged with ischemia and deserve special attention.

Physical Examination

A physical examination guided by history, although often normal, may provide important data to support a diagnosis of cardiac ischemia.

CHEST PAIN

General appearance and vital signs provide important clues as to severity and acuity. Individuals with acute myocardial ischemia may be hyperadrenergic with tachycardia and hypertension. Unequal right and left arm blood pressure is an important clue to thoracic aortic dissection. Careful cardiopulmonary examination may reveal left ventricular failure (rales, ventricular filling gallop [S_3]) or new mitral regurgitation murmur due to papillary muscle dysfunction. If the chest wall is tender, the patient should be asked if palpation reproduces his/her symptoms. Chest wall tenderness may, however, be present with myocardial ischemia.[11] Wheezing may be seen in left ventricular failure, but focal rales or dullness suggests primary pulmonary disease. A thorough abdominal examination helps in the exclusion of gallbladder disease and abdominal aortic dissection.

The ECG is of critical importance and *should be obtained within 5 minutes after presentation*, and then compared with a previous ECG, when available. In a recent report of more than 2000 patients with acute chest pain, the prevalence of AMI was 80% among patients with 1 mm or more of new ST-segment elevation, and 20% among patients with ST-segment depression or T-wave inversion not known to be old. In contrast, patients without a previous history of CAD and without these electrocardiographic changes had a frequency of AMI of 2%.[12]

Differential Diagnosis

Evaluation of possible *pulmonary embolism (PE)* begins with a consideration of risk factors. Virchow's triangle of stasis, endothelial trauma, and a hypercoagulable state increase the risk of deep venous thrombosis. Risk factors include recent bed rest, prolonged (>12 hr) air travel, stroke, knee or hip surgery, active cancer, obesity, pregnancy, oral contraceptives, and a previous or family history of thromboembolic disease. Symptoms of PE typically include acute onset of dyspnea and pleuritic chest pain. Other presenting symptoms may include nondescript substernal chest pain, cough, leg pain, hemoptysis, and syncope.[13] Chest pain may be absent. Physical findings in decreasing order of frequency are tachypnea, rales, a loud second heart sound, and tachycardia. Decreased oxygen saturation on pulse oximetry is suggestive when present but is not sufficiently sensitive to be reassuring when absent. Arterial oxygen pressure (PaO_2) is between 85 and 105 mm Hg in approximately 18% of patients with pulmonary embolism, and up to 6% may have a normal alveolar-arterial gradient for oxygen.[14] Nonspecific ECG findings, including tachycardia, nonspecific ST-segment and T-wave changes, right atrial enlargement, and atrial and ventricular ectopy, are common in PE. The classical combination of a prominent S wave in lead I with a deep Q wave and inverted T wave in lead III (S1Q3T3) is seen in only 10% of patients.[15] Chest radiographs may be normal or may reveal focal infiltrates, pleural effusions, atelectasis, or an elevated hemidiaphragm. Less frequently, pleural-based densities (known as Hampton's hump) or dilated pulmonary arteries with diminished parenchymal perfusion (known as Westermark's sign) are seen.[16]

Patients with thoracic *aortic dissection* typically develop penetrating chest discomfort that is severe and tearing in nature. It is more common in older patients (men over 60 years old) and those with Marfan's syndrome. Smaller dissections may cause less severe chest discomfort that starts and stops abruptly. Often, the patient can pinpoint when the pain started. Physical findings may include asymmetrical peripheral pulse deficits (systolic differences between extremities of 20 to 30 mm Hg), cardiac tamponade (muffled heart sounds, hypotension, prominent neck veins), and ischemic myelopathy with posterior column (position and vibratory sense) sparing. ECG findings may include acute myocardial ischemia resulting from proximal dissection to the coronary arteries. Chest radiograph often shows mediastinal widening.[17]

Spontaneous rupture of the esophagus, or Boerhaave's syndrome, generally occurs in patients following persistent vomiting, caustic (i.e., alkaline) ingestion, or upper endoscopy, but also in patients with a history of alcoholism, peptic ulcer disease, esophageal stricture, esophagitis, or neoplasm. Hermann Boerhaave described the syndrome in 1724 after observing, at autopsy, a transmural rupture of the distal esophagus in Admiral Baron John de Wassenaeur of the Dutch Navy. Presenting symptoms include nausea, vomiting, and sharp chest pain. Patients are frequently dyspneic and may sit upright and forward to minimize discomfort. Pertinent physical findings include basilar rales, wheezing, and crepitus along the chest wall (subcutaneous emphysema). Patients may not appear ill on initial presentation, and fever and subcutaneous emphysema are uncommon within the first 12 hours. Hamman's sign (a rasping crackle in cadence with the cardiac sounds) is noted in up to 20% of patients.[18] Atypical presentations are commonly described in the literature. Although many patients have a history of inadvertently performing a Valsalva maneuver, many others do not.[19] Chest radiography is often helpful and may show a pleural effusion, pneumothorax, mediastinal emphysema, or mediastinal widening. Diatrizoate meglumine (Gastrografin) esophagram confirms the diagnosis in most cases. Treatment is generally surgical repair and irrigation.

Acute pericarditis is generally seen in younger patients, who present with substernal chest pain, pericardial friction rub, and concordant ST-segment elevation on ECG. It often occurs after viral illness but can be seen in many autoimmune, inflammatory, infectious, or malignant diseases. Frequently, no underlying cause is found. The patient is usually febrile, and the pain may be mild or severe. It is typically exacerbated by inspiration and relieved by leaning forward. On physical examination, a one-, two-, or three-part cardiac rub may be intermittently heard in early diastole, late diastole, and systole. Signs of tamponade are unusual. The chest radiograph may be normal, or the heart shadow may be slightly enlarged. Pleural effusions may be noted, but the presence of pulmonary congestion suggests associated myocarditis. The ECG typically shows generalized ST-segment elevation, with subtle PR interval depression in some cases. The QRS is normal unless there is a large pericardial effusion.[20] Evaluation and treatment generally consist of an echocardiogram to confirm the diagnosis and exclude tamponade, and nonsteroidal anti-inflammatory treatment with outpatient follow-up.

Primary spontaneous pneumothorax is a relatively rare, potentially serious cause of chest pain. It typically occurs in healthy, tall, thin patients between the ages of 10 and 30 years and rarely presents after the age of 40. It is more common in males than females in a ratio of 4:1. Smoking cigarettes increases the risk of primary spontaneous pneumothorax in men by as much as a factor of 20 in a dose-dependent manner.[21] Case reports also suggest an association with marijuana use, as might be expected with repeated prolonged Valsalva maneuver.[22] Patients generally present with ipsilateral pleuritic chest pain or acute dyspnea. Chest pain may be minimal or severe, and may progress from "sharp" to a "steady ache." Pain often resolves within 24 hours, even if the pneumothorax remains untreated and does not resolve. Tachycardia is the most common physical finding. In patients with a large pneumothorax, the findings on examination may include hyperresonant percussion, diminished fremitus, and decreased or absent breath sounds on the affected side. Patients with a small pneumothorax (<15%) may have normal findings on physical examination. Pulse oximetry will show decreased saturation if the pneumothorax is large. The diagnosis is confirmed by chest radiography. The average rate of recurrence is 30%.[23]

Panic disorder is a common cause of chest pain. A review of the literature reveals that panic disorder is present in more than 30% of patients with chest pain who have no or minimal CAD.[24] It also may coexist with CAD. The symptoms of acute panic attack include chest pain, shortness of breath, palpitations, sweating, depersonalization, and a sense of impending doom that may be overwhelming. The chest discomfort may closely mimic that of acute coronary syndrome, and the diagnosis often can be confirmed only after stress testing has shown the absence of significant coronary disease. Panic disorder has been found to respond to cognitive/behavioral therapy, as well as to selective serotonin reuptake inhibitors (SSRIs) or tricyclic antidepressants.

Pleurisy is a symptom complex that includes respirophasic lower chest pain that may be associated with viral symptoms. Chest radiograph is typically normal but may reveal a small pleural effusion.

Gastroesophageal reflux disease (GERD) may cause substernal chest discomfort that is either burning or dull, and sometimes severe. These patients may relate a history of heartburn, regurgitation, and nocturnal

CHEST PAIN

cough. Occasionally, patients with GERD complain of a dull, background chest ache that lasts for hours at a time. Reflux symptoms may start 20 to 30 minutes after a meal and are occasionally exertional.

Musculoskeletal pain is generally sharp, localized, position dependent, and worse with breathing or moving, with localized tenderness and an antecedent history of acute injury.

 ## PHONE TRIAGE ◄─────────────────

Patients in acute distress with severe chest pain, abnormal vital signs, or difficulty breathing should call Emergency Services to be transported to the nearest emergency department. Most patients will be less severely ill and will need assessment over the phone. Secretaries should be trained to transfer chest pain calls to nurses or physicians, who are qualified to assess risk. This evaluation of chest pain requires a careful limited history. Life-threatening diagnoses, particularly coronary artery disease, are the primary concern. Risk factors for coronary disease must be considered, as outlined earlier. Patients with multiple risk factors must be evaluated more aggressively. A careful history of the pain must include location, quality, duration, radiation, what precipitates and relieves it, and associated symptoms. Other potentially life-threatening causes of pain should also be kept in mind, particularly pulmonary embolism. Associated symptoms, including pleuritic chest pain, shortness of breath, and leg pain or swelling, are particularly worrisome in a patient with risk factors such as a history of malignancy, recent surgery, bed rest, or pregnancy.

CHEST PAIN

Decisions regarding site and timing of evaluation are based on the history obtained. Patients with acute ongoing pain typical of coronary ischemia, and with one or more risk factors, should be told to chew an aspirin tablet and arrange ambulance or Fire Rescue transport to the nearest emergency department. Those whose pain has some high-risk features, but who are without risk factors (e.g., a 35-year-old healthy woman with exertional chest pain), should have same-day appointments in the office. Same-day appointments should also be given to those with atypical pain but multiple risk factors (e.g., a 50-year-old diabetic man with burning chest discomfort at rest). Those with no risk factors and atypical pain, or patients with recurrences of previously diagnosed pain, are candidates for a therapeutic trial and office evaluation within a few days. For example, a 25-year-old man with substernal burning pain after meals might be tried on H_2 blockers in the coming week. It is generally prudent to respect patients' requests for same-day or urgent appointments because they may not be able to articulate the severity of their symptoms.

Initial Management

For all patients with active chest pain who are at risk for significant morbidity or mortality (e.g., those whose history, physical, ECG, and chest radiograph suggest ongoing myocardial ischemia, pulmonary embolism, aortic dissection, or esophageal rupture), call 911 first; then administer supplemental oxygen, apply a cardiac monitor, and establish a peripheral IV. If pulse oximetry is available, deliver supplemental oxygen to maintain saturations above 95%.

Myocardial Ischemia. For all patients with ongoing ischemic chest discomfort, administer 325 mg of aspirin if the patient is not allergic. Give one 0.4-mg tablet of nitroglycerin every 5 minutes (up to three doses) for active chest pain. Hold the nitroglycerin for a systolic blood pressure below 90 mm Hg.

Equipment and Medications

- Oxygen tank
- Nasal prong oxygen tubing
- 100% non-rebreathing oxygen mask: Adult, pediatric, and infant
- Cardiac monitor: With adult- and child-size chest electrodes
- 20-, 18-, and 16-gauge IV catheters
- 22- and 24-gauge IV catheters for pediatric use
- Saline locks, including saline flush
- 5- or 10-mL syringes
- Alcohol and povidone-iodine swabs
- Tourniquet
- 325-mg aspirin tablets
- Children's chewable aspirin tablets
- 0.4-mg nitroglycerin tablets
- Electrogardiographic machine
- Pulse oximeter
- Defibrillator: Adult- and child-size paddles

Disposition and Transfer

Patients with normal physical examination, and without evidence of AMI on ECG, may still require hospital admission. In patients with myocardial infarction, physical examination is generally normal unless there is cardiac failure. A completely normal ECG is reassuring but does not exclude unstable angina. One prospective study found that 4% of chest pain patients with a normal ECG had unstable angina.[11] If one includes patients without ST-segment elevation or depression, but with nonspecific T-wave changes, the percentage with unstable angina may be as high as 30%.[25] Therefore, patients with typical pain and risk factors should receive aspirin and be transported to the hospital by ambulance for admission.

All patients with active chest pain who are at risk for significant morbidity or mortality (e.g., those with identified or suspected ongoing myocardial ischemia, pneumothorax, pulmonary embolism, aortic dissection, or esophageal rupture) should be transported by an Advanced Life Support (ALS) ambulance to an emergency department, preferably the closest emergency department equipped to manage such disorders.

If acute ischemic heart disease and other life-threatening diagnoses seem unlikely to be the cause of the chest pain, the possibility of pulmonary, GI, and musculoskeletal conditions, as well as pericarditis and other cardiovascular causes, should be investigated, generally in the outpatient setting by the patient's primary care physician.

Epidemiology and Pathophysiology

Acute Myocardial Ischemia. Coronary artery occlusion develops from the rupture of an atherosclerotic plaque, which causes coronary spasm, intraplaque hemorrhage, and thrombosis.[26] Acute myocardial infarction proceeds in a "wavefront" from subendocardium to subpericardium, with more than 70% of transmural necrosis occurring within 6 hours.[27] The extent of myocardial necrosis occurring during AMI is affected, in part, by the delay before implementation of reperfusion therapy. Aspirin inhibits platelet aggregation by preventing the formation of thromboxane A_2.

Pulmonary Embolism. Obstruction of the pulmonary vascular bed from a migrating thrombus leads to a sudden increase in pulmonary artery pressure and right ventricular work. High right ventricular pressures lead to ventricular dilation, tricuspid insufficiency, bulging of the interventricular septum, decreased left ventricular compliance, and diminished cardiac output. Ventilation-perfusion mismatching, intrapulmonary shunting, and alveolar hypoventilation each may contribute to low arterial oxygen pressure (PaO_2) levels. Platelets release serotonin and histamines that may cause localized bronchoconstriction and wheezing.

Thoracic Aortic Dissection. Hypertension is a risk factor. Over time, an aperture forms in the aortic intima, causing a hematoma in the media. Once the false lumen is created, ongoing dissection is favored by hypertension and a rapid rise in pressure over time (i.e., dP/dT). Consequently, diminishing blood pressure and dP/dT are critical in the medical treatment of aortic dissection. Proximal dissection may lead to stroke, myocardial ischemia, aortic insufficiency, and cardiac tamponade.

Pneumothorax. Pneumothorax is a collection of air between the parietal and visceral pleurae. Spontaneous pneumothoraces are caused by subpleural blebs. Spontaneous pneumothoraces are more common among males 20 to 40 years old. These patients are usually tall and thin and smoke tobacco. About 30% of spontaneous pneumothoraces recur within 2 years, usually on the same side.[21]

Esophageal Perforation. Esophageal perforation following severe retching (Boerhaave's syndrome) usually occurs in the distal left esophagus. The result is gastric content in the left hemithorax, leading to mediastinitis, empyema, sepsis, shock, and respiratory insufficiency, frequently among alcoholic patients. Esophageal manipulation (e.g., upper endoscopy) is another relatively common cause of esophageal perforation. Caustic ingestion is less common but similarly leads to esophageal perforation.

Pediatric Chest Pain

Chest pain is a frequent complaint in the pediatric age group and can be a physically and emotionally distressing symptom, but it rarely represents an office emergency. History and physical examination are often sufficient for diagnosis. Laboratory studies, chest radiography, and ECG have limited use.[28] Studies including 457 children with chest pain have shown musculoskeletal/costochondral chest pain to be the most common occurrence, with exercise-induced asthma, GI causes, and psychogenic causes seen less frequently. Pain of cardiac origin is rare (less than 4% in these series).[28, 29] Young children are more likely to have cardiorespiratory problems. Organic disease is more likely with pain of acute onset, abnormal physical examination results, pain that awakens the child from sleep, or the presence of fever. Laboratory tests are rarely helpful. An abnormal ECG was related to the cause of pain in less than than 1% of patients. Psychogenic pain is more likely in children with chronic pain, those older than 12 years of age, and those with a family history of heart disease or chest pain. In patients with rare, life-threatening illnesses (such as congenital heart disease, Kawasaki's disease with coronary aneurysm, and cocaine abuse in older adolescents), stabilization with oxygen, cardiac monitoring, peripheral IV access, and transport to the emergency department should proceed as they do in adults.

CHEST PAIN

References

1. Pope JH, Aufderheide TP, Ruthazer R, et al: Missed diagnoses of acute cardiac ischemia in the emergency department. N Engl J Med 342:1163, 2000.
2. Klinkman MS, Stevens D, Gorenflo DW: Episodes of care for chest pain: A preliminary report from MIRNET. Michigan Research Network. J Fam Pract 38:345, 1994.

3. Goyal RK: Changing focus on unexplained esophageal chest pain. Ann Intern Med 124:1008, 1996.
4. Martina B, Bucheli B, Stotz M, et al: First clinical judgment by primary care physicians distinguishes well between nonorganic and organic causes of abdominal or chest pain. J Gen Intern Med 12:4590, 1997.
5. Luke LC, Cusack S, Smith H, et al: Non-traumatic chest pain in young adults: A medical audit. Arch Emerg Med 7:183, 1990.
6. Pryor DB, Harrell FE, Lee KL, Califf RM: Estimating the likelihood of significant coronary artery disease. Am J Med 75:771, 1983.
7. Mittleman MA, Mintzer D, Maclure M, et al: Triggering of myocardial infarction by cocaine. Circulation 99:2737, 1999.
8. Kanitz MG, Giovannucci SJ, Jones JS, Mott M: Myocardial infarction in young adults: Risk factors and clinical features. J Emerg Med 14:139, 1996.
9. Panju AA, Hemmelgarn BR, Guyatt GH, Simel DL: Is this patient having a myocardial infarction? JAMA 280:1256, 1998.
10. Ros E, Armengol X, Grande L, et al: Chest pain at rest in patients with coronary artery disease. Myocardial ischemia, esophageal dysfunction, or panic disorder? Dig Dis Sci 42:1344, 1997.
11. Lee TH, Cook F, Weisberg M, et al: Acute chest pain in the emergency room. Identification and examination of low-risk patients. Arch Intern Med 145:65, 1985.
12. Lee TH, Goldman L: Primary care: Evaluation of the patient with acute chest pain. N Engl J Med 342:1187, 2000.
13. Riedel M: Acute pulmonary embolism. 1. Pathophysiology, clinical presentation, and diagnosis. Heart 85:229–240, 2001.
14. Ely EW, Smith JM, Haponik EF: Pulmonary embolism and normal oxygenation: Application of PIOPED-derived likelihood ratios. Am J Med 103:541, 1997.
15. Stein PD, Terrin ML, Hales CA, et al: Clinical laboratory, roentgenographic, and electrocardiographic findings in patients with acute pulmonary embolism and no pre-existing cardiac or pulmonary disease. Chest 100:598, 1991.
16. Worsely DF, Alavi A, Aronchick JM, et al: Chest radiographic findings in patients with acute pulmonary embolism. Radiology 189:133, 1993.
17. Flachskampf FA, Daniel WG: Aortic dissection. Cardiol Clin 18:807, 2000.
18. Curci JJ, Horman MJ: Boerhaave's syndrome: The importance of early diagnosis and treatment. Ann Surg 183:401, 1976.
19. Brauer RB, Liebermann-Meffert D, Stein HJ, et al: Boerhaave's syndrome: Analysis of the literature and report of 18 new cases. Dis Esoph 10:64, 1997.
20. Oakley CM: Myocarditis, pericarditis and other pericardial diseases. Heart 84:449, 2000.
21. Sahn SA, Heffner JE: Spontaneous pneumothorax. N Engl J Med 342:868, 2000.
22. Feldman AL, Sullivan JT, Passero MA, Lewis DC: Pneumothorax in polysubstance-abusing marijuana and tobacco smokers: Three cases. J Subst Abuse 5:183, 1993.
23. Schramel FM, Postmus PE, Vanderschueren RG: Current aspects of spontaneous pneumothorax. Eur Respir J 10:1372, 1997.
24. Fleet RP, Dupuis G, Marchand A, et al: Panic disorder, chest pain and coronary artery disease: Literature review. Can J Cardiol 10:827, 1994.
25. Norell M, Lythall D, Cheng A, et al: Limited value of the resting electrocardiogram in assessing patients with recent onset chest pain: Lessons from a chest pain clinic. Br Heart J 67:53, 1992.
26. Falk E: Plaque rupture with severe pre-existing stenosis precipitating coronary thrombosis: Characteristics of coronary atherosclerotic plaques underlying fatal occlusive thrombi. Br Heart J 50:127, 1983.
27. Reimer KA, Lowe JE, Rasmussen MM, et al: The wavefront phenomenon of ischemic cell death. 1. Myocardial infarct size vs duration of coronary occlusion in dogs. Circulation 56:786, 1977.
28. Selbst SM, Ruddy RM, Clark BJ, et al: Pediatric chest pain: A prospective study. Pediatrics 82:319, 1988.
29. Evangelista JA, Parsons M, Renneburg AK: Chest pain in children: Diagnosis through history and physical examination. J Pediatr Health Care 14:3, 2000.

Chapter 5

Acute Shortness of Breath

Roger J. Zoorob

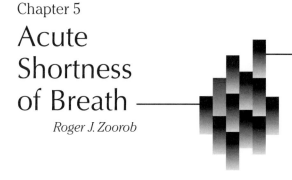

Dypsnea can be described as unpleasant or uncomfortable respiratory sensations that, according to the definition of the American Thoracic Society, derive from interactions among physiologic, psychological, social, and environmental factors.[1] The underlying disorders of dyspnea range from relatively simple to more serious emergencies that should be treated in the emergency department. The most important step is determining whether the condition is a result of a pulmonary, cardiac, or other cause.[2]

 ## CLINICAL RECOGNITION

First, a history should be obtained with concurrent examination of the patient to enable determination of the extent of the emergency. It is important for the clinician to assess the patient's airway, ability to speak, breathing pattern, cardiac rhythm, and mental status. Family physicians can obtain vital signs while asking the patient or family about the duration of the dyspnea and any underlying cardiac or pulmonary disease. A focused history should be taken, including the medications taken; the presence of cough, fever, and chest pain; and any incident of trauma.[3] The clinician should continue the physical examination by observing the skin color and listening to breath sounds and the heart.

Once an emergency situation is excluded and the need for intubation or oxygenation is determined, an expanded history should be obtained and testing performed that is appropriate to the differential diagnosis for acute dyspnea (Box 5–1).

41

> ### Box 5–1. *Differential Diagnosis of Acute Dyspnea*
>
> | | |
> |---|---|
> | Cardiac | Congestive heart failure, CAHD, arrhythmia, pericarditis, acute MI |
> | Central | Neuromuscular causes, pain |
> | Endocrine | Metabolic acidosis, drugs |
> | Pediatric | Bronchiolitis, croup, epiglottitis, asthma, foreign body aspiration |
> | Pulmonary | COPD, asthma, pneumonia, pneumothorax, pulmonary embolism, pleural effusion, metastatic disease, GERD |
> | Psychogenic | Panic attacks, hyperventilation, pain, anxiety |
> | Upper airway obstruction | Epiglottitis, foreign body, croup, Epstein-Barr virus |
>
> CAHD, coronary artery heart disease; COPD, chronic obstructive pulmonary disease GERD, gastroesophageal reflux disease; MI, myocardial infarction.

History

Emphasis should be placed on cardiac and pulmonary symptoms.[4] Cardiac and pulmonary causes may coexist and are the most common reason for shortness of breath.[5] Patients should be questioned about the onset of dyspnea, its duration, and its occurrence at rest or exertion.

The presence of cough may imply asthma or pneumonia.[6] Cough associated with dyspnea and change in the character of sputum may be due to exacerbation of chronic obstructive pulmonary disease (COPD).[7] Fever associated with dyspnea usually implies an infectious cause, such as pneumonia,[6] croup, or bronchiolitis in children.[8] Acute epiglottitis needs to be ruled out when severe sore throat is associated with acute dyspnea.[9]

Chest pain may be due to coronary or pleural conditions, depending on the quality and description of the pain. Pleuritic chest pain could be due to pericarditis, pulmonary embolism, pneumothorax, or pleuritis. Dyspnea or tachypnea with pleuritic chest pain occurs in 97% of patients who have clinically apparent pulmonary embolism.[10] Some authors, however, have questioned the use of clinical presentation for the accurate prediction of pulmonary embolism.[11]

Spontaneous pneumothorax should be considered in patients with COPD, cystic fibrosis, or acquired immunodeficiency syndrome (AIDS).[12, 13] Although rare, catamenial pneumothorax should be considered in a menstruating female with spontaneous symptoms.[14] If the patient is a diver, barotrauma is a possibility.[15] Chest pain is almost universal in spontaneous pneumothorax, with dyspnea described as the second most common symptom.[16]

Anginal chest pain accompanied by shortness of breath may signify ischemia associated with left ventricular dysfunction. Paroxysmal dyspnea or pulmonary edema may be the only clinical presentation in 10% of patients with myocardial infarction.[17] A history of orthopnea, pedal edema, and nocturnal paroxysmal dyspnea is important, as these may suggest congestive heart failure (CHF).[18]

Indigestion or dysphagia may signify reflux or aspiration.[19] Anxiety symptoms may imply a psychogenic cause. However, hyperventilation of psychogenic origin should be diagnosed only after organic disease has been ruled out.[20]

Physical Examination

General Appearance and Vital Signs

The patient's respiratory effort, use of accessory muscles, mental status, and ability to speak help the clinician to determine severity of the dyspnea. A rectal temperature may be taken if necessary because airflow may decrease the oral temperature. Pulsus paradoxicus may exist in COPD, asthma, and cardiac tamponade.[21] Stridor is indicative of an upper airway obstruction.[8]

Neck Examination

Neck veins should be examined. Distention may imply congestive heart failure, cor pulmonale due to severe COPD, or cardiac tamponade. Physicians should check for thyroid enlargement and to determine if the trachea is in the midline.

Cardiac and Pulmonary Examination

The chest should be palpated for subcutaneous emphysema and crepitus, and percussed for dullness (which indicates consolidations and effusions) and hyperresonance (which is noted in pneumothorax and bullous emphysema).

The heart and lungs should be auscultated for absent breath sounds. This may be consistent with pneumothorax or pleural effusion.[22] Wheezing most often suggests obstructive lung disease but could indicate pulmonary edema. Rales exist in pulmonary edema or pneumonia.[23]

A ventricular filling gallop (S_3) suggests left ventricular systolic dysfunction in congestive heart failure (CHF). An atrial gallop (S_4) may suggest left ventricular dysfunction or ischemia but can be normal. An irregular heart rhythm may signify arrhythmia, such as atrial fibrillation. A loud pulmonic second heart sound (P_2) suggests pulmonary hypertension or cor pulmonale.

ACUTE SHORTNESS OF BREATH

The physician should listen for murmurs, which can be an indirect sign of CHF, and for distant heart sounds in cardiac tamponade.[24]

Abdominal Examination

Hepatomegaly and ascites may indicate CHF. Hepatojugular reflux may be used as a bedside maneuver in the diagnosis of congestive heart failure in acutely dyspneic patients.[25]

Extremities

Edema or swelling of the lower extremities or other signs consistent with deep vein thrombosis suggest pulmonary embolism as a cause of the dyspnea.[26] Clubbing and cyanosis of the digits can also be useful signs.

Table 5–1 displays the possible physical and diagnostic findings in the common disease entities that cause acute shortness of breath.

Table 5–1. Physical and Diagnostic Findings of Diseases Presenting with Acute Dyspnea

Disease	Physical Findings	Chest/Neck Radiograph	Pulse Oximetry/ Spirometry	Other Office Tests
Acute asthma	Wheezing, pulsus pardoxicus, accessory muscle use	Hyperinflated lungs	Decreased oxygen saturation, decreased PEFR & FEV_1	
COPD exacerbation	Wheezing, clubbing, barrel chest, decreased breath sounds	Hyperinflated lungs	Decreased oxygen saturation and FEV_1	
Pneumonia	Fever, crackles, increased fremitus	Infiltrates; effusion consolidation	Normal or decreased oxygen saturation	Normal or high WBC count
Congestive heart failure/ pulmonary edema	Edema, neck vein distention, S_3, S_4 hepatojugular reflux, wheezing, murmurs, rales, hypertension/ hypotension	Interstitial edema, cardiomegaly, pleural effusion	Decreased oxygen saturation	ECG:LVH, ischemia, arrhythmia, nonspecific Hb: Anemia
Pneumothorax	Absent breath sounds; hyperresonance	Collapsed lung, mediastinal shift	Decreased oxygen saturation	
Croup	Inspiratory stridor, rhonchi, retractions	Subglottic narrowing by anteroposterior plain film or computed tomography scan	Decreased or normal oxygen saturation	
Epiglottitis	Stridor, drooling, fever	Enlarged epiglottis	Decreased or normal	High WBC

Table 5–1. Physical and Diagnostic Findings of Diseases Presenting with Acute Dyspnea *(Continued)*

Disease	Physical Findings	Chest/Neck Radiograph	Pulse Oximetry/ Spirometry	Other Office Tests
Foreign body aspiration	Stridor, wheezing, persistent pneumonia	Visualization of foreign body, air trapping, hyperinflation	oxygen saturation Decreased or normal oxygen saturation	Normal or high WBC
Bronchiolitis	Wheezing, flaring, retractions, apnea	Hyperinflation, atelactasis	Decreased or normal oxygen saturation	WBC: Normal, respiratory syncytial virus
Hyperventilation	Sighing	Normal	Normal	

COPD, chronic obstructive pulmonary disease; ECG, electrocardiogram; FEV$_1$, forced expiratory volume in 1 second; Hb, hemoglobin; LVH, left ventricular hypertrophy; PEFR, peaked expiratory flow rate; WBC, white blood cells. Data from references 2, 6, 8, 21–30, and 39.

LABORATORY RECOGNITION

The work-up varies according to what diagnostic modalities are available in the office. If available, pulse oximetry should be performed to determine level of oxygenation. A chest radiograph should be obtained in suspected cases of pneumothorax, pneumonia, COPD, pulmonary edema, and CHF.[27] A lateral neck radiograph should be done in stridor or upper airway obstruction such as foreign body aspiration, epiglottitis (enlarged epiglottis), and subglottic edema (narrowed antero-posterior [AP] tracheal air column).[28] If any of these is suspected, the patient should be directed to the emergency department.

An electrocardiogram (ECG) should be performed to enable detection of ischemia, left ventricular hypertrophy,[23] or arrhythmia. Bedside spirometry and peak expiratory flow rate (PEFR) are useful in detecting exacerbations of asthma or COPD.[29, 30] A complete blood count can help when infection or anemia is suspected.

A patient suspected of having pulmonary embolism usually requires evaluation in a hospital setting. Negative rapid and standard enzyme-linked immunosorbent assay (ELISA) D-dimer tests (not considered an office procedure), whether performed alone or in conjunction with normal alveolar dead-space fraction, can help exclude pulmonary embolism.[31, 32] Spiral computed tomography (CT) also has a role in the diagnostic work-up of pulmonary embolism in the hospitalized patient, especially when the ventilation-perfusion V/Q scan is nondiagnostic. Spiral CT may eventually replace pulmonary angiography.[33]

ACUTE SHORTNESS OF BREATH

PHONE TRIAGE

Protocols and clearly written office procedures for staff are recommended to promote proper care and minimize risk for patients calling about dyspnea.[34] Figure 5–1 presents a triage algorithm an office nurse may use for acute dyspnea.

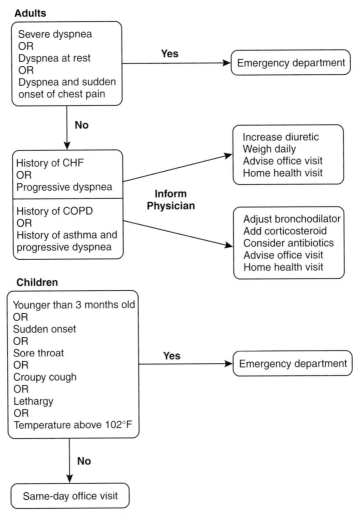

CHF: congestive heart failure.
COPD: chronic obstructive pulmonary disease.

Figure 5–1. Telephone triage algorithm for acute dyspnea, for use in the office.

When an adult patient calls with a chief complaint of shortness of breath, triage nurses may ask the following questions:
- Have you been short of breath for less than an hour?
- Is it sudden?
- Are you short of breath at rest?
- Is your shortness of breath severe?[2, 35]
- Do you have chest pain? Describe the pain.[11]

Sudden shortness of breath at rest is suggestive of pulmonary embolism or pneumothorax. Severe dyspnea over 1 to 2 hours suggests CHF or asthma.[36] If the answer to any of the previous questions is yes, the patient should be advised to proceed directly to the emergency department or call 911. If all answers are no, proceed to the following questions:
- What chronic illnesses do you have?
- Do you have asthma, COPD, CHF, or anxiety?
- Is your shortness of breath mild or moderate?

If the answer to the last question is yes and the patient has a known illness, refer the call to a physician or nurse practitioner for decision making.

At this point, depending on the clinical situation, possible triage options for this scenario include:
1. Office visit
2. Home health nurse visit
3. Physician house call
4. Adjustment of medication (e.g., increase diuretic, start corticosteroid)

Pediatric Triage

- Is the baby younger than 3 months of age?
- Is the shortness of breath sudden?
- Does the baby have a sore throat?
- Is there croupy cough?
- Is the child not playful, not feeding well, not arousable?
- Is the fever above 102°F?
- Is the shortness of breath severe?

If the answer is yes to any of the previous questions, advise the parent to take the child to the emergency department or call 911. In the pediatric age group, the main worry is foreign body aspiration. If fever and sore throat are reported, epiglottitis should be considered. If the answer is no to all of the previous questions, ask the following questions:
- Is the child alert, awake, eating well, and playful?
- Is the dyspnea progressive and not sudden?
- Is there history of asthma or a known predisposing illness?

If the answer is yes to the previous questions, advise the parent to visit the office that same day.

Initial Management of Unstable Patients in the Office

Management of acute dyspnea is targeted toward initial evaluation, stabilization, and resuscitation. Provision of definitive care is dependent on the specific diagnosis and follows the stabilization phase. The following initial quick assessment of the patient should be performed to determine if the patient is unstable:

1. Assess airway patency and listen to the lungs
2. Observe pattern of breathing, including use of accessory muscles
3. Put on the monitor (defibrillator or ECG machine may be used as a monitor)
4. Measure vital signs and pulse oximetry
5. Obtain history of cardiac or pulmonary disease or history of trauma
6. Evaluate mental status

Unstable patients present with one or more of the following clinical pictures: respiratory rate above 40, retractions, cyanosis, hypoxia, hypotension, unstable arrhythmia, altered mental status, stridor, breathing effort without air movement (suspect upper airway obstruction), unilateral tracheal deviation, hypotension, or unilateral breath sounds (suspect tension pneumothorax). Health care professionals should call 911 for these patients.

For any of the previously mentioned patients, depending on what is available in the office and the patient's condition:

1. Administer oxygen
2. Establish an intravenous (IV) access line and start fluids
3. Consider intubation
4. Perform needle tracheostomy in tension pneumothorax
5. Administer nebulized bronchodilator therapy if obstructive pulmonary disease is known
6. Administer IV or IM furosemide if pulmonary edema is noted

Disposition and Transfer

After the patient has been stabilized, disposition and transfer depend on the diagnosis or differential diagnosis. If the patient remains unstable, transfer him or her to the closest emergency department by ambulance for stabilization and resuscitation. Trained health care personnel should accompany the patient in the ambulance and continue to provide management measures until care is transferred to the emergency department personnel. Table 5–2 displays management and disposition options for patients who were initially stabilized in the office and did not require emergency transfer to the emergency department.

ACUTE SHORTNESS OF BREATH

Table 5–2. Management and Disposition of Common Disease Entities Presenting with Acute Shortness of Breath

Disease	Management	Disposition
COPD exacerbation	Oxygen: 1–2 L. β_2 agonist and ipratropium bromide aerosol. IV access. Steroids PO or IV	Lung exam clears: Home on bronchodilators ± prednisone ± antibiotics
No response: Wheezing, low pulse oximetry, working to breathe	Antibiotics Repeat bronchodilator Rx	Admit for respiratory monitoring. Intensive aerosol Rx. IV steroids. Ipratropium bromide. Possible antibiotics. Possible theophylline.
Acute asthme attack	Oxygen. Bronchodilator aerosol q 20–60 min x3 IV steroid. Antibiotics only if complicating bacterial pneumonia	Patient does not respond; PEFR still < 40% of predicted, or FEV_1 < 15%–45%: Admit. PEFR between 40% & 70%, may watch for 12 h and reevaluate. PEFR > 70%: Home on maximum Rx.
Pneumonia	Antibiotics, oxygen, fluids	If increased age, leukopenia, bacteremia, multilobular involvement, hypoxia, metastatic infection, comorbid illness: Admit.
Decompensated CHF, pulmonary edema (with a previously known diagnosis)	Oxygen, IV or IM furosemide, control BP, control arrhythmia, ECG to rule out MI or ischemia; correct electrolyte imbalance	No hypoxia, clear lungs, back to baseline, no ischemia: Home on medical Rx, adjust meds. If hypoxia, lungs not clear, or cardiac ischemia: admit.
Decompensated CHF, acute pulmonary edema new diagnosis	Oxygen, IV morphine 2–5 mg, furosemide 20–60 mg IV. Control BP, control arrhythmia. ECG to rule out MI or ischemia	Admit for diuresis, oxygenation and determine etiology. Rule out MI
Pulmonary embolism (suspected)	Oxygen, IV access, coagulation studies. Chest radiograph, pulse oximetry: Anticoagulate.	Emergency department or direct admission for stat blood gas, ECG, and V-Q scan
Pneumothorax	< 15%–20% oxygen, IV access, > 20%: Chest tube, sclerotherapy	Admit for further observation
Croup	Rule out epiglottitis: Lateral neck radiograph. Oxygen, hydration, humidified air, racemic epinephrine, IV dexamethasone	Hypoxia, fatigue, cyanosis, RR > 40/min, significant retractions: Admit. Responds and remains stable for 3 hours: Home.
Epiglottitis	Do not examine the throat. Do not take child from mother. 100% oxygen. If stridor: Nasotracheal intubation or tracheostomy. IV ceftriaxone	Emergency department for stabilization and admission
Foreign body aspiration Adequate ventilatory function.	Oxygen. Remove proximal foreign body by laryngoscope	Distal foreign body: Consult Foreign body removed: Send home
Bronchiolitis	Hydration, oxygen, albuterol aerosol. Ribavirin for high risk only	RR < 50, playful, alert, normal oxygen saturation, feeding well, no underlying disease: Home. Others: Admit
Hyperventilation	Rule out organic disease (i.e., metabolic acidosis), reassure	Home, education, counseling. Rx of anxiety or depression

BP, blood pressure; CHF, congestive heart failure; COPD, chronic obstructive pulmonary disease; ECG, electrocardiogram; FEV, forced expiratory volume; IM, intramuscular; IV, intravenous; MI, myocardial infarction; PEFR, peak expiratory flow rate; PO, by mouth; RR, respiratory rate; Rx, treatment; V = Q, ventilation perfusion.
Data from references 7, 8, 13, 22, 28, 29, 31, 37, 38, and 40–46.

ACUTE SHORTNESS OF BREATH

Medications

The medications most commonly used in the office for treatment of acute shortness of breath are listed in Table 5–3. This table also displays pediatric dosing and explains how the drug is supplied.

Table 5–3. Dosages of Common Medications Used in Acute Dyspnea in the Office Setting

	Dosage	Pediatric Dosage	Labeling
Adenosine	6 mg IV bolus. Repeat 12 mg in 1–2 min	0.1 mg/kg rapid IV push. May increase dose by 0.05 mg/kg increments every 2 min to a max of 0.25 mg/kg until termination of arrhythmia or maximum dose of 12 mg is reached	3 mg/mL (2 mL)
Albuterol rotacaps	200 µg every 4–6 hr PRN	Rotacaps 200 µg every 4–6 hr	200 µg/Rotacap
Albuterol puffs	2 puffs may repeat every 20–60 min x3	Albuterol puffs: 1–2 puffs (90–180 µg) every 4–6 hr	90 µg actuation. 200 actuations/17-g canister
Albuterol nebulized solution	2.5 µg may repeat every 20–60 min x3	Neonate, infant: 0.05–0.15 mg/kg/dose 1–5 years: 1.25–2.5 mg/dose 5–12 years: 2.5 mg/dose	0.5% 5 mg/mL. Prediluted: 2.5 mg in a 3-mL vial (0.083%)
Ceftriaxone	1–2 g IV or IM	50–75 mg/kg every 24 hr in 1 or 2 divided doses	250 mg, 500 mg, 1-g vials
Diltiazem	0.25 mg/kg IV. No response: 0.35 mg/kg in 15 min		5 mg/mL in 5-mL vials
Epinephrine (racemic)	0.05 mL/kg diluted to 3 mL with saline nebulizer over 15 min q 1–2 hr. Max dose— 0.5 mL	0.05 mL/kg diluted to 3 mL with saline nebulizer over 15 min q 1–2 hr. Max dose 0.5 mL	2.25% solution in 15- or 30-mL ampules
Furosemide	20–80 mg IV or IM	Infants and children: 0.5 mg–2 mg/kg dose IV push or IM	10 mg/mL (2–10-mL vials)
Methyl-prednisolone	Status asthmaticus: 60–125 mg IV bolus	Status asthmaticus: Load with 2 mg/kg dose IV	40 mg, 125 mg, and 500 mg/mL
Nitroglycerin sublingual	0.2–0.6 mg sublingual 5 min for a max of 3 doses		Sublingual tabs: 0.15, 0.3, 0.4, and 0.6 mg
Verapamil	2.5–5.0 mg IV followed by IV doses of 5–10 mg. Max dose 20 mg	0.1–0.3 mg/kg/dose given over 3 min. Max first IV dose is 5 mg. Repeat dose of max 10 mg can be given in 30 min	2.5 mg/mL (2- and 4-mL vials)

Data from reference 46

Pediatrics

Many causes are associated with acute shortness of breath in the pediatric age group. The most common causes in children are acute asthma, pulmonary infection, and upper airway obstruction. Some causes, such as epiglottitis, croup, and myocarditis, are serious and may be fatal. Foreign body aspiration is also an important cause of dyspnea in the pediatric age group. Nonrespiratory causes in children include anemia, acidosis such as diabetic ketoacidosis, and drug poisoning.[37, 38]

References

1. American Thoracic Society: Dyspnea. Mechanisms, assessment, and management: A consensus statement. Am J Respir Crit Care Med 159:321–340, 1990.
2. Michelson E, Hollrah S: Evidence based emergency medicine: Evaluation and diagnostic testing. Emerg Med Clin North Am 17:221–227, 1999.
3. Janssens JP, de Muralt B, Titelion V: Management of dyspnea in severe chronic obstructive pulmonary disease. J Pain Symptom Manage 19:378–392, 2000.
4. Silvestri GA, Mahler DA: Evaluation of dyspnea in the elderly patient. Clin Chest Med 14:393–404, 1993.
5. Cockcroft A, Adams L, Guz A: Assessment of breathlessness. Q J Med 72:669–676, 1989.
6. Fang GD, Fine M, Orloff J, et al: New and emerging etiologies for community-acquired pneumonia with implications for therapy: A prospective multicenter study of 359 cases. Medicine 69:307–316, 1990.
7. Aboussouan LS: Acute exacerbation of chronic bronchitis: Focusing management for optimum results. Postgrad Med 99:89–102, 1996.
8. Godden CW, Campbell MJ, Hussey M, Cogswell JJ: Double blind placebo controlled trial of nebulised budesonide for croup. Arch Dis Child 76:155–158, 1997.
9. Deeb ZE: Acute supraglottitis in adults: Early indicators of airway obstruction. Am J Otolaryngol 18:112–115, 1997.
10. Stein PD: Acute pulmonary embolism. Dis Mon 40:467–523, 1994.
11. Hoffman GM, Lee A, Grafton ST, et al: Clinical signs and symptoms in pulmonary embolism. A reassessment. Clin Nucl Med 19:803–808, 1994.
12. Mahler D: Dyspnea: Diagnosis and management. Clin Chest Med 8:215–229, 1987.
13. Van Schil PE, Vercauteren SR, Vermeire PA, et al: Catamenial pneumothorax caused by thoracic endometriosis. Ann Thorac Surg 62:585–586, 1996.
14. Russi EW: Diving and the risk of barotrauma. Thorax 53(suppl 2):S20–S24, 1998.
15. Sasson CS: The etiology and treatment of spontaneous pneumothorax. Curr Opin Pulm Med 1:331–338, 1995.
16. Sahn SA: Spontaneous pneumothorax: A common emergency. J Respir Dis 4:12–21, 1983.
17. Lusiani L, Perrone A, Pesavento R, Conte G: Prevalence, clinical features, and acute course of atypical myocardial infarction. Angiology 45:49–55, 1994.
18. Ciocon JO, Fernandez BB, Ciocon DG: Leg edema: Clinical clues to the differential diagnosis. Geriatrics 48:34–40, 1993.
19. Siegel PD, Katz J: Respiratory complications of gastroesophageal reflux disease. Prim Care 23:433–441, 1996.
20. Saisch SG, Wessly S, Gardner WN: Patients with acute hyperventilation presenting to inner-city emergency room. Chest 110:952–957, 1996.
21. Cokcroft DW: Management of acute severe asthma. Ann Allergy Asthma Immunol 75:83–89, 1995.
22. Abolnik IZ, Lossos IS, Gillis D, Breuer R: Primary spontaneous pneumothorax in men. Am J Med Sci 305:297–303, 1993.
23. Gillespie ND, McNeill G, Pringle T, et al: Cross sectional study of contribution of clinical assessment and simple cardiac investigations to diagnosis of left ventricular dysfunction in patients admitted with acute dyspnea. BMJ 314:936–940, 1997.

24. Rich MW: Epidemiology, pathophysiology, and etiology of congestive heart failure in older adults. J Am Geriatr Soc 45:968–974, 1997.
25. Marantz PR, Kaplan MC, Alderman MH: Clinical diagnosis of congestive heart failure in patients with acute dyspnea. Chest 97:775–781, 1990.
26. Worsley DF, Palevsky HI, Alavi A: A detailed evaluation of patients with acute pulmonary embolism and low or very low probability lung scan interpretations. Arch Intern Med 154:2737–2741, 1994.
27. Butcher BL, Nichol KL, Parenti CM: High yield of chest radiography in walk-in clinic patients with chest symptoms. J Gen Intern Med 8:115–119, 1993.
28. Frantz TD, Rasgon BM, Quesenberry CP: Acute epiglottitis in adults: Analysis of 129 cases. JAMA 272:1358–1360, 1994.
29. Brenner B, Kohn MS: The acute asthmatic patient in the ED: To admit or discharge. Am J Emerg Med 16:69–75, 1998.
30. Members of the Cardiopulmonary Diagnostics Guidelines Committee: American Association of Respiratory Care Clinical Practice Guideline—Spirometry. Respir Care 36:1414–1417, 1991.
31. Kline JA, Israel EG, Michelson EA, et al: Diagnostic accuracy of a bedside d-dimer assay and alveolar dead-space measurement for rapid exclusion of pulmonary embolism: A multicenter study. JAMA 285:761–768, 2001.
32. Oger E, Leroyer C, Bressollette L, et al: Evaluation of a new, rapid, and quantitative d-dimer test in patients with suspected pulmonary embolism. Am J Respir Crit Care Med 158:65–70, 1998.
33. Paterson DI, Schwartzman K: Strategies incorporating spiral CT for the diagnosis of acute pulmonary embolism: A cost-effectiveness analysis. Chest 119:1791–1800, 2001.
34. Robinson DL, Anderson MM, Erpenbeck PM: Telephone advice: New solutions for old problems. Nurs Pract 22:179–180, 183–186, 1997.
35. Mahler DA, Harver A: Do you speak the language of dyspnea? Chest 117:928–929, 2000.
36. Accident and emergency medicine. Acute dyspnea. Austral Fam Phys 24:663–670, 1995.
37. Levy BT, Garber MA: Respiratory syncytial virus infection in infants and young children. J Fam Pract 45:473–481, 1997.
38. Morgan WC, Hodge HL: Diagnostic evaluation of dyspnea. Am Fam Phys 57:711–716, 1998.
39. Thompson WH, Nielson CP, Carvalho P, et al: Controlled trial of oral prednisone in outpatients with acute COPD exacerbation. Am J Respir Crit Care Med 154:407–412, 1996.
40. Van Zwieten PA: Current and newer approaches in the drug treatment of congestive heart failure. Cardiovasc Drugs Ther 10:693–702, 1997.
41. Hull RD, Raskob GE, Ginsberg JS, et al: A non-invasive strategy for the treatment of patients with suspected pulmonary embolism. Arch Intern Med 154:289–297, 1994.
42. Senkaya I, Sagdic K, Gebitekin C, et al: Management of foreign body aspiration in infancy and childhood. A life-threatening problem. Turk J Pediatr 39:353–362, 1997.
43. Small GW, Feinberg DT, Steinberg D, Collins MT: A sudden outbreak of illness suggestive of mass hysteria in schoolchildren. Arch Fam Med 3:711–716, 1994.
44. Emerman CL, Cydulka RK: A randomized comparison of 100 mg vs. 500 mg methylprednisolone in the treatment of acute asthma. Chest 107:1559–1563, 1995.
45. Pomilla PV, Brown RB: Outpatient treatment of community acquired pneumonia in adults. Arch Intern Med 154:1793–1802, 1994.
46. Physicians' Desk Reference. Montvale, NJ, Medical Economics Company Inc, 2000.

Chapter 6

Hypertensive Urgencies

Zachary F. Meisel
Iris M. Reyes

Hypertension is a highly prevalent chronic illness that affects nearly 25% of all adults in the United States. The devastating role of chronically elevated blood pressure in cardiovascular disease, stroke, renal failure, and thus, overall morbidity and mortality in this country has been well documented and is largely understood by the medical community. The National Heart, Lung, and Blood Institute estimates that hypertension accounts for more than $259 billion in health care costs per year.[1] Because hypertension is a modifiable risk factor for such serious illnesses, the management of hypertension has been reported to be the leading indication for visits to physicians and for the use of prescription drugs in the United States.

Because of the high prevalence of hypertension, as well as increased awareness about high blood pressure among both patients and health care providers, it is not uncommon for health care providers to encounter acutely elevated blood pressure in the office setting. It is important for clinicians to realize that the greatest impact of hypertension results from its *chronic effects*; a rarer and much more select group of patients who present to the physician's office with high blood pressure require immediate intervention. The goal of this chapter is to provide information about identifying, treating, and generating a proper disposition on such patients with hypertensive "urgencies" and "emergencies."

Classification

In 1997, the National Heart, Lung, and Blood Institute's Joint National Committee (JNC) published its sixth report on the "Prevention, Detection, Evaluation, and Treatment of High Blood Pressure" (JNC VI).[1] This consensus report noted that blood pressure greater than 135/85 mm Hg should be considered elevated. Hypertension was categorized by the JNC to be classified into three stages as follows: *stage 1* comprises blood pressures of (140–159)/(90–99), *stage 2* includes (160–179)/(100–109), and

53

stage 3 refers to values of (≥180)/(≥110). Management should be based on the clinical impact of the elevated blood pressure on the patient. The health care provider must remember to treat the patient, not the number on the sphygmomanometer. Overzealous treatment of acute hypertension can significantly worsen a patient's condition.

Hypertensive Emergency

Hypertensive emergency is defined by JNC as clinical situations that "require immediate blood pressure reduction (not necessarily to normal ranges)" to limit end-organ damage. These are rare situations in which target organs, specifically, the brain, heart, kidneys, and eyes, are damaged, often irreversibly, by acutely elevated blood pressure. Examples of hypertensive emergencies include:
• Hypertensive encephalopathy
• Intracerebral bleeding
• Stroke
• Acute renal failure
• Acute left ventricular heart failure with pulmonary edema
• Acute coronary syndrome/myocardial infarction
• Aortic dissection
• Eclampsia of pregnancy

These situations require rapid identification and intervention. Definitive intervention should be performed in an emergency department and then in an intensive care unit setting. One of the primary goals of the office-based clinician is to identify patients with such emergencies and then arrange for immediate transport to the nearest health care facility, where advanced care can be provided.

Hypertensive Urgency

JNC VI defines *hypertensive urgency* as "those situations in which it is desirable to reduce blood pressure within a few hours." Included in this category is hypertension with:
• upper limit stage 3 hypertension
• severe perioperative hypertension
• optic disc edema (stage 4 hypertensive retinopathy)
• progressive target organ complications.

This category is less clearly defined than that of hypertensive emergencies. Available literature on the diagnosis and management of hypertensive urgencies is limited. Of note, the current JNC VI diagnostic approach and classification for patients in "hypertensive urgency" significantly differ from previous recommendations from the JNC. As with hypertensive emergencies, management is directed by the clinical scenario, not by the number on the sphygmomanometer.

Asymptomatic Acute Hypertension

Asymptomatic acute hypertension is any elevated blood pressure in the absence of symptoms or new/progressive target organ damage. These scenarios *rarely* require emergency therapy.[2] A substantial and growing body of literature has demonstrated significant adverse ischemic effects caused by the routine use of rapid-acting antihypertensive medications for nonemergent/nonurgent hypertension (especially with the use of short-acting nifedipine).[3] JNC VI notes that the "upper levels of stage 3 hypertension"—greater than 210/120 (classified as stage 4 by the 5th JNC in 1994)—may be considered hypertensive urgency. Therefore, even in the absence of symptoms, a patient with a severely elevated blood pressure is to be considered eligible for blood pressure reduction within a few hours. This recommendation is controversial and vague at best, however. No study to date has demonstrated that lowering the blood pressure of an *asymptomatic* patient within hours prevents complications.

 CLINICAL RECOGNITION ◀

Identifying isolated hypertension is not difficult. Medical office staff or patients with home sphygmomanometers will identify and may be alarmed by elevated blood pressure readings. As was discussed earlier, because asymptomatic hypertension rarely requires urgent intervention, the focused history and physical examination should be aimed at determining if a patient is currently (or will shortly be) suffering end-organ damage from his or her hypertension. Also, the evaluation should aim to identify any possible specific causes of the elevated blood pressure; in addition to untreated or undertreated essential hypertension, other causes of elevated blood pressure include:

- *Toxicologic causes*—cocaine or amphetamine ingestion; simultaneous use of monoamine oxidase (MAO) inhibitor antidepressants and tyramine-containing foods or α-agonist–containing decongestants[4]
- *Iatrogenic causes*—for example, commonly used exogenous glucocorticoid therapy can precipitate Cushing's syndrome and hypertension. Various weight loss medications (both prescription and over-the-counter) contain stimulants that can elevate blood pressure. Anabolic steroids, lead, cadmium, bromocriptine, and erythropoietin have also been implicated in hypertension[5]

- *Withdrawal*—especially from antihypertensive medications such as clonidine and β-adrenergic antagonists; often causes hypertension and tachycardia
- *Acute central and renovascular causes*—stroke and acute renal failure can be the causes as well as the effects of elevated blood pressure owing to the loss of the autoregulation process, which would otherwise maintain blood pressure in an individual with a healthy brain or kidneys, respectively[6]

Identification of any of these secondary causes of hypertension is important because it may serve to guide treatment and disposition.

Acute end-organ damage nearly always manifests in specific symptoms. These are listed in the "Phone Triage" section of this chapter.

The medical history must also include asking all women of child-bearing age if they are, could be, or recently have been pregnant. Preeclampsia and eclampsia are associated with elevations in blood pressure.

Antihypertensive medication use (or cessation) must be elicited to identify (1) if the patient is presenting with new or previously diagnosed hypertension, and (2) if the patient may be suffering from a withdrawal syndrome.

Use of illegal stimulants such as cocaine or amphetamines must be asked. Herbal weight loss products or cold remedies may contain ephedrine, which can acutely raise blood pressure. St. John's Wort, an herbal medicine advertised to treat depression, has intrinsic MAO inhibitory properties. Its use should be identified in patients with elevated blood pressure.[7]

The physical examination, like the history, should be focused on identifying any signs of target organ damage associated with hypertension. First, an elevated blood pressure should be confirmed by repeat measurements in all four limbs using cuffs of proper size. Manual measurements have been shown to be more accurate than those attained with automated blood pressure cuffs. Other vital sign abnormalities that occur in conjunction with hypertension may point to evidence of end-organ damage. Tachycardia, tachypnea, and fever are frequent sequelae of cardiopulmonary or central nervous system (CNS) injury. Evidence of CNS compromise may be elicited by a careful neurologic examination, including a mental status analysis. Weakness, visual field cuts, and/or speech difficulties can indicate stroke. Headache can point to a subarachnoid hemorrhage. Confusion and elevated blood pressure might mark hypertensive encephalopathy. The pulmonary and cardiovascular examination should focus on identifying heart failure and pulmonary edema: tachycardia, an S_3 sound, and lung rales can indicate this condition. Differences in upper and lower extremity blood pressures might assist the clinician in diagnosing aortic dissection, although the absence of this finding should not be used to rule out a dissection. A funduscopic examination should be performed to evaluate the optic discs. Papilledema or blurred optic discs can indicate advanced hypertensive retinopathy.

Pregnant women with hypertension may be found to have edema on physical examination. This finding can indicate preeclampsia. Eclampsia is defined as the presence of hypertension, edema, proteinuria, and seizures of no other apparent cause in a woman who has reached 20 weeks of pregnancy or who has delivered within the previous week.[8] Eclampsia is a true hypertensive emergency and is associated with a high mortality rate if not treated emergently.

 PHONE TRIAGE ◄———————————————————————

The patient who calls with a complaint of high blood pressure will often have a home sphygmomanometer or may have had his or her blood pressure taken at a health fair or mall. Blood pressures that are stage 2 (179/109) or lower in the absence of symptoms reflecting end-organ damage may not need to be evaluated urgently. Stage 3 hypertension (equal to or greater than 180/110) should be confirmed in the office and evaluated with a history and physical examination, as well as ancillary testing.[1] Acute end-organ damage symptoms include the following:

Central nervous system compromise
- Headache
- Visual disturbances
- Weakness
- Confusion
- Seizures

Cardiovascular compromise
- Chest pain
- Dyspnea
- Tearing back pain
- Palpitations
- Syncope

Acute renal compromise
- Decreased urine output
- Bloody or foamlike urine
- Vague abdominal pain
- Malaise

Stress and anxiety are well-known stimulants of elevated blood pressure. Patients checking their blood pressure at home may become anxious by elevated readings. This can lead to a cycle of hypertension and emotional stress. Patients with nonurgent, asymptomatic hypertension should be encouraged to check their blood pressure no more than twice daily. Medication compliance should be emphasized and relaxation techniques such as deep breathing can be encouraged on the phone.

Patients who call and note symptoms consistent with hypertensive urgency or emergency (discussed earlier) should be referred immediately to the nearest emergency department. If the patient is complaining of chest pain reflective of ischemic cardiac disease, he or she can chew an aspirin tablet. Otherwise, the patient should refrain from eating or taking any medicine but should be sure to bring his or her medications to the hospital.

 LABORATORY RECOGNITION ◄—————————

A limited number of ancillary office tests can be helpful in addressing potential hypertensive emergencies or urgencies. Laboratory testing for patients with asymptomatic or chronic nonurgent hypertension is not discussed in this chapter.

Women who are of child-bearing age and present with hypertension should undergo a urine human chorionic gonadotropin (hCG) check in the office. Although preeclampsia/eclampsia does not usually present until the second or third trimester of gestation, it is important not to miss this diagnosis. All patients with hypertension should have a urine dipstick analysis. New or severe proteinuria, hematuria, or red blood cell casts in urine may be indicative of acute renal failure. An electrocardiogram (ECG) should be performed if cardiac ischemia or an arrhythmia is suspected. A plain chest radiograph can be helpful in assessing for left ventricular heart failure or aortic dissection (possibly showing pulmonary edema and a wide mediastinum, respectively).[9]

It should be emphasized that rapid triage and transfer should not be delayed for the sake of in-office testing for patients who present with hypertension and signs or symptoms of end-organ injury.

Treatment and Disposition

Unlike with treatment of chronic hypertension, the office setting has a limited role in the treatment of acute hypertension. As has been discussed, there is no evidence to support the short-term treatment of nonemergent hypertension; but patients should receive appropriate long-term antihypertensive therapy. Thus, the office-based practitioner should be focused on differentiating hypertensive emergencies from nonurgent episodes of acute hypertension. Generating the proper disposition for these patients is also essential. Once a hypertensive urgency or emergency has been potentially identified, the patient should be immediately transferred via an Advanced Cardiac Life Support (ACLS)-certified patient transport unit to the emergency facility—most commonly this involves activating the local emergency medical service. Intravenous access can be initiated, and all pertinent records and test results should be transferred with the patient to the hospital. A phone call informing the emergency facility of the patient's imminent arrival is appropriate.

Blood pressure reduction in hypertensive emergencies is to be performed in the emergency or intensive care unit setting. The treatment goal in most of these emergencies is the reduction of mean arterial pressure [MAP = $\frac{1}{3}$ (SBP − DSP) + DSP, where MAP is mean arterial pressure, SBP is systolic blood pressure, and DSP is diastolic blood pressure] by 20% to 25% over 60 minutes. Close monitoring and the use of easily titratable IV medications are most appropriate for this purpose. A few exceptions exist; these are discussed in the following paragraphs.

Stroke and Intracranial Hemorrhage

Patients may present with weakness, aphasia or visual field cuts, facial droop, or dysarthria. Reduction of hypertension in cerebral ischemia may limit cerebral perfusion pressure and exacerbate the stroke. It is important that the clinician not attempt blood pressure reduction for these patients in the outpatient setting. If they are deemed to be candidates for thrombolysis, an inpatient neurology team may carefully bring the blood pressure to 185/110 using IV agents.[10] Intracranial hemorrhage (ICH) may require blood pressure reduction but is often indistinguishable from ischemic stroke in the outpatient setting. Once an ICH has been identified, often by computed tomographic (CT) scan or lumbar puncture, nicardipine and/or nitroprusside should be initiated for reduction of vasospasm and for blood pressure control.[11] Aspirin should be avoided for all patients with potential stroke (because it can complicate thrombolysis). If possible, transfer to a specialized stroke center should be arranged.

Hypertensive Encephalopathy

In addition to hypertension, nonspecific CNS signs and symptoms such as nausea, vomiting, severe headache, confusion, blurry vision, or seizures may be evident. Rapid transfer to an acute setting is mandatory because this condition can rapidly progress. Because this syndrome may

HYPERTENSIVE
URGENCIES

be difficult to distinguish from ischemic stroke, antihypertensive medication should be avoided in the outpatient setting. Intravenous sodium nitroprusside (0.5 mcg/kg/min) is the hospital treatment of choice once this diagnosis has been confirmed.[6]

Left Ventricular Heart Failure/Pulmonary Edema/Acute Coronary Syndromes

The increased peripheral vascular resistance that occurs in hypertension may precipitate pulmonary edema by way of left-sided heart failure. This can also lead to acute ischemic coronary syndromes. Vasodilatation and rapid blood pressure reduction can bring rapid relief to these patients. Definitive treatment for hypertension with pulmonary edema is hospital-based intravenous nitroglycerin, diuretics, and possibly angiotensin-converting enzyme (ACE) inhibitors and/or morphine sulfate. Sublingual nitroglycerin (0.4 mg tablet or spray), repeated up to 3 times while blood pressure is being closely monitored, *may be safely used in the outpatient setting* while the patient is being prepared for transfer to a higher level of care setting. One aspirin to be chewed should be provided before transfer to all eligible patients with potential acute coronary syndromes.[12]

Aortic Dissection

Shearing forces related to hypertension can result in this potentially devastating event in which a tear in the intima of the aorta dissects into the lumen of the great vessel. Tearing chest pain radiating to the back or abdomen and associated with high blood pressure may first identify this condition. Definitive care comprises reduction of the shearing forces and surgical evaluation and correction, depending on the location of the dissection. Office-based care includes rapid transfer to an emergency facility with surgical support, intravenous access, and supportive/ACLS care. Combination intravenous therapy to reduce shearing forces includes β-adrenergic blockade and sodium nitroprusside therapy.[7]

Acute Renal Failure

Patients may present with hematuria, oliguria, anuria, and sudden elevations in blood urea nitrogen (BUN) and creatinine. Transfer to an emergency department is appropriate for blood pressure reduction (usually with sodium nitroprusside), evaluation, and admission.

Hypertensive Retinopathy

Patients may present with blurred vision and edematous optic discs seen on funduscopic examination. Treatment is similar to that described for hypertensive encephalopathy.

Preeclampsia/Eclampsia

Pregnant (or recently postpartum) women with hypertension, edema, and proteinuria have preeclampsia. If they develop seizures, they have eclampsia, which is a life-threatening hypertensive emergency. Definitive care for these conditions includes delivery, magnesium sulfate, and hydralazine and/or labetalol. ACE inhibitors and angiotensin-receptor blockers are to be avoided in pregnancy owing to their teratogenicity. Office-based care for these patients includes transfer to the nearest emergency facility, preferably with obstetric care available and alerted. (See Chapter 15 on emergencies associated with third trimester pregnancy.)[8]

Pediatrics

Children with hypertension should be evaluated in a similar fashion to adults. Of note, hypertension is significantly more rare in children, and a lower threshold should be used to make an urgent referral. In addition, toxicologic causes of hypertension should be examined more closely in children because they are predisposed to ingestion, depending on the age of the child. The technique for measuring blood pressure in children should be emphasized here: The cuff bladder should completely encircle the arm and cover 75% of its length. The child should be seated and calm during measurement, and the fifth Korotkoff sound (muffling) should be used to determine the diastolic pressure.

Conclusion

Hypertensive emergencies are uncommon and have multiple causes and sequelae. One of the primary roles of the office-based practitioner is to identify hypertensive emergencies based on high blood pressure and a constellation of signs and symptoms and laboratory tests. Disposition for these diagnoses is to an acute care facility for intensive monitoring and treatment. Office-based medical treatment for acute severe hypertension is rarely indicated. If the patient has evidence of end-organ injury, treatment should involve intravenous medication and intensive care unit–style monitoring. If the patient has no evidence of end-organ injury, rapid lowering of blood pressure using oral medications offers no proven benefit and may cause complications.

References

1. National Heart, Lung, and Blood Institute (NHLBI)—National Institutes of Health: The sixth report of the Joint National Committee (JNC) on Prevention, Detection, Evaluation and Treatment of High Blood Pressure. Arch Intern Med 157:2413–2446, 1997.

2. Thach A, Schultz P: Nonemergent hypertension: New perspective for the emergency medicine physician. Emerg Med Clin North Am 13:1009–1035, 1995.
3. Fagan TC: Acute reduction of blood pressure in asymptomatic patients with severe hypertension: An idea whose time has come and gone. Arch Intern Med 149:2169–2170, 1989.
4. Nelson L, Perrone J: Herbal and alternative medicine. Emerg Med Clin North Am 18:709–722, 2000.
5. Grossman E, Messerli FH: High blood pressure: A side effect of drugs, poisons and food. Arch Intern Med 155:450–460, 1995.
6. Gifford RW Jr: Management of hypertensive crises. JAMA 266:829–835, 1991.
7. Murphy C: Hypertensive emergencies. Emerg Med Clin North Am 13:973–1007, 1995.
8. National High Blood Pressure Education Program Working Group on High Blood Pressure in Pregnancy: Report of the National High Blood Pressure Education Program Working Group on High Blood Pressure in Pregnancy. Am J Obstet Gynecol 183:S1–S22, 2000.
9. Kaplan NM: Management of hypertensive emergencies. Lancet 344:1335–1338, 1994.
10. Lewandowski C, Barsan W: Treatment of acute ischemic stroke. Ann Emerg Med 37:202–216, 2001.
11. Haley ED Jr, Kassell NF, Torner JC: A randomized controlled high dose intravenous nicardipine in aneurysmal subarachnoid hemorrhage. J Neurosurg 78:537–547, 1993.
12. Varon J, Marik P: The diagnosis and management of hypertensive crises. Chest 118:214–227, 2000.

Chapter 7

Vascular Emergencies

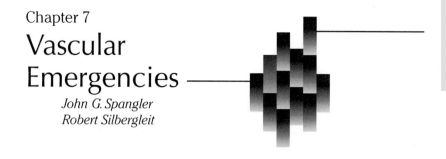

John G. Spangler
Robert Silbergleit

Aortic Dissection

Aortic dissection is a life-threatening condition requiring early recognition and management. Owing to its catastrophic potential, this condition should always be considered in any patient presenting with chest pain. Dissection begins as a transverse tear through the intima and into the media where blood then dissects proximally (retrograde dissection) or distally (antegrade dissection) along the aorta.[1]

 ## CLINICAL RECOGNITION ◄

History

Patients with aortic dissection usually present with the abrupt onset of tearing or ripping anterior chest pain that is maximally intense from its onset[1]; except among patients with altered mental status, pain is universally present.[2] Proximal dissections (type A) are most commonly associated with anterior chest pain; distal dissections (type B) have a higher rate of interscapular pain and pain radiating down the back into the hips.[1,3] Classically, aortic dissection occurs in the hypertensive male between 50 and 70 years of age[1,3]; although the male/female ratio is 3:1, there is an association with third trimester pregnancy among women.[3] Disorders that weaken the aorta and are also associated with aortic dissection include Marfan's syndrome, Ehlers-Danlos syndrome, congenital heart disease, coarctation of the aorta, Turner's syndrome, and trauma.

As dissection progresses, major arteries may become occluded, giving rise to symptoms of myocardial infarction, stroke, mesenteric ischemia, acute renal failure, limb ischemia, and spinal artery occlusion with paraplegia.[1] Proximal dissections disrupting the aortic valve are disastrous, causing sudden aortic insufficiency with pulmonary edema (15%), syncope or stroke (6%), hemopericardium with tamponade (10%), and hemothorax (6%, usually left-sided).[2]

Physical Examination

Signs of arterial or venous compression may be present with diminished pulses, venous engorgement, or neurologic deficits. A new murmur of aortic insufficiency occurs in up to 60% of patients with proximal dissection.[2] Leakage of blood may lead to hemothorax or a pericardial friction rub, the latter of which is an ominous sign of impending tamponade (Box 7–1). Rupture is the most frequent terminal event. Most patients (50% to 75%) are hypertensive[2] at presentation, but 25% to 30% of patients are hypotensive, indicating aortic rupture, severe aortic insufficiency, pericardial tamponade, or cardiogenic shock. Blood pressure should be measured in both arms, as well as the legs, to rule out pseudohypotension from occluded subclavian arteries.[2, 4] A difference of greater than 20 mm Hg in blood pressure between the arms with diminished pulses greatly increases the likelihood of aortic dissection.[2]

**Box 7–1. *Acute Aortic Dissection: Clinical Features **
*(Always Consider in any Patient with Chest Pain)***

Chest pain (90%): Sudden, excruciating, migrating (70%)[†]
   Anterior chest or face (type A); interscapular (type B)
Hypertension (70%; in 2% of hypertensives)
Arterial or venous compression (50% type A, 15% type B)
   Pulse deficits, bruits, venous distention
   Neurologic deficit (30%); Horner's syncope, etc.
   Coronary-visceral ischemia (10%)
Other compression: Hoarseness, dysphagia
Aortic incompetence (25%, 60% type A)
Extravasation
   High risk: pleural cavity or mediastinum
   Ominous: pericardial rub, hemoptysis, hematemesis

---

*Male female 3:1; age 40 to 70 years old; Marfan's (11%); Musculoskeletal, (100%); family history (85%); ocular (70%); cardiovascular (98%.
[†] Pain and/or migration active dissection.
Reproduced from Fuster V, Halperin JL: Aortic dissection: A medical perspective. J Card Surg 9: 713–728, 1994.

Laboratory data do not help the clinician to establish the diagnosis of aortic dissection. If available, an electrocardiogram (ECG) should be obtained to help in the determination of whether myocardial infarction is present[3] (Box 7–2). A chest radiograph may reveal a widened mediastinum or a left pleural effusion, but transport should not be delayed for this study because it is only remotely reliable.

Box 7–2. *Acute Aortic Dissection: Office Management*

ECG monitoring, Foley, monitor airway
Hypertensive patients
   Trimethaphan (Arfonad)* IV, 1 to 2 mg/min to maintain a systolic
      BP in the range of 110 mm Hg, or lowest level that maintains a
      urinary output of 20 to 30 mL/hr
OR

   Sodium nitroprusside[†] IV, 1 mcg/kg/min can be used in place of
      trimethaphan
PLUS

   Propranolol[‡] IV, 0.5 mg initially, then 1 mg every 15 minutes to a
      pulse rate of 60 to 70; then 1 to 2 mg every 4 to 6 hr IV or 20 to
      40 mg orally every 6 hours to maintain a heart rate of about
      60 beats/min.
Normotensive patients
   Propranolol IV, 1 to 2 mg every 4 to 6 hr

---

*Antihypertensive and lowers shearing forces, labetalol as alternative.
[†] Calcium channel antagonists as an alternative.
[‡] Atenolol or metoprolol as alternatives.
BP, blood pressure; ECG, electrocardiogram.
Adapted from Fuster V, Halperin JL: Aortic dissection: A medical perspective. J Card Surg 9: 713–728, 1994.

Initial Management

Office staff should call 911 to transport the patient; the physician in the emergency department who will be receiving the patient should be notified as well (Fig. 7–1). Attention to airway, breathing, and circulation (ABCs) and vital signs is essential. The patient must maintain an airway; supplemental oxygen should be applied, and the clinician must be prepared to assist ventilations if needed. A large-bore peripheral IV should be started, the patient should be attached to a cardiac monitor, and a Foley catheter should be inserted so that urine output can be followed, if indicated and available. An ECG should be obtained; if myocardial ischemia is present, aspirin and nitroglycerin should be administered. Vital signs should be repeated frequently until paramedics arrive. Hypotension must be treated aggressively with volume replacement.[1]

While awaiting emergency transport, the clinician should treat hypertension aggressively to a goal of systolic blood pressure 100 to 120 mm Hg achieved within 5 to 10 minutes. Sodium nitroprusside, 1 mcg/kg/min intravenously, titrated to systolic blood pressure 100 to 120 mm Hg (see Box 7–2), is the treatment of choice for blood pressure control. Cyanide and thiocyanate toxicity can develop after more than 48 hours of continuous use. Because nitroprusside increases arterial shearing forces, it should not be used *without simultaneous administration of a β-adrenergic blocking*

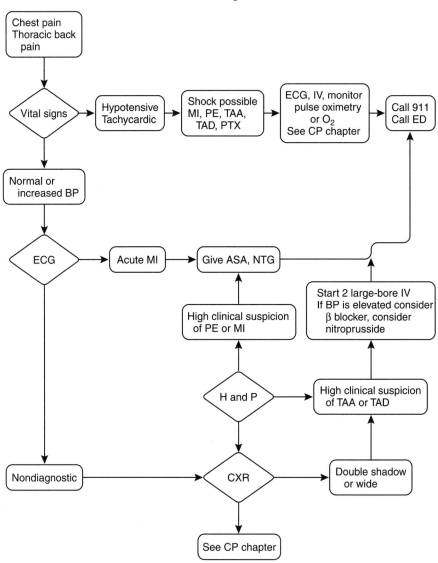

Figure 7–1. Aortic dissection flow diagram. ASA, aspirin; BP, blood pressure; CP, chest pain; CXR, chest X-ray; ECG, electrocardiogram; ED, emergency department; H and P, history and physical examination; MI, myocardial infarction; NTG, nitroglycerin; PE, pulmonary embolism; PTX, pneumothorax; TAA, thoracic aortic aneurysm; TAD, thoracic aortic dissection.

agent. Traditionally, propranolol has been used in aortic dissection and has been administered intravenously 0.5 mg initially, followed by 1 mg every 15 minutes until the pulse rate is 60 to 70 beats per minute, then 1 to 2 mg intravenously every 4 to 6 hours. Ultra–short-acting esmolol is also extremely useful because it can be withdrawn quickly in intolerant patients (e.g., those with asthma, chronic obstructive pulmonary disease, or heart failure). Patients who cannot tolerate nitroprusside or β blockers can be given trimethaphan camsylate (Arfonad) IV 1 to 2 mg/min to maintain a systolic blood pressure in the range of 110 mm Hg or a urine output of 20 to 30 mL/hr. This drug has the disadvantage of rapid tachyphylaxis. Use of labetalol, with both α-adrenergic and β-adrenergic blocking properties, is another option.[6]

If the office does not have these antihypertensive medications in stock, sublingual nitroglycerin tablets or nitroglycerin paste should be administered to achieve a systolic blood pressure of 100 to 120 mm Hg. Oral clonidine (0.2-mg tablet) may also be administered, but onset of antihypertensive effect can be delayed (up to 2 hours). Intravenous furosemide may be used in conjunction with other antihypertensive agents at doses of 10 to 40 mg. Keep in mind that hypertensive crises are vasoconstrictive events and that diuretics by themselves may not be effective or may produce profound hypotension once definitive antihypertensive therapy has been initiated in the emergency department. **The use of sublingual nifedipine is strongly condemned[5] because of the potential for uncontrolled and precipitous drops in blood pressure, leading to severe cerebral, myocardial, and renal ischemia.**

The patient must be transported quickly for definitive diagnosis and treatment. Among imaging procedures, contrast-enhanced computed tomography is available in most hospitals, is rapidly performed, and has high diagnostic accuracy.[3] If available, transesophageal echocardiography is considered by many to be the noninvasive diagnostic procedure of choice.[7–9] This procedure can be performed within minutes at the bedside with a diagnostic accuracy approaching 100%.[10]

Aneurysms

True aneurysms involve all layers of the aorta, with dilatation of the lumen at least one and one half times normal. Risk factors for aneurysms include cigarette smoking, atherosclerosis, collagen disorders, trauma, and, less commonly today, syphilis.[1]

Thoracic Aneurysms

Aneurysms within the thorax can be classified as ascending, transverse, descending, thoracoabdominal, or traumatic; the descending type is the most common.[1] Most thoracic aneurysms are asymptomatic and are noted incidentally on chest radiography.[11] When symptoms occur, they relate to position.[1, 11, 12] Proximal aneurysms have a high incidence of aortic insufficiency and heart failure. Aneursysms of the aortic arch may compress the trachea, bronchi, left recurrent laryngeal nerve, or other mediastinal structures, producing hoarseness and dyspnea. Descending aneurysms may produce only deep chest pain.[11] Traumatic aneurysms are often fatal at the scene and are associated with other major trauma[1]; patients would not present to the primary care office. Immediate referral to a medical center capable of open heart surgery is necessary for all symptomatic thoracic aneurysms or "stable" aneurysms that exhibit a change on chest radiography. Office management includes fluid resuscitation for the hypovolemic patient[11] and immediate transport to the emergency department.

Abdominal Aortic Aneurysms

Abdominal aortic aneurysms (AAAs) are common, occurring in about 5% of people over the age of 60 years.[13] Men are affected 6 times more frequently than women, with 95% of AAAs located infrarenally.[1] The typical patient is an older hypertensive male who smokes; other risk factors include atherosclerosis, cystic medial necrosis, Ehlers-Danlos syndrome, and syphilis.[13] Seventy-five percent of AAAs are silent and are found incidentally on physical examination.[13] AAAs typically grow at a rate of 5 mm/yr; once they reach 6 cm, their potential for rupture increases exponentially.[1, 13]

 CLINICAL RECOGNITION ←

History
Symptomatic AAA indicates rupture or impending rupture. Patients present with abrupt onset of any type of chest, abdominal, back, or flank pain, classically associated with a pulsatile abdominal mass and low blood pressure.[1] The differential diagnosis is extensive (Box 7–3), but because of the high associated mortality, AAA should always be suspected in an elderly patient with back, chest, or flank pain.

Physical Examination
A pulsatile mass is usually found on abdominal examination and may be tender to palpation, especially if it is rupturing. Palpate femoral, popliteal, dorsalis pedis, and posterior tibial pulses bilaterally.

Initial Management
Office staff should call 911 immediately to transport the patient; the physician in the emergency department that will be receiving the patient

Box 7–3. *Differential Diagnosis of Abdominal Aortic Aneurysm*

Myocardial infarction
Renal colic
Ischemic bowel
Pancreatitis
Perforated ulcer
Appendicitis
Diverticulitis
Biliary colic
Internal hernia

Reproduced from Semashko DC: Vascular emergencies. MT Sinai J Med 64: 316–322, 1997.

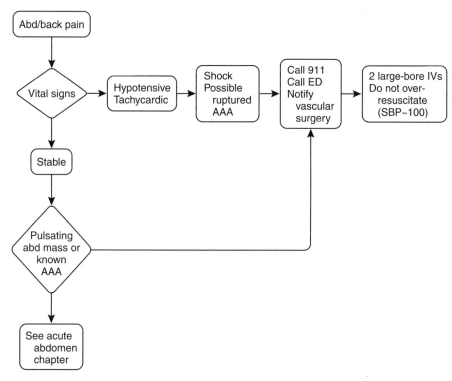

Figure 7–2. Aortic aneurysm flow diagram. AAA, abdominal aortic aneurysm; Abd, abdominal; ED, emergency department; SBP, systolic blood pressure.

should also be called. These patients are usually taken directly to the operating suite. Vital signs should be repeated often until the paramedics arrive (Fig. 7–2). Attend to ABCs and vital signs. Make sure the patient is maintaining an airway, give supplemental oxygen, and be prepared to assist with ventilations if necessary. Begin a large-bore IV line, and support blood pressure with fluids if necessary.

Less urgent repair of AAA can be considered for the asymptomatic patient who is a low surgical risk and who has either an aneurysm of 5 cm or greater, or who has a smaller aneurysm (4 cm or more) that has enlarged by 0.5 cm or more over the previous 6 months. Patients who are high surgical risks (e.g., those with poor left ventricular function, severe coronary artery disease, or severe chronic obstructive pulmonary disease) should be monitored serially until their aneurysms become 7 cm or larger, or until they become symptomatic.[13] Most asymptomatic patients should be managed by elective surgery.[13–15]

Peripheral Arterial Thromboembolic Disease

Peripheral artery occlusion from in situ thrombosis or embolization causes critical limb ischemia. Thrombosis occurs in the setting of endothelial injury (e.g., atherosclerosis) or systemic low-flow states. Embolization results from thrombi or atherosclerotic plaques that break off, or from foreign bodies or tumors. Emboli from thrombi usually lodge at arterial bifurcations owing to the change in size of blood vessels. Atherosclerotic plaque emboli are usually small and lodge distally (e.g., in the digits).[1]

 CLINICAL RECOGNITION ◄────────────────

History

Acute peripheral arterial occlusion, classically resulting from embolization, causes coolness of the extremity, pallor, pain, paresthesias, diminished pulses, and reduced motor function. Painful, cyanotic toes with palpable pulses ("blue toe syndrome") is a common presentation.[1] The typical patient with embolism has a history of atrial fibrillation, myocardial infarction, atherosclerosis, or valvular heart disease. Thrombosis classically occurs in patients with long-standing pain, usually in the form of claudication, from established peripheral vascular disease. Collateral flow is often well developed, and patients have signs of chronic arterial insufficiency (diminished pulses, hair loss, thickened toe nails, shiny skin). Patients with critical limb ischemia are usually in their seventh decade, with diabetes, smoking, and hypertension being the most common associated risk factors; three quarters of patients present urgently with rest pain or ulceration.[16]

Initial Management

Start an IV and administer oxygen. Elevate the ischemic limb (usually the leg) if it is edematous.[2] Emergent vascular surgery consultation is imperative. Refer promptly to a medical center for appropriate invasive and noninvasive imaging (i.e., angiogram and Doppler examination), angioplasty, surgical embolectomy, anticoagulation, or fibrinolytic therapy. Medical centers with a team approach to management of critical limb ischemia can achieve a limb salvage rate of 75% to 80%, but in-hospital mortality remains around 10%.[16, 17] Owing to other cardiovascular risk factors in these patients, 5-year survival in patients with critical limb ischemia is around 46%.[18]

Stroke

Stroke is defined as rapidly developing signs of focal or global cerebral dysfunction of vascular origin, lasting longer than 24 hours or leading to death. A transient ischemic attack (TIA) is an acute, focal loss of cerebral function lasting less than 24 hours caused by temporary reduction in blood supply. The most common causes of stroke or TIA are vascular occlusion and thrombosis. Occlusive strokes occur with large or small artery thrombosis, or from emboli, vasculitis, atherosclerosis, or hypercoagulable states. Watershed occlusive strokes occur in border areas between arterial territories during episodes of hypotension. Lacunar strokes are due to occlusion of penetrating branches of the major cerebral arteries, resulting from miniature atherosclerotic plaques or from degenerative vasculopathy of small vessels. Hemorrhagic stroke occurs in subarachnoid hemorrhage, ruptured arteriovenous malformation, or hemorrhagic metastasis.[19]

 ## CLINICAL RECOGNITION ◄————————————————

For optimal outcome, treatment of stroke by tissue plasminogen activator (t-PA) within 3 hours of symptom onset is crucial.[20–22] This necessitates recognition of stroke symptoms by family members, primary care office personnel, Emergency Medical Services (EMS) dispatchers and workers, and primary care physicians. Office staff members must be aware of the signs and symptoms of stroke so that they can rapidly triage patients. Any sudden numbness, tingling, or weakness in the face, arm, or leg may be an early sign of stroke. Other signs include the sudden loss (or slurring) of speech, sudden visual field cuts, sudden dizziness, sudden headache, or sudden loss of consciousness. Patients who call the office with these symptoms should be instructed to call EMS or to proceed to a medical center with 24-hour availability of stroke expertise, high-resolution cranial imaging, and experience in the administration of t-PA.[20]

Initial Management

The most important factor for office management of acute stroke is rapid transfer of the patient to a medical center with expertise in the evaluation of stroke and administration of t-PA.[20] The office staff should call 911 to transport the patient; the physician in the emergency department who will be receiving the patient should be notified as well (Fig. 7–3). Attend to ABCs and vital signs. Make sure the patient is maintaining an airway, provide supplemental oxygen, and be prepared to assist with ventilations if needed. Start a large-bore IV, attach the patient to a cardiac monitor, and insert a Foley catheter to monitor urine output, if indicated and available. Calculate the National Institutes of Health (NIH) Stroke Scale (Table 7–1). Vital signs should be repeated frequently until the paramedics arrive. Treat hypotension with IV fluids; monitor cardiac status carefully. If diastolic blood pressure is very high (>110 to 120 mm Hg), consider using sodium nitroprusside 0.5 mcg/min, labetalol 10 to 20 mg IV push over 1 to 2 minutes, or nitroglycerin (sublingual tablets, topical paste, or infusion, if available at 5 to 100 µg/min IV).

Obtain historical information regarding the exact time of onset and a description of symptoms, as well as information on any preceding events such as trauma or seizures. Other diagnoses to ask about include previous TIAs, migraines, and conditions associated with stroke such as smoking, hypertension, diabetes mellitus, arrhythmias, valvular heart disease, postpartum state, and hypercoagulable conditions (e.g., lupus anticoagulant, hyperviscosity syndromes, and oral contraceptive pills). In patients with epilepsy, postictal paralysis (Todd's paralysis) may occur. Patients with subarachnoid hemorrhage may complain of sudden onset of excruciating headache, usually with neck stiffness and nausea.[23]

A brief physical examination should focus on evidence of trauma and neurologic function. Assess and monitor a patient's level of consciousness, evidence of seizure activity, and patterns and character of facial and limb movement. If rapidly available, obtain an ECG and pulse oximetry, instituting arrhythmia or oxygen therapy as appropriate. Check blood glucose level in patients with diabetes or other risk for hypoglycemia. Transport the patient to a medical center as rapidly as possible for definitive evaluation and treatment.[23]

Risk Factors

The major risk factor for stroke is age, but smoking and hypertension each confer a fourfold increase in risk as well. A patient who both smokes and has hypertension incurs a 20-fold increase in risk for stroke.[22] Other risk factors include diabetes mellitus, hypercholesterolemia, oral contraceptive use (especially of preparations with >50 µg of estrogen), obesity, and cardiac disease (e.g., atrial fibrillation, congenital heart disease, large anterior myocardial infarction, and valvular disease).[23]

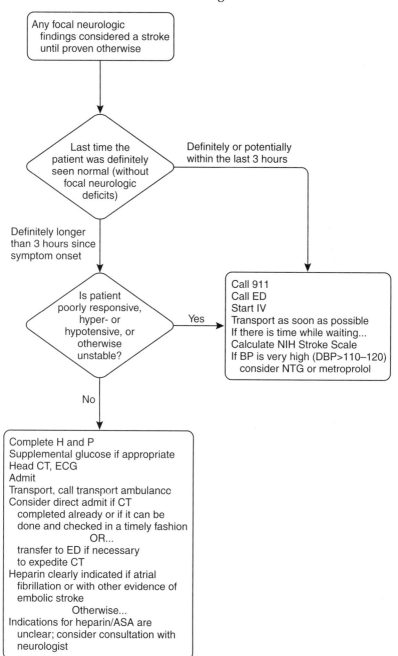

Figure 7–3. Stroke flow diagram. ASA, acetylsalicylic acid; BP, blood pressure; CT, computed tomography; DBP, diastolic blood pressure; ECG, electrocardiogram; ED, emergency department; H and P, history and physical examination; NIH, National Institutes of Health; NTG, nitroglycerin.

Table 7–1. National Institutes of Health Stroke Scale

Category	Patient Response	Score
1a. Level of consciousness (LOC)	Alert	0
	Drowsy	1
	Stuporous	2
	Coma	3
1b. LOC Questions	Answers both corectly	0
	Answers one correctly	1
	Answers none correctly	2
1c. LOC Commands	Obeys both correctly	0
	Obeys one correctly	1
	Obeys none correctly	2
2. Best Gaze	Normal	0
	Partial Gaze Palsy	1
	Forced Deviation	2
3. Best Visual	No visual loss	0
	Partial hemianopsia	1
	Complete hemianopsia	2
4. Facial Palsy	Normal	0
	Minor facial weakness	1
	Partial facial weakness	2
	No facial movement	3
5. Best Motor Arm	No drift after 10 seconds	0
	Drift	1
	Cannot resist gravity	2
	No effort against gravity	3
6. Best Motor Leg	No drift after 5 seconds	0
	Drift	1
	Cannot resist gravity	2
	No effort against gravity	3
7. Limb Ataxia	Absent	0
	Present in upper or lower extremities	1
	Present in both upper and lower	2
8. Sensory	Normal	0
	Partial Loss	1
	Dense Loss	2
9. Neglect	No Neglect	0
	Partial Neglect	1
	Complete Neglect	2
10. Dysarthria	Normal articulation	0
	Mild to Moderate dysarthria	1
	Near unintelligible or worse	2
11. Best Language	No aphasia	0
	Mild to Moderate Aphasia	1
	Severe Aphasia	2
	Mute	3

A rapid, reproducible neurologic evaluation of patients with stroke. (Modified from Brott T, Adams HP Jr, Olinger CP, et al. Measurements of acute cerebral infarction: A clinical examination scale. Stroke 1989; 20(7): 864–870.)

Differential Diagnosis

The differential diagnosis of stroke is extensive because many phenomena produce focal or global attenuation of cerebral function (Table 7–2). As many as 10% of patients initially diagnosed as victims of "stroke" ultimately are found to have another disorder.[23]

Table 7–2. Differential Diagnosis of Ischemic Stroke

Disorder	Comments
Hypotension	
Migraine, with or without headache	Family history of migraine helpful
Labyrinthine disorders (e.g., acoustic neuroma, benign positional vertigo, etc.)	
Postictal (Todd's) paralysis	Patient usually has a history of seizures
Infection (e.g., meningitis, encephalitis, brain abscess, neurosyphilis)	
Drug intoxication (e.g., alcohol, opiates, barbiturates, benzodiazepines)	
Metabolic disorders (e.g., hypoglycemia, hyperglycemia, myxedema coma, electrolyte imbalances)	
Subdural hematoma	Up to 50% of patients give a history of falling
Demyelinating disorders (e.g., multiple sclerosis)	Patients are usually <40 years old with subacute onset of symptoms
Subarachnoid hemorrhage	Sudden onset of excruciating headache, neck stiffness, and nausea

From Scearce T: Stroke. In Mengert TJ, Eisenberg MS, Copass MK (eds): Emergency Medical Therapy, 4th ed. Philadelphia, WB Saunders, 1996, pp 752–765.

Venous Thromboembolism

Venous thromboembolism, which includes deep venous thrombosis (DVT) and pulmonary embolism (PE), is a common, serious, and often fatal disorder. Early initiation of treatment is necessary to reduce the risk of fatal PE. Because most patients who present with suspected DVT or PE do not have these conditions,[24] and because the diagnosis cannot be made on clinical grounds alone, objective testing is necessary to confirm or exclude the presence of these disorders.

Deep Venous Thrombosis

 CLINICAL RECOGNITION ◄——————————

Certain clinical conditions greatly increase the likelihood that a patient will develop DVT[25] (Box 7–4). Elderly, chronically ill patients who are immobilized for prolonged periods, postoperative and trauma patients, and patients with previous DVT are more likely to develop

---

Box 7-4. *Risk Factors for Venous Thromboembolism*

Age >60 yr
Extensive surgery*
Previous venous thromboembolism
Marked immobility, preoperative or postoperative
   Hip surgery
   Major knee surgery
Fracture of pelvis, femur, or tibia
Surgery for malignant disease
Postoperative sepsis
Major medical illness
   Heart failure
   Inflammatory bowel disease
   Sepsis
   Myocardial infarction

*Risk of postoperative thrombosis is increased by patient's age, presence of varicose veins, obesity, and length of surgery.
Reproduced from Hirsh J, Hoak J: Management of deep venous thromboembolism and pulmonary embolism: A statement for healthcare professionals. Circulation 93: 2212–2245, 1996.

DVT. In addition, certain patients (those with protein C or S deficiencies, antithrombin III deficiency, homocystinuria, hyperviscosity syndromes, adenocarcinoma, and patients on oral contraceptive pills) may have hypercoagulability, predisposing them to developing DVT, especially when their lower extremities are immobilized.[25, 26] Patients with suspected DVT should be categorized into low-, intermediate-, and high-risk groups based on associated conditions[25] (Table 7–3). These categorizations impact on diagnosis and treatment (see "Initial Management," later). In addition, patients with lower extremity pain and swelling who have suspected DVT should be questioned regarding shortness of breath, chest pain, apprehension, and other symptoms of PE.

A distinction often is made between distal DVT (i.e., thrombosis of calf veins only) and proximal DVT (i.e., thrombosis above the knee). Studies suggest that up to 20% of calf vein DVT will extend into more proximal veins within 2 weeks of presentation.[24–27] Thus some authorities recommend initiation of anticoagulation therapy for patients with calf vein DVT; others recommend serial outpatient studies (i.e., impedance plethysmography or compressive ultrasonography with or without D-dimer testing), which reveal whether or not extension has developed.[24–39] Thrombosis of superficial veins on the legs, often occurring in varicose veins, is usually a self-limited condition; however, sometimes it can extend into deeper veins, giving rise to PE.[25]

Table 7–3. Risk Categories for Venous Thromboembolism

Thrombolic Event	Category 1, Low Risk	Category 2, Moderate Risk*	Category 3, High Risk
	Patient younger than 40 hr	General surgery in patient older than 40 yr	Hip and major knee surgery
	Uncomplicated surgery (e.g., hysterectomy), minimal immobility	Acute myocardial infarction	Previous venous thrombosis
		Chronic illness	Surgery for extensive malignant disease
		Leg fracture in a patient younger than 40 yr	
Calf vein thrombosis	≈2%	10%–20%	40%–70%
Proximal vein thrombosis	≈0.4%	2%–4%	10%–20%
Fatal pulmonary embolism	<0.02%	0.2%–0.5%	1%–5%

*Risk increased by patient's age, length of surgery, obesity, varicose veins, chronic illness, and postoperative sepsis.
Reproduced from Hirsch J, Hoak J: Management of deep venous thromboembolism and pulmonary embolism: A statement for healthcare professionals. Ciculation 93: 2212–2245, 1996.

Upper extremity DVT was once thought to produce minimal morbidity. Recent studies, however, indicate that from 17% to 36% of upper extremity DVTs are associated with PE.[40, 41] Further, postthrombotic complications in the upper extremity are common.[41]

Differential Diagnosis

A variety of lower extremity conditions that can mimic DVT[42] are listed in Box 7–5; these include ruptured Baker's cysts, venous stasis problems, cellulitis, and musculoskeletal injuries.

Box 7–5. *Differential Diagnosis of Deep Venous Thrombosis*

Baker's cyst
Cellulitis
Knee injury
Hematoma
Lymphangitis
Lymphatic obstruction
Muscle strain
Muscle tear
Postphlebitic syndrome
Vasomotor changes in a paralyzed leg

From Mengert TJ: Deep venous thrombosis and pulmonary embolism. In Mengert TJ, Eisenberg MS, Copass MK (eds): Emergency Medical Therapy, 4th ed. Philadelphia, WB Saunders, 1996, pp 337–349.

Physical Examination

Carry out a directed physical examination to evaluate possible concurrent PE or other conditions that can mimic DVT. Monitor vital signs for tachycardia (>100 beats/min), tachypnea (>16 breaths/min), and fever. Inspect the skin for cyanosis or diaphoresis, and for erythema of the lower extremities. Auscultate the heart for an accentuated S_2, or an S_3 or S_4 gallop, and the lungs for rales.[42]

Up to 50% of patients with DVT do not have typical lower extremity signs or symptoms of this disorder. Classically, however, patients present with unilateral leg or calf pain and swelling; if the femoral or iliac veins are involved, the whole leg may be swollen and tender. Homans' sign (pain at the back of the knee or calf when the ankle is slowly and gently dorsiflexed with the knee slightly bent) may be present but is not highly sensitive or specific. A "cord" (tender, inflamed, slightly indurated vein) may be palpable in the distribution of the thrombosis. **It must be emphasized that clinical signs and symptoms are unreliable in the diagnosis of DVT**. Because 50% of DVT will result in clinically significant PE,[24] objective testing is mandatory.

Initial Management (Fig. 7–4)

Arrange for patients with suspected DVT to undergo objective testing as soon as possible. If coexisting symptoms of PE are present, urgently transfer the patient to a medical center that is capable of diagnosis and treatment of this disorder (see "Pulmonary Embolism," later).

The most sensitive noninvasive test for DVT is compressive venous ultrasonography, but this test can miss some calf vein thrombi (which potentially can extend proximally during the 2 weeks after presentation).[24, 25] Contrast venography is the gold standard for the diagnosis of DVT, but this test is invasive, requires technical expertise, can induce DVT in a small percentage of cases,[25] and is sometimes painful. Impedance plethysmography, a second noninvasive test, is less sensitive and specific for DVT than is compressive ultrasonography, and it misses most calf thrombi.[25] Magnetic resonance imaging (MRI) is in the early stages of investigation for use in the diagnosis of DVT; currently, its successful use is institution-dependent.[26]

Patients with low clinical probability of DVT (see Table 7–2) and a negative compressive venous ultrasound are unlikely to have DVT, and no further evaluation or treatment is necessary (see Fig. 7–4). Patients with intermediate or high probabilities of DVT (see Table 7–2) but a negative ultrasound should at least have their ultrasound repeated in 5 to 7 days. Venography may also be performed among those individuals with a high clinical probability of DVT but a negative venous ultrasound. Patients with positive venous ultrasound at presentation should be anticoagulated (see Fig. 7–4).[25] The choice between outpatient anticoagulation with low-

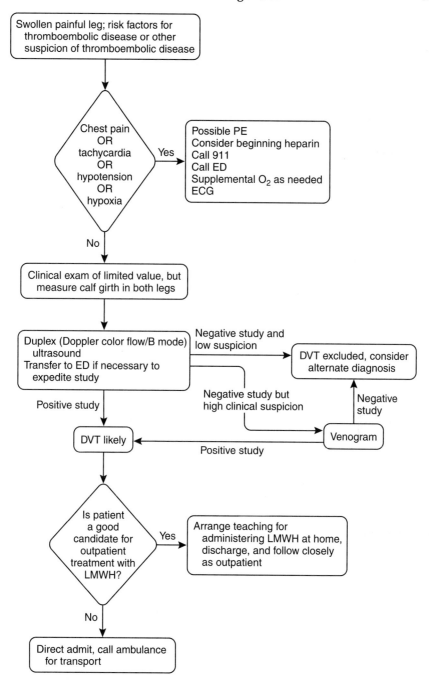

Figure 7–4. Thromboembolic disease flow diagram. DVT, Deep venous thrombosis; ECG, electrocardiogram; ED, emergency department, LMWH, low-molecular-weight heparin; PE, pulmonary embolism.

molecular-weight heparin (LMWH) versus inpatient anticoagulation with unfractionated heparin is based on physician comfort in the use of LMWH, as well as on patient factors such as comorbidities and the physician's ability to purchase and administer LMWH in the outpatient setting.

Recent research has suggested that laboratory determination of the fibrin degradation product D-dimer may aid in the diagnosis of thromboembolic disease.[27, 28, 29] D-Dimer may be used as a screening test for DVT when used alone[30] or in combination with clinical assessment[31, 28, 29] or with ultrasonography.[32, 28, 29] It has also been advocated for screening for PE.[33] Unfortunately, D-dimer is limited by a variable sensitivity that is highly dependent on the laboratory technique used.[27–29] Furthermore, the test takes time and special equipment.[29] New bedside whole blood tests for D-dimer can be used conveniently in the primary care physician's office, but the accuracy and usefulness of these tests need to be corroborated before their use can be recommended.[28, 29]

Recommendations for treatment of DVT are changing rapidly with the development of low-molecular-weight heparins. These compounds are at least as effective as unfractionated heparin, are administered subcutaneously without laboratory monitoring of the activated partial thromboplastin time, and have fewer bleeding complications.[24, 25, 43, 44] Although good data support the treatment of patients at home with subcutaneous low-molecular-weight heparin,[36, 37] clinical guidelines for such use have not yet been defined.[45]

Pulmonary Embolism

Pulmonary embolism occurs when a thrombus, air bubble, or foreign body lodges in the pulmonary vascular bed. This disorder can be asymptomatic or symptomatic; large PE can be fatal.

 CLINICAL RECOGNITION ◄————————————

History
The clinical features of PE, like those for DVT, are nonspecific, and must be confirmed by objective testing. Classically, patients present with the sudden onset of sharp, localized, pleuritic chest pain associated with hemoptysis. Small thrombi may produce transient symptoms. Larger thrombi, in addition to producing prolonged symptoms, may be associated with shortness of breath. Many patients with PE are apprehensive and diaphoretic and complain of cough (Table 7–4).[24, 25, 42, 45] Risk factors and clinical conditions associated with PE are similar to

Table 7–4. Clinical Findings Possibly Associated with Pulmonary Embolism*

Clinical situation	Elderly or chronically ill (e.g., malignancy) Prolonged immobility Postoperative time Trauma Prior venous thromboembolism Prothrombic disorder (e.g., factor V Leiden, prothrombin [factor II] variant 20210 G to A, hyperhomocystinuria, protein C or S deficiency, antithrombin III deficiency)	Chest radiograph	Elevated hemidiaphram (loss of lung volume) Infiltrate Pleural effusion Atelectasis
Symptoms	Dyspnea Chest pain (pleuritic) Hemoptysis Syncope Apprehension Cough Diaphoresis	Electrocardiogram[†]	Sinus tachycardia $S_1Q_3T_3$ Rightward QRS axis Transient Right bundle branch block T-wave inversion, ST-segment depression in right precordial leads P pulmonale pattern ST-segment elevation in lead III
Signs	Tachypnea Tachycardia Evidence of lower extremity DVT Hypotension Fever Crackles Loud P_2 Gallop rhythm		

*Within each category, findings are listed in approximate order of positive predictive value based on expert opinion.
[†] changes found in less than 10% of cases of PE.
DVT, deep venous thrombosis.
Adapted from Venous Thromboembolism Guideline Team, University of Michigan Health System: Guidelines for clinical care: Venous thromboembolism. Ann Arbor, Mich, Office of Clinical Affairs, University of Michigan Health System, 1998.

those associated with DVT; they include elderly or chronically ill patients who are immobilized for prolonged periods, postoperative and trauma patients, and patients with previous DVT or PE (see Box 7–4).[25, 26] In addition, certain patients (those with protein C or S deficiencies, antithrombin III deficiency, homocystinuria, hyperviscosity syndromes, adenocarcinoma, and patients on oral contraceptive pills) may have hypercoagulability, predisposing them to developing DVT and subsequently PE.[24, 25, 42, 45]

Differential Diagnosis

The differential diagnosis of PE is extensive and includes a variety of musculoskeletal, cardiac, and pulmonary conditions (Box 7–6).[42] Herpes zoster can also produce chest pain as can some abdominal processes (e.g., pancreatitis, gallbladder disease, peptic ulcer disease).[42]

Physical Examination

A directed physical examination should be carried out to look for tachypnea, tachycardia, evidence of lower extremity DVT, hypotension, fever, rales, an accentuated S_2, or an S_3 or S_4 gallop.[45]

Box 7–6. *Differential Diagnosis of Pulmonary Embolism*

Acute myocardial infarction
Angina
Anxiety attack
Asthma
Chronic obstructive pulmonary disease exacerbation
Congestive heart failure
Costochondritis
Herpes zoster infection
Hyperventilation
Lung cancer
Musculoskeletal pain
Pancreatitis
Pericarditis
Pleurisy
Pneumonia
Pneumothorax
Rib fracture
Tuberculosis

From Mengert TJ: Deep venous thrombosis and pulmonary embolism. In Mengert TJ, Eisenberg MS, Copass MK (eds): Emergency Medical Therapy, 4th ed. Philadelphia, WB Saunders, 1996, pp 337–349.

Initial Management

The office staff should call 911 to transport the patient; the physician in the emergency department that will be receiving the patient should be notified as well. Office personnel should instruct patients who call with complaints of chest pain associated with shortness of breath, hemoptysis, or diaphoresis to activate EMS and be taken immediately to the emergency department. Patients in the office with suspected PE must also be transferred urgently to a medical center capable of diagnosis and treatment of this disorder.

Attend to ABCs and vital signs and make sure the patient is maintaining an airway (see Fig. 7–4). Apply supplemental oxygen, and monitor oxygenation status by pulse oximetry if available. Be prepared to assist with ventilations if needed. Attach the patient to a cardiac monitor, insert a large-bore IV, and treat hypotension with fluid. Insert a Foley catheter to follow urine output, if indicated and available. Perform an ECG; specific signs of PE on ECG are present in less than 10% of patients (e.g., sinus tachycardia, transient right bundle branch block, P pulmonale pattern, rightward axis, etc.).[45] If patient transport will not be delayed, obtain a chest radiograph. Radiographic signs of PE are nonspecific and include an elevated hemidiaphragm, infiltrate, pleural effusion, and atelectasis.[45] Vital signs should be repeated often until the paramedics arrive.

Discussion of definitive diagnosis and treatment of PE is beyond the scope of this chapter. Diagnostic studies for pulmonary embolism typically include ventilation-perfusion (V/Q) lung scans and pulmonary angiography. Although helical chest computed tomography is now being used at some centers to screen for,[46] or confirm the diagnosis of, PE,[47] the true sensitivity, specificity, and accuracy of this technique remain controversial.[28, 29, 48, 49] D-Dimer use has also been advocated in the diagnosis of PE,[28, 29, 49, 50] but it should be reserved for use in combination with imaging techniques. Some form of diagnostic imaging must be available at the medical center to which the patient is transported. Treatment protocols for DVT and PE are currently undergoing change with the advent of low-molecular-weight heparins, which have equal or superior antithrombotic efficacy and fewer bleeding complications compared with unfractionated heparins.[24, 25, 43, 44, 51]

Epidemiology

Approximately 600,000 PEs occur in the United States yearly, leading to 60,000 deaths and contributing to another 100,000 deaths.[25] PE is the most frequent cause of maternal death[52]; overall, women are more frequently affected by PE than men.[25] The mortality of untreated PE is substantial (30%), with a significant percentage of deaths occurring within 60 minutes of the event.[42] Diagnosis and treatment of PE significantly reduces mortality.[24, 25]

Pediatrics

Vascular emergencies are rare among children, but they can occur. Venous thromboembolism is increasingly being recognized as a complication of life-threatening illnesses in children.[53] Central venous catheters, including those used in neonates, are the most common risk factors for venous thromboembolism among children. Other risk factors include congenital and acquired prothrombotic diseases (e.g., protein C or S deficiencies, lupus), surgery, and trauma.

Kawasaki's disease (KD) is an idiopathic vasculitis of small and medium-sized vessels. Children with KD usually present with a fever, conjunctivitis, rash, and lymph node adenopathy, all of which can be confused with a simple viral infection. The characteristic features that set KD apart are "strawberry tongue" and desquamation of the fingers and hands. The most significant morbidity of KD results from coronary artery aneurysms. These can be found in about 25% of children with KD and can cause myocardial ischemia or sudden cardiac death. Any child suspected of having KD should be transferred to the ED or directly admitted for consideration of intravenous γ-globulin therapy and salicylates or nonsteroidal anti-inflammatory drugs (NSAIDs).

Stroke is very uncommon among children, but it does occur in patients with sickle cell anemia, moyamoya syndrome (see later), and certain embolic conditions. Sickle cell anemia is the most common cause of pediatric stroke in the United States, and children who develop focal neurologic symptoms consistent with stroke should be immediately transferred to the hospital for treatment and admission. Exchange transfusion is often indicated for these patients. Moyamoya syndrome is an idiopathic intracranial vasculopathy found most frequently (but not exclusively) in Asian girls just younger than 10 years of age. It can cause ischemic or hemorrhagic stroke and is identified by the "puff of smoke" sign on angiography.

Thromboembolic disease in children is also very rare. Unlike adults, who generally form thromboemboli from deep venous thromboses in the legs, most thromboemboli in children are formed from valvular or structural abnormalities in the heart. Right-sided cardiac abnormalities can cause pulmonary emboli; left-sided abnormalities can cause stroke or peripheral arterial occlusion. Any child with embolic disease should be admitted to the hospital and anticoagulated. If fever is present, septic emboli should be considered and the patient should be started on an antibiotic before transport.

Aortic aneurysmal disease and dissection are almost absent among children. Coarctation of the aorta is potentially life threatening in neonates, but it can be picked up as an incidental finding on physical examination in older kids who present with decreased groin and lower extremity pulses and a heart murmur. These findings can often be worked up in the office on an outpatient basis. The office physician must stay alert for these rare but potentially devastating vascular diseases in children.

References

1. Semashko DC: Vascular emergencies. Mt Sinai J Med 64:316–322, 1997.
2. Sornsin SM: Diseases of the aorta and peripheral arteries. In Schwartz GR, Cayten CG, Mangelsen MA, et al (eds): Principles and Practice of Emergency Medicine, 3rd ed. Philadelphia, Lea and Febiger, 1992, pp 1376–1390.
3. Fuster V, Halperin JL: Aortic dissection: A medical perspective. J Card Surg 9:713–728, 1994.
4. Izzat MB, Jones AJ, Angelini GD: Acute aortic dissection. Br J Hosp Med 52:523–528, 1994.
5. Varon J, Marik PE: The diagnosis and management of hypertensive crises. Chest 118:214–227, 2000.
6. Grubbs BP, Sirio C, Zelis R: Intravenous labetalol in acute aortic dissection. JAMA 258:78–79, 1987.
7. Sanderson JE, Chan WW: Transesophageal echocardiography. Postgrad Med J 73:137–140, 1997.
8. Blanchard DG, Kimura BJ, Dittrich HC, DeMaria AN: Transesophageal echocardiography of the aorta. JAMA 272:546–551, 1994.
9. Nienaber CA, von Kodolitsch Y, Nicholas V, et al: The diagnosis of thoracic aortic aneurysm by non-invasive imaging procedures. N Engl J Med 328:1–9, 1993.
10. Cohn LH: Aortic dissection: New aspects of diagnosis and treatment. Hosp Pract 29:47–56, 1994.
11. Lindsay J, Garcia JM: Thoracic aneurysm. In Schwartz GR, Cayten CG, Mangelsen MA, et al (eds): Principles and Practice of Emergency Medicine, 3rd ed. Philadelphia, Lea and Febiger, 1992, pp 1374–1375.
12 Coselli JS, de Figueiredo LF: Natural history of descending and thoracoabdominal aortic aneurysms. J Card Surg 12:285–289, 1997.
13. Santilli JD, Santilli SM: Diagnosis and treatment of abdominal aortic aneurysms. Am Fam Physician 56:1081–1090, 1997.
14. Karmody AM, Leather RP, Goldman M, et al: The current position of non-resective treatment for abdominal aortic aneurysm. Surgery 94:591–597, 1983.
15. Cutter TAM: Abdominal aortic aneurysm: Use of screening programs. Am Fam Physician 56:1040–1048, 1997.
16. Varty K, Nydahl P, Butterworth M, et al: Changes in the managment of critical limb ischemia. Br J Surg 83:953–956, 1996.
17. Wolfe JHN: Defining the outcome of critical limb ischaemia: A one year prospective study [abstract]. Br J Surg 73:321, 1986.
18. Dormandy JA, Thomas PRS: What is the natural history of a critically ischemic patient with and without his leg? In Greenhalgh RM, Jamieson CW, Nicholaides AN (eds): Limb Salvage and Amputation for Vascular Diseases. Philadelphia, WB Saunders, 1988, pp 11–26.
19. Johnson CJ: Cerebrovascular disease. In Barker LR, Burton JR, Zieve PD (eds): Principles of Ambulatory Medicine, 4th ed. Baltimore, Williams and Wilkins, 1995, pp 1229–1239.
20. Broderick JP: Practical considerations in the early treatment of ischemic stroke. Am Fam Physician 57:73–80, 1998.
21. The National Institute of Neurological Disorders and Stroke rt-PA Stroke Group Study: Tissue plasminogen activator for acute ischemic stroke. N Engl J Med 333:1581–1587, 1995.
22. Zivin JA, Mazzarella V: Tissue plasminogen activator plus glutamate antagonist improves outcome after embolic stroke. Arch Neurol 48:1235–1238, 1991.
23. Scearce T: Stroke. In Mengert TJ, Eisenberg MS, Copass MK (eds): Emergency Medical Therapy, 4th ed. Philadelphia, WB Saunders, 1996, pp 752–765.
24. Ginsberg JS: Management of venous thromboembolism. N Engl J Med 335:1816–1828, 1996.
25. Hirsh J, Hoak J: Management of deep venous thromboembolism and pulmonary embolism: A statement for healthcare professionals. Circulation 93:2212–2245, 1996.

26. Hull RD, Pineo GF: Prophylaxis of deep venous thrombosis and pulmonary embolism. Med Clin North Am 82:477–493, 1998.

27. Becker DM, Philbrick JT, Bachhuber TL, Humphries JE: D-Dimer testing and acute venous thromboembolism: A shortcut to accurate diagnosis? Arch Intern Med 156:939, 1996.

28. ACCP Consensus Committee on Pulmonary Embolism: Opinions regarding the diagnosis and management of venous thromboembolic disease. Chest 113:499–504, 1998.

29. Baker WF: Current concepts of thrombosis: Prevalent trends for diagnosis and management. Med Clin North Am 82:459–476, 1998.

30. Wildberger JE, Vorwerk D, Kilbinger M, et al: Bedside testing (SimpliRED) in the diagnosis of deep vein thrombosis: Evaluation of 250 patients. Invest Radiol 33:232–235, 1998.

31. Wells PS, Anderson DR, Bormanis J, et al: SimpliRED d-dimer can reduce the diagnosis of deep vein thrombosis. Lancet 351:1405–1406, 1998.

32. Bernardi E, Prandoni P, Lensing AW, et al: D-Dimer testing as an adjunct to ultrasonography in patients with clinically suspected deep vein thrombosis: Prospective cohort study. BMJ 317:1037–1040, 1998.

33. Oger E, Leroyer C, Bressollette L, et al: Evaluation of a new, rapid, and quantitative D-dimer test in patients with suspected pulmonary embolism. Am J Resp Crit Care Med 158:65–70, 1998.

34. Lagerstedt CI, Olsson CG, Fagher BO, et al: Need for long-term anticoagulant treatment of symptomatic calf-vein thrombosis. Lancet 2:515–518, 1985.

35. Hull RD, Hirsh J, Carter CJ, et al: Diagnostic efficacy of impedance plethysmography for clinically suspected deep-venous thrombosis: A randomized trial. Ann Intern Med 102:21–28, 1985.

36. Huisman MV, Buller HR, ten Cate JW, et al: Management of clinically suspected acute venous thrombosis in outpatients with serial impedance plethysmography in a community hospital setting. Arch Intern Med 149:511–513, 1989.

37. Huisman MV, Buller HR, ten Cate JW, Vreeken J: Serial impedance plethysmography for suspected deep-venous thrombosis in outpatients. N Engl J Med 314:823–828, 1986.

38. Heijboer H, Buller HR, Lensing AWA, et al: A comparison of real-time compression ultrasonography with impedance plethysmography for the diagnosis of deep-vein thrombosis in symptomatic outpatients. N Engl J Med 329:1365–1369, 1993.

39. Hull RD, Carter CJ, Jay RM, et al: The diagnosis of acute, recurrent, deep-vein thrombosis: A diagnostic challenge. Circulation 67:901–906, 1983.

40. Hingorani A: Upper extremity versus lower extremity deep venous thrombosis. Am J Surg 174:214–217, 1997.

41. Prandoni P: Upper-extremity deep vein thrombosis. Risk factors, diagnosis, and complications. Arch Intern Med 157:57–62, 1997.

42. Mengert TJ: Deep venous thrombosis and pulmonary embolism. In Mengert TJ, Eisenberg MS, Copass MK (eds): Emergency Medical Therapy, 4th ed. Philadelphia, WB Saunders, 1996, pp 337–349.

43. Levine M, Gent M, Hirsh J, et al: A comparison of low-molecular weight heparin administered primarily at home with unfractionated heparin administered in the hospital for proximal deep-vein thrombosis. N Engl J Med 334:677–681, 1996.

44. Koopman MMW, Prandoni P, Piovella F, et al: Treatment of venous thrombosis with intravenous unfractionated heparin administered in the hospital as compared with subcutaneous low-molecular weight heparin administered at home. N Engl J Med 334:682–687, 1996.

45. Venous Thromboembolism Guideline Team, University of Michigan Health System: Guidelines for clinical care: Venous thromboembolism. Ann Arbor, Mich, Office of Clinical Affairs, University of Michigan Health System, 1998.

46. Mayo JR, Remy-Jardin M, Muller NL, et al: Pulmonary embolism: Prospective comparison of spiral CT with ventilation-perfusion scintigraphy. Radiology 205:447–452, 1997.

47. Drucker EA, Rivitz SM, Shepard JA, et al: Acute pulmonary embolism: Assessment of helical CT for diagnosis. Radiology 209:235–241, 1998.

48. Hansell DM, Padley SP: Continuous volume computed tomography in pulmonary embolism: The answer, or just another test? Thorax 51:1–2, 1996.

49. Lipchik RJ, Goodman LR: Spiral computed tomography in the evaluation of pulmonary embolism. Clin Chest Med 20:731–738, 1999.

50. Kline JA, Johns KL, Colucciello SA, Israel EG: New diagnostic tests for pulmonary embolism. Ann Emerg Med 35:168–180, 2000.
51. Simonneu G, Sors H, Charbonnier B, et al: A comparison of low-molecular weight heparin with unfractionated heparin for acute pulmonary embolism. N Engl J Med 337:663–669, 1997.
52. Kaunitz AM, Hughes JM, Grimes DA, et al: Causes of maternal mortality in the United States. Obstet Gynecol 65:605–612, 1985.
53. Streif W, Andrew ME: Venous thromboembolic events in pediatric patients: Diagnosis and management. Hematol Oncol Clin North Am 12:1283–1312, 1998.

Chapter 8

Coma and Altered Mental Status

Victor Caraballo
Matthew H. Rusk

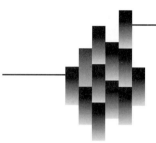

Alteration in a patient's state of consciousness can be characterized by agitation and fluctuating levels of psychomotor activity, also known as delirium, or it can be characterized by decreased levels of awareness and responsiveness. These depressed mental states occur in a spectrum of severity, progressing from lethargy to stupor to coma.[1] Lethargy is defined as a global depression of self and the environment in a wakeful patient; stupor is an unresponsive state from which the patient can be aroused only with noxious stimuli. Coma then is a state of unresponsiveness from which the patient cannot be aroused.

These disease states can progress at different rates, wherein those with a more fulminant onset are generally associated with more severe disease. However, a rapid onset is also generally associated with a treatable and reversible cause. Although it is equally disconcerting to family members, mental status change occurring over longer periods is generally less acutely life-threatening, but it is also less likely to have a treatable cause. Dementia is an example of such a disorder.

Although acute mental status change is related to many causes, the underlying pathophysiology is related to either bilateral cerebral cortical disease or suppression of the brain stem reticular activating system.[2] Bilateral cortical involvement generally occurs as a result of toxic-metabolic processes such as hypoglycemia, hypoxia, and acute renal or hepatic failure. Structural lesions generally do not cause mental status changes on the basis of cortical disease because both cortices would need to be affected. The large size of such a lesion would most likely first cause mental status change by disruption of the reticular activating system as a result of brain stem herniation caused by elevated intracranial pressure. In fact, all intracranial masses or hemorrhages cause mental status disruption by this mechanism.

For purposes of discussion, the various pathophysiologic causes of altered mental status are treated separately here. However, it must be emphasized that these pathophysiologic states are not static, and they do progress across a continuum. Also, the initial assessment and treatment approaches for these disorders are the same. Altered mental states with depressed consciousness and psychomotor activity, such as lethargy, stupor, and coma, are discussed under the general heading of coma.

 ## Clinical Recognition ◄————

Dementia

Dementia is characterized by a progressive loss of intellectual function, wherein patients demonstrate significant deterioration of both long- and short-term memory. They also exhibit impaired abstract thinking and judgment, and gross personality changes. Dementia is caused by widespread neuronal degeneration and is most often caused by Alzheimer's disease, which accounts for 50% to 90% of all cases.[3] Other causes include multi-infarct dementia, chronic alcoholism, and a variety of chronic conditions such as human immunodeficiency virus (HIV). Patients with dementia are typically both alert and aware until late in the disease. Dementia tends to be slowly progressive and unremitting.

The treatable causes of dementia fall into three categories: CNS structural lesions, metabolic and systemic illness, and neuropsychiatric disease. Space-occupying lesions may be associated with signs of elevated intracranial pressure on physical examination but are usually difficult to diagnose without the benefit of computed tomography or magnetic resonance imaging techniques. Dementia may be the presenting complaint of patients with a variety of metabolic disorders or systemic diseases, including chronic liver or renal failure, vitamin B_{12} deficiency, malignancy, and hypothyroidism. Depression is a common neuropsychiatric disorder that can mimic a dementia-like picture.

Delirium ◄————

Delirium, originally described by Hippocrates, is an acute confusional state characterized by global cognitive impairment. Other features include attention abnormalities, decreased level of consciousness, fluctuating psychomotor activity, hallucinations, and disruption of the normal sleep-wake cycle.[4]

Psychomotor disturbances can be hyperactive or hypoactive in nature. Although hyperactivity may be more apparent to the evaluating physician, hypoactivity is actually more common. Patients frequently exhibit enhanced somnolence during the day and agitation at night. Those who are frail and elderly are at increased risk for delirium, especially if they have dementia.[5] Hospitalization is also commonly associated with delirium, either as a result of the precipitating disorder, or as a result of underlying advanced age and dementia. The mortality rate of hospitalized patients with acute delirium is eight times greater than that of age-matched controls.[6]

While dementia is typically a permanent progressive condition; delirium is generally a transient event from which most patients recover fully.[7] Delirium is a clinical diagnosis that can be caused by a wide range of medical or surgical conditions. Although virtually any disease process can precipitate delirium, its common causes can be categorized as either primary cerebral disease or systemic illness.

Primary brain disorders include head injury, stroke, increased intracranial pressure, central nervous system (CNS) infection, and seizure disorders. Systemic disorders include toxic-metabolic, infectious, cardiopulmonary, and environmental causes.

The most common cause of delirium is drug-induced toxicity.[8] Any drug may induce delirium; however, the agents most often implicated include anticholinergic medications, sedative-hypnotics, narcotics, digitalis, propranolol, steroids, lithium, anticonvulsants, aspirin, nonsteroidal anti-inflammatory drugs, H_2 blockers, penicillin, cephalosporins, and sulfonamides. Other drug-induced causes of delirium include drugs of abuse, such as alcohol, cocaine, hallucinogens, and other illicit substances.

Coma ◄——————————————————————————

The numerous causes of altered mental states with depressed consciousness can be summarized by the mnemonic AEIOU-TIPS (Box 8–1). Another way to organize these disorders is into the categories of toxic-metabolic, infectious, and CNS causes.

Toxic-metabolic causes dominate as a cause for depressed mental status change. Hypoglycemia or hyperglycemia and hypoxia are important reversible causes that should be ruled out immediately after assessment of the patient's airway, breathing, and circulation (ABCs). Hepatic and renal failure can cause mental status change through multiple metabolic mechanisms. The primary care physician's knowledge of the patient's medical history can help in assessment of the probability of these potential causes. Other electrolyte disorders, especially of calcium and sodium, can also cause depressed mental status.

Box 8–1. *Mnemonic for Causes of Coma*

A— Alcohol, drugs, and toxins
E— Endocrine: Hypothyroidism-hyperthyroidism, Adrenal disease
   Exocrine: Liver disease—hepatic encephalopathy
   Electrolyte disorders
   Epilepsy
I— Insulin: Hypoglycemia-hyperglycemia
O— Oxygen: Hypoxia
   Opiates
U— Uremia, other renal causes such as hypertensive
   encephalopathy
T— Trauma
   Temperature disorders: Hypothermia
   Thiamine deficiency in alcoholics
I— Infection
P— Psychiatric causes
S— Space-occupying central nervous system lesion, stroke
   Sepsis

Numerous toxic ingestions, especially ethanol, can lead to coma syndromes. History, current medications, and information from family can be used along with toxicologic screening to make this diagnosis.

Infections, especially of the CNS, can cause depressed mental status change via multiple mechanisms. The elderly in particular are susceptible, even with apparently minor infections such as simple urinary tract infections. The underlying affected system may be the basis for mental status change, such as hypoxia in pneumonia, and other factors such as dehydration or hypotension from sepsis can also contribute. Hypoglycemia or hyperglycemia can also result from infectious processes. CNS infections such as meningitis or encephalitis should be aggressively pursued, particularly when no other apparent cause can be discerned.

Central nervous system processes, which cause depressed mental status, include tumor, stroke, hemorrhage, hypertensive encephalopathy, and seizure. Patients with no previous history of seizure should be suspected of having another primary process.

 PHONE TRIAGE ◄

Changes in mental status should always be evaluated with at least a complete office visit. When the change occurs suddenly and suggests a CNS infection, stroke, or head trauma, the patient should be seen immediately in an emergency department. In general, sudden mental status changes suggest more dangerous disease processes. Fever and headache with neck stiffness suggests meningitis, which requires immediate intravenous antibiotics. If symptoms of a stroke are noted, such as weakness, numbness, or garbled speech, a computed tomography (CT) scan should be done immediately so that emergency therapies such as thrombolytics can be considered, if appropriate. A CT scan should also be considered in patients with head trauma and mental status changes to ensure that there has been no intracranial bleeding.

Chronic changes in mental status should be evaluated first in the office with a complete history and physical. During the office visit, the clinician will determine which laboratory studies and radiographic images are appropriate.

Initial Management

The initial management of a patient with altered mental status should begin with assessment of the ABCs: airway, breathing, and circulation. The examiner should look, listen, and feel for air movement and institute appropriate airway measures as required, such as the chin lift or jaw thrust. The patient should then be assessed for adequate ventilatory function and supported as necessary with a bag-valve mask device. Patients in coma require endotracheal intubation. In these cases, rapid transport to the emergency department is required. Finally, the clinician should assess circulation by palpating the patient's pulse and measuring blood pressure. One should always be alert for occult trauma. Altered mental status associated with trauma (including syncope) mandates the use of cervical spine precautions during assessment.

Once the patient's ABCs have been assessed and stabilized, rapidly reversible causes of altered mental status should be explored. Specific measures include blood glucose measurement, application of oxygen for hypoxia, and treatment with naloxone hydrochloride (Narcan) for those with suspected narcotic overdose. In alcoholics, thiamine should be given along with glucose administration. In most cases, transport to the closest emergency department via a unit with Advanced Life Support (ALS) capabilities should be arranged.

Equipment and Medications

- Bag-valve mask
- Oral airways

- Oxygen
- Glucometer
- Dextrose ampule: 50 mL 25% solution
- Thiamine
- Pulse oximeter
- Ceftriaxone
- Vancomycin

Disposition and Transfer

If the patient arrives with fever and a stiff neck, immediate intravenous access should be obtained and IV antibiotics started, if available. Waiting for CT scanning or lumbar puncture should not delay the initiation of antibiotics. Patients should receive 2 g of ceftriaxone (Rocephin) and 1 g of vancomycin. In the case of head trauma and mental status changes, an IV line should be placed, and the patient should be kept calm and closely monitored while he or she awaits transfer to an emergency department. Cervical spine precautions should be observed at all times by placement of the patient in a cervical collar and in a flat supine position. The patient's head should be taped down, if necessary. Management of patients with possible stroke should be similar while they await immediate transfer.

Chronic mental status changes generally can be evaluated on an outpatient basis as long as the patient is closely watched by family members and is in a safe environment. The most common cause of chronic dementia, Alzheimer's disease, may be accompanied by agitation. If the diagnosis is fairly certain, this can be controlled with low doses of haloperidol (typically .5 to 1 mg every 12 hr) while the work-up is completed.

It is imperative that the office-based clinician convey knowledge of the patient's current condition and medical history to the receiving emergency physician.

References

1. Henry GL: Coma and altered states of consciousness. In Tintinalli JE, Ruiz E, Krome RL, American College of Emergency Physicians (eds): Emergency Medicine: A Comprehensive Study Guide, 4th ed. New York, McGraw-Hill, 1996, pp 150–158.
2. Peterson J: Coma. In Rosen P (ed): Emergency Medicine: Concepts and Clinical Practice, 3rd ed. St. Louis, Mosby, 1992, pp 1728–1750.
3. Schneider S: Altered mental status. In Bosker G (ed): The Elderly in Emergency Medicine. Atlanta, American Health Consultants, 2000, pp 1033–1044.
4. Sacktor N, Mayeux R: Symptoms of neurologic disorders. In Rowland L (ed): Merrit's Textbook of Neurology, 9th ed. Baltimore, Williams and Wilkins, 1995, pp 1–7.
5. Lipowski ZJ: Update on delirium. Psychiatr Clin North Am 15:335–346, 1992.
6. Francis J, Martin D, Kapoor WN: A prospective study of delirium in hospitalized elderly. JAMA 263:1097–1101, 1990.
7. Sirois F: Delirium: 100 cases. Can J Psychiatr 33:375–378, 1988.
8. Purdie FR, Honigman B, Rosen P: Acute organic brain syndrome: A review of 100 cases. Ann Emerg Med 10:455–461, 1981.

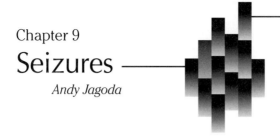

Chapter 9

Seizures

Andy Jagoda

Classification

The classification of seizures is based on behavioral and electrophysiologic features (Box 9–1). When focal seizures (partial seizures) generalize, they are called partial seizures with secondary generalization; when they involve altered mental status, they are called complex partial seizures. Epilepsy refers to a condition of recurrent unprovoked seizures.

Box 9–1. *Classification of Seizures*

I. Partial seizures
  A. Simple partial
  B. Complex
II. Generalized seizures
  A. Primary generalized
    1. Nonconvulsive (absence)
    2. Convulsive
  B. Secondary generalized
III. Status epilepticus
  A. Convulsive generalized
    1. Primary generalized
    2. Secondary generalized
  B. Convulsive focal
  C. Nonconvulsive

 CLINICAL RECOGNITION

The "aura" experienced by many patients is a focal seizure, which can remain focal or can spread. Patients with primary generalized seizures do not have an aura because they do not have a focus. Not all seizures involve the motor cortex; instead they may involve only the areas of the brain concerned with sensory or autonomic function. The clinical presentation of a seizure includes not only convulsive

95

motor activity, but also altered mental status, sensory or psychic experiences, and autonomic disturbances. Patients who seize for longer than 30 minutes or who have had repeated convulsions without a return to baseline are in status epilepticus and in need of emergent management because prognosis worsens in relation to length of the event.[1]

PHONE TRIAGE ◄—————————————————————

Most telephone calls related to seizures are from family members who have witnessed a friend or family member who has had a motor event. If the patient is actively seizing, tell the caller to protect the patient from hurting himself or herself by laying the patient on the floor, putting a pillow under the head, and removing objects that the patient might hit. Nothing should be placed in the patient's mouth (the patient will not swallow his or her tongue), and the caller should call 911. If the patient is a diabetic, the caller should put granulated sugar under the patient's tongue. If the patient has a known seizure disorder, inquire if there is an established plan that has been worked out with a physician that needs to be activated, such as administering rectal diazepam gel (see later under "Initial Management"). Once the seizure is over, the patient should be turned onto his or her side while awaiting arrival of the Emergency Medical Services (EMS); make sure that the caller understands that the patient is at risk for having another event. Tell the caller to collect any available medications or medical records; these should be brought to the hospital with the patient.

Differential Diagnosis

Several conditions can be misinterpreted as a seizure. Because misdiagnosis can have significant impact on patient care, some key points must be emphasized. Up to 40% of patients with syncope have some motor activity, most commonly involving tonic extension of the trunk or myoclonic jerks of the extremities.[2] This activity usually occurs if the patient is kept in a sitting position. These events are termed convulsive syncope and usually are not associated with tonic-clonic movements, tongue biting, cyanosis, incontinence, or postictal amnesia.

Cardiac dysrhythmias can cause hypotension with central nervous system (CNS) hypoperfusion, resulting in symptoms that are potentially confused with convulsive or nonconvulsive seizures.[3] A careful history often reveals preceding cardiac symptoms such as palpitations, light-headedness, or diaphoresis. The diagnosis frequently requires Holter monitoring, continuous cardiac loop monitoring, and head-up tilt table testing.

Decerebrate posturing has been mistaken for tonic seizures, resulting in misdiagnosis and delay in provision of potentially lifesaving interventions for increased intracranial pressure.[4] This posturing results in both upper and lower extremity extension. Tonic seizures are rare in adults; when they do occur, they are usually of short duration with upper extremity abduction.

Psychogenic seizures are nonepileptic events that are "functional" in cause.[5] They are often long-lasting with no postictal period, and patients often, but not always, recall events during the seizure. Incontinence and physical injury can occur but are characteristically uncommon. Classically, patients with psychogenic motor events have asynchronous extremity movements, forward pelvic thrusting movements, and head turning from side to side; they avoid noxious stimuli, although no one feature is pathognomonic.[6] Diagnostically, patients with psychogenic motor events do not develop a metabolic acidosis despite prolonged seizure activity, nor do they manifest an elevation in serum prolactin levels.

History

A careful description of the event and associated circumstances is fundamental to management of the seizure patient. Key historical features include whether an "aura" is present, progression of the clinical pattern, and duration of the event, including the postictal period. In treatment of patients with epilepsy, it is important for the clinician to establish if there is a change in the disorder's characteristics. All anticonvulsants that the patient uses, dosage scheduling, and compliance must be determined.

Systemic infections, intracranial lesions, fatigue, stress, pregnancy, new medication use, and various toxins, including alcohol and cocaine, can precipitate seizures (Box 9–2). The identification of one of these factors directs management toward eliminating the stressor instead of initiating or increasing anticonvulsant dosing. A careful medical history and review of systems will help to identify factors that may be essential to management.

Physical Examination

To complete a thorough physical examination, assess the patient's vital signs, mental status, and pupil position and reactivity. If the patient is actively seizing, describe the motor activity: Muscles that are in extension are "tonic," and those that are in flexion are "clonic"; "tonic-clonic" are muscles that have alternating flexion and extension. Myoclonus is characterized by rapid involuntary muscle contractions, predominantly in flexor muscles. Patients with underlying seizure foci often have tonic eye deviation toward the focus. Note the presence of "automatisms"; these are repetitive,

SEIZURES

Box 9–2. *Etiologies of Seizures**

Idiopathic causes
Vascular event
   Subarachnoid hemorrhage
   Subdural hemorrhage
   Epidural hemorrhage
   Stroke
   Vasculitis
Infection
Tumor
Metabolic disorder[†]
Toxin[‡]
Eclampsia

---

* Hypoglycemia is the most common metabolic cause of seizures.
† Hyponatremia is a rare cause of seizures except in infants younger than 6 months.
‡ Consider alcohol, cocaine, sympathomimetics, and anticolinergics.

---

stereotypical motor events, such as lip smacking, that are seen in complex partial seizures. The presence of automatisms in a patient with altered mental status may be the only indication that the patient's altered behavior is secondary to seizure activity.

Examine the patient for signs of trauma. The neurologic examination identifies focal deficits that may represent an old lesion, new intracranial disease, or a postictal motor or sensory deficit, termed "Todd's paralysis." Document the patient's mental status and talk with family members or friends to compare it with the patient's baseline. Complex partial status epilepticus can present with behavioral changes that are recognized only by persons familiar with the patient and thus their concerns must be taken seriously.[7]

Indicators that a patient has had a seizure include hyperreflexia and upgoing toes (that resolve during the postictal period), incontinence, and evidence of fractures, lacerations, or dislocations. Absence of these findings does not eliminate the possibility that the patient had a motor seizure, but their presence is suggestive.

 LABORATORY RECOGNITION ◄──────────────────

Diagnostic Studies

Hypoglycemia is by far the most common metabolic cause of seizures, making an immediate glucose determination critical in every seizing patient.[8] Controversy exists about which laboratory tests are indicated for patients presenting after having had a first-time seizure who are alert and oriented and have no clinical findings. At a minimum, these patients need a serum glucose determination and electrolytes, and women of child-bearing age require a pregnancy test.[8] A drug of abuse screen should be considered. All other laboratory tests are of very low yield in this group of patients. However, patients who are on dialysis, malnourished, or taking diuretics, and those who have underlying significant medical disorders need comprehensive testing including complete blood count (CBC), blood urea nitrogen (BUN), creatinine, calcium, phosphate, magnesium, and urinalysis.

Patients with a known seizure disorder, who had a "typical" event while taking medications but who are asymptomatic, alert, and oriented at the time of evaluation, need only a serum anticonvulsant level unless they have other underlying disease, such as diabetes, that could result in metabolic derangement. For these patients, the clinician must investigate potential precipitants such as infections or new medications that might have contributed to the event.

Neuroimaging

The indications and timing of neuroimaging are directed by the patient's history and physical examination.[9] An emergent computed tomogram of the head is indicated in patients with persisting altered mental status or focal neurologic deficits, or in those whose history is suspicious for an intracranial event such as stroke or subdural hematoma. Otherwise, an elective magnetic resonance image is the preferred diagnostic modality.

Initial Management

Patients Who Are Actively Seizing. Office management of the convulsing patient is directed toward securing the airway, maintaining oxygenation, and protecting the patient from injury. Secure intravenous access in case the seizure persists, and have suction available in case the patient vomits. Fortunately, a majority of seizures are of short duration and, in most cases, little else needs to be done. The use of a padded tongue blade is contraindicated because it may induce emesis or break a tooth; a nasal trumpet can be used to help maintain the airway when needed. Perform an immediate blood sugar determination or, if not available, give empirical dextrose. When the seizure stops, remain prepared for a second event; do not allow patients to be placed in a position in which they might fall and hurt themselves.

If the seizure continues for longer than several minutes, give lorazepam 2 mg intravenously every minute up to a maximum of 10 mg, or diazepam

SEIZURES

Box 9–3. *Management of the Seizing Patient*

Stabilization
- Protect the patient; do not place anything in the mouth
- Prepare equipment (see Table 9–1)
- Secure the airway; intubate if evidence of ineffective respirations/oxygenation
- Establish intravenous access with nondextrose solution if seizure persists longer than 3 to 5 minutes

Initial Interventions
- Dextrose, if hypoglycemic, 50 mL of 50% glucose; in children, 2 mL/kg of 25% glucose; thiamine, 100 mg IV or IM before glucose, if malnourished
- Lorazepam, 0.1 mg/kg at 2 mg/min to a maximum of 10 mg; or diazepam, 0.2 mg/kg at 5 mg/min to a maximum of 20 mg
- Ceftriaxone, 100 mg/kg up to 2 g IV, if meningitis suspected

Persisting seizures
- Phenytoin, 18 mg/kg IV at 25 mg/kg in patients with cardiac disease, otherwise 50 mg/min; in children, 1 mg/kg/min

OR
- Fosphenytoin 20 PE/kg IV at 150 mg/min

OR
- Phenobarbital 20 mg/kg at 100 mg/min IV

PE, phenytoin equivalents.

---

5 mg every minute up to a maximum of 20 mg. Lorazepam is the preferred benzodiazepine because its anticonvulsant duration of action is up to 12 hours versus less than 30 minutes for diazepam.[10, 11] If intravenous access is not available, give intramuscular midazolam 0.1 to 0.3 mg/kg, or rectal diazepam (Box 9–3). Rectal diazepam 0.5 mg/kg, up to 20 mg, is effective in terminating seizures and in decreasing their frequency in patients subject to seizure clusters.[12]

Patients who do not stop seizing after a full dose of a benzodiazepine most likely have a serious underlying problem.[13] Management options include phenytoin or phenobarbital. Phenytoin is dosed at 20 mg/kg; phenobarbital is an acceptable alternative, although it is associated with respiratory depression. The dose of phenobarbital is 100 mg per minute up to 20 mg/kg. Phenytoin is prepared in a propylene glycol vehicle and has a pH of 11. Intravenous loading can result in infusion site irritation, hypotension, confusion, and ataxia. It is recommended that infusions always be passed through a large vein to minimize sclerosis from the alkaline pH, at a rate no faster than 25 mg/min in patients with cardiac disease to minimize cardiovascular complications, and 50 mg/min in other patients. Patients who are known to be taking phenytoin but whose level is unknown can be given a half-load of phenytoin, or they can be loaded with phenobarbital.

A new preparation of phenytoin, fosphenytoin, which is a phosphate ester of phenytoin, has recently become available.[14] Fosphenytoin is water soluble, obviating the need for the propylene glycol vehicle. It can be given intramuscularly or intravenously with 100% bioavailability. Fosphenytoin is less of a tissue irritant than the phenytoin/propylene glycol preparation; pruritus and paresthesias are the most common side effects. Minimal cardiotoxic effects are associated, although hypotension has been reported with rapid infusions. Fosphenytoin has a peak serum level within 1 hour after intramuscular administration and at 6 minutes after intravenous loading. The loading dose is 20 phenytoin equivalents (PE)/kg given intramuscularly or intravenously.

Patients Who Have Seized and Have Persisting Altered Mental Status. These patients are most likely postictal; however, other diagnoses must be considered. In one study, 14% of patients treated for convulsive status epilepticus continued to have evidence of ongoing nonconvulsive status epilepticus on electroencephalographic (EEG) monitoring.[15]

In patients with altered mental status after a seizure, the serum glucose must be checked, and one must ensure that they are oxygenating well, ideally through the use of pulse oximetry. A nasal trumpet is helpful in patients with sonorous respirations; intubation is indicated in patients without a swallow reflex. A careful physical examination must be performed; evidence of trauma or increased intracranial pressure should be sought. The C-spine should be immobilized if there is concern about trauma preceding or during the seizure. Establish intravenous access, place the patient on a cardiac monitor, and provide transport to an emergency department via an Advanced Life Support (ALS) unit.

Patients Who Have Seized and Have Returned to Baseline. This group of patients can be placed into two categories—those who have had a first-time seizure and those who have a known seizure disorder.

New-Onset Seizures. The initial focus in the management of patients with new-onset seizures is to ensure that there are no correctable underlying causes that need to be addressed, such as a CNS lesion or drug toxicity. Patients who are alert, oriented, and asymptomatic will need a neuroimaging study and an EEG before a final management decision can be reached. Initiation of anticonvulsant therapy pending the diagnostic work-up is dependent on assessing the risk/benefit ratio. The incidence of seizure recurrence after a first unprovoked event is dependent on the patient's age and the seizure's underlying cause, with an average recurrence rate across all ages of 42%.[16] Seizure cause combined with EEG findings is the best predictor of recurrence; when no cause is identified and the EEG is normal, the recurrence rate is 24% at 2 years.

Seizures in Patients with a Known Seizure Disorder. Anticonvulsant medication noncompliance is the most common cause of seizure recurrence in patients with epilepsy.[17] Patients who have subtherapeutic antiepileptic drug (AED) serum levels despite compliance could have seized owing to being physically stressed secondary to an infection, pregnancy, sleep deprivation, and so forth, in which case management focuses on removing the stressor and not necessarily increasing the anticonvulsant. In those patients on single-day dosing of phenytoin, it has been noted that phenytoin results in a twofold difference between peak and trough serum levels; therefore, consideration can be given to changing the dosing schedule to twice a day.

In patients taking phenytoin, drug loading is based on the serum level. If the serum level is 0, oral loading will result in therapeutic levels within 4 hours; the recommended loading dose is 19 mg/kg in men and 23 mg/kg in women given in a single dose.[18] Intramuscular dosing of fosphenytoin gives predictable therapeutic levels within 1 hour.

In general, seizure management is best accomplished with monotherapy with anticonvulsants taken to levels that cause toxicity; therapy is not necessarily guided by the serum level.[19]

Equipment and Medications

Table 9–1 lists the equipment and medications needed to manage the seizing patient. As in all emergencies, equipment for securing cardiovasuclar and pulmonary function is essential. Because hypoglycemia is the most common metabolic cause of both altered mental status and seizures, a glucometer or glucose chemistry testing strips are extremely valuable.

Of all the treatments potentially useful in the seizing patient, oxygen, dextrose, and a benzodiazepine are the most essential. As has been discussed, lorazepam is the preferred anticonvulsant because it has the longest antiseizure effect; when lorazepam is used, addition of a longer-acting agent such as phenytoin or phenobarbital is not immediately necessary.

Disposition and Transfer

Patients who have had a first-time seizure but have returned to baseline with a nonfocal examination, and who are not at risk for an intracranial process (e.g., anticoagulation, cancer, dialysis), do not necessarily need transport to the hospital and can be evaluated as outpatients. Patients who have a seizure history, have the capacity to care for themselves, and feel comfortable with self-managing their disorder may also be managed as outpatients. Seizure patients in status epilepticus, patients with altered mental status, patients who have had a first-time seizure who have

Table 9–1. Equipment and Medications Needed to Manage the Seizing Patient

Equipment

Airway
  Oxygen
  Suction
  Nasal trumpets, various sizes
  Oral airways, various sizes
  Bag-valve mask
Intravenous cannulation
  Angiocatheters
  Normal saline
Glucometer or glucose reagent testing strips

Medications (preparations for intravenous administration)

	Refrigeration	Shelf Life	Cost (average wholesale)
Dextrose (D_{50})	No	24–36 months	$210.00/case of 40 syringes
Lorazepam	Yes	Varies with storage temperature	$125.00/1 mg/tubex: box of 10
Diazepam	No	24–36 months	$35.00/5 mg/mL: box of 10
Diazepam rectal gel (Diastat)	No	24 months	$70–$90/10-mg dose
Midazolam	No	24 months	$41.00/2 mg/2mL vial: box of 10
Phenytoin	No	24 months	$1.00/500-mg vial
Fosphenytoin	Yes	18 months	$20.00/500-mg vial

SEIZURES

undergone a focal examination or are at risk for intracranial disease, and those patients with a change in seizure pattern require transport to an emergency department. Precautions must be taken during transport in case the patient has a second event.

Admission. Admission is considered for all patients with a first-time seizure, for patients in whom the cause of the seizure is uncertain or secondary to a systemic disorder, or when there is concern that the patient will not receive a timely outpatient work-up. Patients who were in status epilepticus, regardless of cause, require admission for monitoring of potential delayed sequelae.

Epidemiology and Pathophysiology

The incidence of epilepsy is estimated to be 1.2% of the population through age 24, increasing to 4.4% by age 85.[20] The incidence of epilepsy is high in the first year of life, decreases throughout childhood, and then increases in older age, coinciding with the increase in degenerative, neoplastic, and vascular disorders.

Any process that destabilizes CNS electrical homeostasis can result in a seizure. Seizures result from either recurrent excitatory connections in the cerebral cortex or a loss of synchronization between aggregates of neurons. The excitability can be due to positive feedback loops or lack of inhibitory pathways. At the neuronal level, hyperexcitability can occur from hypoxic or hypoglycemic impairment of the Na-K pump. Glutamic acid is thought to be an excitatory transmitter and γ-amino butyric acid (GABA) an inhibitory transmitter. Disturbance in the balance between these two transmitters results in seizures. Seizure threshold is a function of genetic predisposition, environmental factors, and metabolic and structural conditions.

Systemically, in convulsive seizures, blood pressure, serum lactate, serum glucose, and white blood cell count increase (which is a leukemoid reaction without bands).[21] Body temperature is frequently elevated. Acidosis due to elevated lactate occurs within 60 seconds of a convulsive event and normalizes within 1 hour postictus. A transient cerebrospinal fluid (CSF) pleocytosis has been reported to occur in 2% of patients with motor events and in 18% of patients in status epilepticus.[22] After approximately 30 minutes, the body loses many of its autoregulatory mechanisms and seizing patients are at increased risk of hypotension, as well as decreased cerebral perfusion. Consequently, the morbidity and mortality associated with seizures increase over time.

Pediatrics

Several seizure types are associated with infants and children, including absence seizures, infantile spasms, Lennox-Gastaut syndrome, and febrile seizures. *Absence* (petit mal) *seizures* usually begin between the ages of 5 and 10 and are characterized by a sudden onset of unresponsiveness, without a preceding aura or a subsequent postictal period. The average duration of an absence event is 10 seconds, with patients having no awareness that it has occurred. Treatment of choice is ethosuximide unless the child also has motor seizures, in which case valproic acid is recommended.[23]

Infantile spasms (West's syndrome) begin before 12 months of age and are associated with mental retardation. These seizures consist of sudden single jerks, often accompanied by a short cry and awakening the child from sleep. The symptoms can be misdiagnosed as colic. When this disorder is suspected, children need referral to a pediatric neurologist.

Lennox-Gastaut syndrome is characterized by a mixture of diverse seizure types and is usually seen in children with mental retardation or behavior problems. These seizures tend to be refractory to anticonvulsant therapy. Use of empirical glucose is contraindicated in patients with Lennox-Gastaut because they are frequently maintained on a ketogenic diet. Glucose will reverse the ketosis, thereby exacerbating the seizure disorder.[24]

Febrile seizures occur between 6 months and 5 years of age. They are associated with fever and have no identifiable underlying cause. Simple febrile seizures are generalized tonic-clonic events with no focality lasting less than 15 minutes with a short postictal period. Complex febrile seizures last longer than 15 minutes or occur in a series, or they have a focal onset or a prolonged postictal period.

The management of simple febrile seizures focuses on parental education. Good evidence is available that simple febrile seizures do not predispose children to long-term intellectual or behavioral sequelae.[25] A diagnostic work-up, even for first-time events, is not indicated when they occur in children older than 18 months who have not been on antibiotics.[26] Diagnostic studies are guided by general fever protocols. In patients younger than 18 months, the signs of meningitis may be subtle or absent; thus lumbar puncture must be strongly considered. In patients with simple febrile seizures, laboratory evaluation of serum electrolytes, calcium, phosphorus, magnesium, or glucose; CBC; and neuroimaging are not routinely necessary.[25] Complex febrile seizures necessitate a complete diagnostic work-up so the clinician may explore underlying precipitating causes.

References

1. Working Group on Status Epilepticus: Treatment of convulsive status epilepticus: Recommendations of the Epilepsy Foundation of America's Working Group on Status Epilepticus. JAMA 270:854–859, 1993.
2. Lin J: Convulsive syncope in blood donors. Ann Neurol 11:525–528, 1982.
3. Linzer M, Grubb B, Simon H, et al: Cardiovascular causes of loss of consciousness in patients with presumed epilepsy: A cause of increased sudden death rate in people with epilepsy. Am J Med 96:146–154, 1994.
4. Haines S: Decerebrate posturing misinterpreted as seizure activity. Am J Emerg Med 6:173–177, 1988.
5. Ozkara C, Dreifuss F: Differential diagnosis in pseudoepileptic seizures. Epilepsia 34:294–299, 1993
6. Gates J, Ramani V, Whalen S, Loewenson R: Ictal characteristics of pseudoseizures. Arch Neurol 42:1183–1187, 1985.
7. Tomson T, Lindbom U, Nilsson B: Nonconvulsive status epilepticus in adults: Thirty-two consecutive patients from a general hospital population. Epilepsia 33:829–835, 1992.
8. American College of Emergency Physicians: Clinical policy for the initial approach to patients presenting with a chief complaint of seizure, who are not in status epilepticus, Ann Emerg Med 22:875–883, 1993.
9. American Academy of Neurology: Neuroimaging in the emergency patient presenting with seizures. Ann Emerg Med 28:114–118, 1996.
10. Treiman D: Pharmacokinetics and clinical use of benzodiazepines in the management of status epilepticus. Epilepsia 30:4–10, 1989.
11. Leppik I, Derivan A, Homan R, et al: Double-blind study of lorazepam and diazepam in status epilepticus. JAMA 249:1452–1453, 1983.
12. Dreifuss F, Rosman P, Cloyd J, et al: A comparison of rectal diazepam gel and placebo for acute repetitive seizures. N Engl J Med 338:1869–1875, 1998.
13. Jagoda A, Riggio S: Refractory status epilepticus in adults. Ann Emerg Med 22:1337–1348, 1993.
14. Wilder BJ (ed): The use of parental antiepileptic drugs and the role for fosphenytoin. Neurology 46:S1–S28, 1996.
15. DeLorenzo R, Waterhouse E, Towne A, et al: Persistent nonconvulsive status epilepticus after the control of convulsive status epilepticus. Epilepsia 39:833–840, 1998.

16. Berg A, Shlomo S: The risk of seizure recurrence following a first unprovoked seizure: A quantitative review. Neurology 41:965–972, 1991.
17. DeLorenzo R, Hauser W, Towne A, et al: A prospective, population based study of status epilepticus in Richmond, Virginia. Neurology 46:1029–1035, 1996.
18. Ratanakorn D, Kaojarern S, Phuapradit P, et al: Single oral loading dose of phenytoin: A pharmacokinetic study. J Neurol Sci 147:89–92, 1997.
19. French J: The long-term therapeutic management of epilepsy. Ann Intern Med 120:411–422, 1994.
20. Rich S, Lee J, et al: Risk of recurrent seizures after two unprovoked seizures. N Engl J Med 338:429–434, 1998.
21. Simon R: Physiologic consequences of status epilepticus. Epilepsia 26(suppl 1):58–66, 1985.
22. Aminoff M, Simon R: Status epilepticus: Causes, clinical features and consequences in 98 patients. Am J Med 69:657–666, 1980.
23. Turnbull T, Vanden Hoed T, Howes D, Eisner R: Utility of laboratory studies in the emergency department patient with a new-onset seizure. Ann Emerg Med 19:373–377, 1990.
24. Vining E: Pediatric seizures. Emerg Med Clin North Am 12:973–988, 1994.
25. Verity C, Greenwood R, Golding J: Long-term intellectual and behavioral outcomes of children with febrile convulsions. N Engl J Med 338:1723–1728, 1998.
26. American Academy of Pediatrics: Practice parameters: Febrile seizures. Pediatrics 97:769–775, 1996.

Chapter 10
Psychosis
Iris M. Reyes

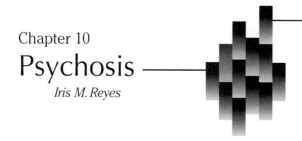

One of the most difficult situations encountered by the primary care practitioner is the patient who presents to the office setting with a change in mental status. The evaluation of a patient with an acute change in behavior or level of consciousness can be quite challenging. Clinicians can simplify this to an extent by becoming familiar with the various causes of these conditions. Acute changes in behavior can be categorized into those caused by dementia, delirium, or psychosis. *Dementia* is a progressive deterioration of mental function caused by organic factors. Both recent and remote memory capabilities are impaired, and typically there is no clouding of consciousness.[1] *Delirium* is an acute, usually reversible, metabolically induced state of fluctuating consciousness. The symptoms are wide ranging and typically cause generalized impairment of cognitive function.[2] Although these descriptions are distinct, there can be a significant amount of crossover with patients who present with elements of each. Patients with dementia or delirium may present with psychotic features.[3]

The term *psychosis* is used to describe a type of behavior in which there is a state of mental dysfunction with a mental capacity that is grossly distorted.[4] This behavioral change manifests with signs and symptoms associated with psychotic conditions.

These include the following:
- Delusions
- Hallucinations
- Disorganized speech
- Disorganized or catatonic behavior

Psychosis is further classified, according to the presumptive underlying pathophysiology, as organic or functional. *Organic* psychosis is as a result of an abnormality of the anatomy, biochemistry, or physiology of the brain. *Functional* psychosis is the term used to describe mental dysfunction in which no clear anatomic, physiologic, or chemical abnormality is found.[5]

Among the most prevalent causes of psychosis of an organic origin is intoxication with or withdrawal from commonly abused substances. Cocaine and amphetamine are commonly associated with psychotic symptoms.[6] Hallucinogens such as lysergic acid diethylamide (LSD), psilocybin, and mescaline can have a similar effect. Withdrawal from benzodiazepines and from alcohol has been associated with an acute psychotic state.[6]

Although most medical conditions that produce psychotic states manifest as delirium, some patients may present with a clear sensorium. The psychosis associated with high-dose steroid treatment such as that used for lupus cerebritis may occur without delirium.[6] Agitated psychosis without delirium has also been noted in patients who present in hyperthyroid states.[6]

 ## CLINICAL RECOGNITION ◄—————————

The evaluation of a patient with suspected acute psychosis requires a careful history and physical examination. Differentiating a functional/ psychiatric disorder from an organic/medical condition is essential for appropriate treatment. This may be difficult to ascertain in patients who present with disorganized thought processes and an inability to have insight into their own conditions. Direct questioning as opposed to open-ended questions is most effective in this scenario. The clinician should recruit the assistance of family members, friends, and care providers to attempt to gain useful insight.

Factors that can assist the health care provider in differentiating the underlying causes include a history of previous mental illness. Determination of the patient's baseline functional status may reveal a chronic psychiatric condition. Patients may also present with acute exacerbations of underlying chronic psychiatric illnesses. It must be recognized, however, that patients with chronic functional psychoses can develop acute decompensation as a result of organic conditions, such as infections, metabolic derangements, medication reactions, and structural lesions. Functional psychosis should be a diagnosis of exclusion in patients with no previous history of psychiatric illness.

Features suggesting an organic cause include[7]:

- Abnormal vital signs—transient vital sign abnormalities such as elevated heart rate or blood pressure are likely to be noted in the acutely agitated patient, but persistent or markedly abnormal signs are usual
- Age older than 40—it is unusual for anyone to develop an acute functional psychosis beyond this age, especially with no previous history of psychiatric illness
- Sudden onset—acute functional psychoses tend to develop over weeks to months
- Loss of consciousness
- Focal neurologic symptoms—point to a structural cerebral lesion as the probable cause of the acute behavioral change

PSYCHOSIS

- Speech difficulties, including incoherent speech
- Confusion/disorientation
- Social immodesty
- Visual hallucinations—auditory hallucinations are common in psychiatric illness, but visual, tactile, and olfactory hallucinations are more commonly associated with organic causes

The *mental status examination*, including an evaluation of cognition and behavior, is helpful in differentiating the various causes of acute psychosis. Included in this is assessment of the following:
- Orientation
- Memory—short and long term
- Affect or mood
- Thoughts
- Recall
- Attention
- Language
- Judgment

A *neurologic examination*, including assessment of cranial nerves, motor and sensory function, reflexes, coordination, and gait, may reveal focal deficits. The discovery of focal deficits should be followed by further evaluation, including computed tomographic (CT) scan of the head or magnetic resonance imaging (MRI).

The *physical examination* should focus on finding the possible causes of an acute deterioration of mental function. The presence of incontinence, fever, or abnormal lung sounds, or abdominal findings may indicate an organic cause of acute psychosis. Evaluation may be limited initially by the patient's noncompliance and possibly by agitated, aggressive behavior, but it should be completed once control of the situation is obtained.

The differential diagnoses of psychosis are listed in Box 10–1.

Box 10–1. *Differential Diagnoses of Psychosis*

Functional
Schizophrenia
Schizophreniform disorder
Schizoaffective disorder
Delusional disorder
Brief psychotic disorder
Shared psychotic disorder

Organic
Central nervous system
- Cerebral infarction
- Seizure

Box 10–1. *Differential Diagnoses of Psychosis* *(Continued)*

- Encephalopathy
- Subarachnoid hemorrhage
- Epidural hematoma
- Subdural hematoma
- Intraparenchymal hemorrhage
- Migraine
- Neoplasms
- Huntington's chorea
- Cerebral abscess
- Concussion

Metabolism
- Drug intoxication or withdrawal
- Hypoxia
- Hypercarbia
- Hypoglycemia
- Electrolyte imbalance

Organ failure
- Addison's disease
- Cushing's disease
- Thyroid disease
- Parathyroid dysfunction
- Pituitary disease
- Diabetic ketoacidosis
- Renal azotemia
- Hepatic encephalopathy
- Shock

Infection
- Sepsis
- Pneumonia
- Meningitis
- Urinary tract infection
- Acquired immunodeficiency syndrome (AIDS)
- Encephalitis

Pharmacologic effects/toxins
- Psychoactive agents/drugs of abuse—PCP, LSD, cocaine, cannabinoids, amphetamines
- Antidepressants
- Anticholinergics
- Antiemetics
- Antihypertensives

PSYCHOSIS

> ## Box 10–1. *Differential Diagnoses of Psychosis* (Continued)
>
> - Anti-inflammatories
> - Antineoplastics
> - Antibiotics
> - Sympathomimetics
> - Antiepileptics
> - Benzodiazepines
> - Procainamide
> - Digoxin
> - Steroids
> - Antihistamines
> - Heavy metals
> - Industrial toxins
> - Carbon monoxide
>
> Substrate deficiency
>
> - Thiamine deficiency—Wernicke-Korsakoff syndrome
> - Niacin deficiency—pellagra
> - Vitamin B_{12} deficiency
> - Folic acid deficiency
> - Hypoglycemia
> - Hypoxia
>
> LSD, lysergic acid diethylamide; PCP, phenylcyclohexyl piperidine.

 PHONE TRIAGE ◄

Patients with an acute psychotic episode are unlikely to call but will more likely arrive with no previous notification. Should a phone call be placed, however, it is imperative that the office staff obtain information regarding the patient's location. The staff member should ask if there is anyone else with the patient, and if so, he or she should ask to speak with that person. The following symptoms should be addressed:

- **Hallucinations**—sensory experiences that exist only in the mind of the person experiencing them. Any sense may be involved; however, they tend to be visual or auditory
- **Delusions**—loss of touch with reality, or beliefs that are clearly implausible and erroneous. They involve a misinterpretation of perceptions. Delusions may be religious, persecutory, or somatic in nature
- **Disorganized speech**—speech pattern includes neologisms, perseverations, word salad, loose associations, or a poverty of content

> • **Disorganized or catatonic behavior**—a lack of awareness of the surrounding environment or difficulty in performing goal-oriented tasks

 ## LABORATORY RECOGNITION ◄————————————

Laboratory evaluation is essential for patients who have a psychosis that is believed to be organic in origin. Those with a clear psychiatric history who present with characteristic symptoms usually do not require laboratory evaluation. The following are commonly ordered tests that can help the clinician to identify the cause of an organic psychosis:
• Pulse oximetry
• Serum glucose
• Serum electrolytes, blood urea nitrogen (BUN), and creatinine
• Complete blood count
• Toxicologic screen/blood alcohol level
• Electrocardiogram (ECG)
• Chest radiograph
• Urinalysis

Those patients with severe, profound alterations in mental status may warrant an expanded evaluation such as:
• Thyroid screening
• Liver function panel
• Pancreatic enzymes
• Serum drug levels
• Blood cultures

If organic causes such as cerebral mass lesions, cerebral infarctions, trauma, or infection are suspected, the following should also be considered:
• Noncontrast CT scan of the head
• Magnetic resonance imaging (MRI)
• Lumbar puncture

Treatment Decision Points

Treatment of acute psychosis should be deferred until differentiation is made between a functional and an organic cause. In the office setting, treatment should be directed at immediately reversible causes such as hypoglycemia and hypoxia. The safety of both the staff and the patient is a priority. If the patient is aggressive or threatening, security personnel or

PSYCHOSIS

local police must be summoned. The use of chemical or physical restraints should be considered as the situation demands.

Disposition and Transfer

Acutely aggressive, violent psychotic patients require rapid and aggressive treatment. This is best determined by the likely cause of the condition. If it is suspected to be organic in nature, transfer to a medical facility equipped to provide urgent intervention, such as an emergency department, is appropriate. If the condition is suspected to be of psychiatric origin, transfer to the nearest psychiatric evaluation center is necessary.

It is essential that the clinician determine the patient's mental capacity to make decisions in the event that he or she refuses treatment and transfer. If it is determined that the patient may be a danger to himself or others, the patient may be held against his will. If the safety of the patient or staff is compromised, the use of either chemical or physical restraints will be necessary to subdue the patient. In the outpatient setting, requesting assistance from the local Emergency Medical Services (EMS) and police authorities trained in physical restraint may be necessary. Chemical restraints commonly used include benzodiazepines such as lorazepam, midazolam, diazepam, and flurazepam. Butyrophenones such as haldol and droperidol represent another type of medication commonly used for rapid sedation. A rapid-acting sedative given intravenously is preferred in the uncooperative, agitated, acutely psychotic patient, but it may be given intramuscularly if no intravenous line has been established.

Not all patients require this level of aggressive treatment. Those with mild agitation may require only transfer for further evaluation and treatment. The patient suspected of being acutely psychotic should not be released without both medical and psychiatric evaluations. Phone contact with the patient's psychiatrist or family physician will likely provide the clinician with greater insight into the underlying cause of the patient's acute deterioration.

Complications

Physical examination of patients presenting with psychosis should never be omitted. The temptation to do this may be great, especially if the patient is being evasive, withdrawn, uncooperative, aggressive, or violent. Medical illnesses can precipitate an acute decompensation of an underlying chronic psychiatric condition.

Patients who present with injuries suspected to be self-induced must be assessed for suicidal ideation. Suicidal threats should always be taken seriously. The risks for suicidality should be evaluated with questions addressing methods, access to weapons, and past attempts. The health

PSYCHOSIS

care provider must be aware that promises, bargains, and negotiations made with suicidal patients do not necessarily prevent a subsequent attempt.

Pediatrics

Evaluation of children and adolescents is essentially the same as for adult patients. Differentiating functional versus organic causes of psychosis will dictate management. Family dynamics and interpersonal interactions at school can play a major role in precipitating acute crises and should be addressed. Schizophrenia frequently has its onset in adolescence, but definitive diagnosis of this condition should be deferred until psychiatric evaluation has occurred.

References

1. Geltmacher DS, Whitehouse PJ: Current concepts: Evaluation of dementia. N Engl J Med 335:330–336, 1996.
2. Meagher DJ: Delirium: Optimising management. BMJ 322:144–149, 2001.
3. Casey DA, DeFazio JV Jr, Vansickle K, Lippmann S: Delirium—quick recognition, careful evaluation, and appropriate treatment. Postgrad Med 100:121–124, 128, 133–134, 1996.
4. Richards CF, Gurr DE: Psychosis. Emerg Med Clin North Am 18:253–262, 2000.
5. American Psychiatric Association: Diagnostic and Statistical Manual of Mental Disorders, 4th ed. Washington, DC, American Psychiatric Association, 1994, pp 579–580.
6. Forster PL, Buckley R, Phelps MA: Phenomenology and treatment of psychotic disorders in the psychiatric emergency service. Psychiatr Clin North Am 22:735–754, 1999.
7. Dubin WR, Weiss KJ, Zeccardi JA: Organic brain syndrome: The psychiatric impostor. JAMA 249:60–62, 1983.

PSYCHOSIS

Chapter 11

Acute Abdominal Pain

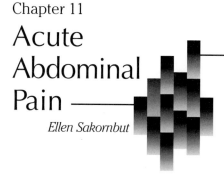

Ellen Sakornbut

Abdominal pain is a common complaint for which patients often seek medical care. This chapter focuses on the following objectives: differentiation of surgical and nonsurgical causes of abdominal pain, and the assessment of urgent causes of abdominal pain that warrant hospitalization or substantive interventions or diagnostic procedures. Rare and unusual causes of abdominal pain are beyond the scope of this chapter, and the management of chronic disorders is not discussed here.

Epidemiology

Abdominal pain is one of the most common complaints of patients seeking care in primary care offices. Most recent-onset abdominal pain seen in an outpatient office represents mild illness and requires few office visits; often a diagnosis is not made.[1-3] The causes of acute abdominal pain vary significantly by age. Significant causes of acute abdominal pain in the young child include intussusception, appendicitis, mesenteric adenitis, and volvulus. In older children, adolescents, and young adults, the most urgent or emergent common causes of acute abdominal pain include appendicitis, abdominal pain from systemic illness (such as diabetic ketoacidosis and sickle cell crisis), and gynecologic problems in young women (such as pelvic inflammatory disease, adnexal torsion, ectopic pregnancy, and ruptured ovarian cyst). Cholelithiasis and diverticulitis are more commonly seen as patients enter middle age, with diverticular disease, volvulus, leaking abdominal aortic aneurysm, and mesenteric infarction occurring more commonly among the elderly. Small-bowel obstruction and appendicitis are seen in patients of all ages.

CLINICAL RECOGNITION ◄————————————————

Because treatment is specific to the cause of abdominal pain, evaluation for seriousness and potential diagnosis should be a matter of top priority. Nonspecific abdominal pain is the most common diagnosis given to patients seen urgently for this problem; however, the clinician should exercise great caution in using this diagnosis in the very young and the older patient. The prevalence of serious illness is higher among elderly patients complaining of acute, severe abdominal pain[4, 5]; they require urgent evaluation and, possibly, emergency department or hospital care. Significant steroid therapy (oral or intravenous) is associated with less specific signs and symptoms of abdominal urgency and requires more vigilance on the part of the evaluator. Patients with human immunodeficiency virus (HIV) may have unusual causes of acute abdomen, such as perforation of the large bowel from cytomegalovirus infection, bowel obstruction secondary to HIV-related malignancies, atypical mycobacteria,[6] or other possibilities.

Patients with acute, substantial abdominal pain and the following types of symptoms or situations are preferably evaluated in a setting with significant resources (including radiologic tools) and potential for surgical intervention:
- Recent, significant trauma potentially involving the abdomen, such as an auto accident or a significant fall
- Collapse, fainting, or inability to stand up from a lying or sitting position
- Acute, severe abdominal pain or any abdominal pain following trauma in pregnancy
- Acute, severe abdominal pain in the elderly
- Bright red blood in vomitus or from the rectum
- Use of heparin or warfarin (Coumadin)
- Use of oral or intravenous, but not inhaled, steroids

If patients who meet these criteria telephone the office, they should generally be directly referred to an emergency room in a hospital setting. If they present to the office, they should receive a quick overview and stabilization as needed; they should then be sent to an emergency department.

Pain Location

The anatomic structures and frequency of various illnesses vary by location. Pain can be considered as generalized or more localized by region:

ABDOMINAL PAIN

- Generalized—gastroenteritis, obstruction/ischemic bowel (in the elderly), diabetic ketoacidosis, sickle cell crisis, toxic ingestion (e.g., methanol)
- Right upper quadrant—hepatitis, cholecystitis, biliary colic, duodenal ulcer, pleurisy, pneumonia
- Right lower quadrant—appendicitis, gynecologic problems
- Epigastric region—ulcers, gastritis, pancreatitis
- Left upper quadrant—pancreatitis, ulcers, ruptured spleen, pneumonia
- Left lower quadrant—diverticulitis, leaking aneurysm, gynecologic problems
- Periumbilical area—appendicitis, small-bowel obstruction
- Pelvis—gynecologic problems, prostatitis

Also, some pains involve or evolve to include more than one location. Characteristic patterns include:
- Right back to right lower quadrant—urethral stone
- Left back to left lower quadrant or groin—urethral stone
- Periumbilical area to right lower quadrant—appendicitis
- Right upper quadrant to right scapula/back or shoulder—gallstones
- Left upper quadrant or left of umbilicus to back—pancreatitis
- Generalized abdominal pain with pain in shoulders—ruptured viscus and free air in the abdomen, such as occurs with perforated ulcer, ruptured spleen, or ruptured ectopic pregnancy
- Radicular or dermatomal distribution—herpetic neuralgia

Physical Examination

The patient presentation also helps with diagnosis and triage. The general appearance and level of distress of the patient should be noted. Patients who lie still and do not wish to move may have peritoneal irritation from a perforated organ, and thus may need surgical intervention. Patients who writhe with pain are more likely to have ureteral stones.

Vital signs are necessary early. Elderly patients may not manifest fever despite surgical causes of abdominal pain, such as appendicitis or cholecystitis. Hypotension suggests the need for urgent intervention. Tachycardia is common with pain and its presence does not particularly help the clinician to identify the cause.

Cardiac and lung examination may be helpful in identifying the cause of abdominal pain, such as right lower quadrant pneumonia. The abdominal examination should be performed systematically. Auscultation for bowel sounds is helpful before palpation. Pain elicited from stethoscope pressure may be helpful in gauging patient responses to palpation by the examining hand. Percussion tenderness should be noted, as should the presence of guarding, whether voluntary or involuntary. Pressure on one side of the abdomen causing pain at another site (referred tenderness) suggests significant disease at the site of pain. Because there may be "rebound" tenderness (i.e., pain causing the patient to wince with sudden release of the examiner's hands), this is best done gently. Unfortunately, some patients with an acute abdomen do not have significant tenderness or rebound tenderness. The elderly patient with abdominal pain may suffer from an acute abdomen without exhibiting typical tenderness; either the absence of tenderness or the presence of generalized, rather than localized, tenderness may be noted instead.

Tenderness resulting from intra-abdominal causes may be distinguished from abdominal wall tenderness by palpation of the abdomen while the patient engages the abdominal muscles and rises part of the way from the supine position. Abdominal muscle rigidity with palpation suggests peritoneal inflammation. This should be differentiated from voluntary muscle contraction due to fear.

The presence of bowel sounds does not exclude an acute abdomen. Acute bowel obstruction is generally represented by abnormal bowel sounds (such as high-pitched tinkling) or absent bowel sounds (especially with necrotic bowel). Abnormal bowel sounds in the elderly are frequently indicative of serious disease.

Rectal examination may demonstrate tenderness in fewer than half of patients with appendicitis. Because the sensitivity of this finding is low, the principal reason for performing a rectal examination in most patients is to determine the presence of occult gastrointestinal bleeding.

The pelvic examination is usually helpful and may be critical in women with lower abdominal pain. For a discussion of pain in pregnant women, see Chapters 14 and 15. Patients should be examined with a speculum, and the presence of bleeding or mucopurulent cervicitis should be documented. The presence or absence of cervical motion tenderness should be documented, along with adnexal tenderness and/or masses.

 ## LABORATORY RECOGNITION ◄————————————

The primary means of diagnosing the acute abdomen is use of information obtained during the history and physical, not data from laboratory or radiologic studies. In keeping with this, laboratory studies should be directed by history and physical findings (e.g., the commonly obtained complete blood count rarely affects the management of acute abdominal pain).[7-9] Amylase and lipase may be helpful in patients with left upper quadrant pain, to assess for pancreatitis, but they are not available immediately in most offices. Urinalysis is helpful when the history is suggestive of a urinary process. The one test that should be done for almost all women of child-bearing age who present with acute abdominal pain is a pregnancy test, whether or not

> the woman has had a tubal ligation. Current urine pregnancy tests are highly sensitive, take only a few minutes, and can be done readily in the office.

Similarly, the classical "three-way" abdominal radiographic series has low sensitivity and low specificity. Occasionally, free air under the diaphragm indicates a ruptured organ not already suspected. The diagnosis of bowel obstruction, either small or large, may be aided by radiographic evaluation. Key findings with obstruction include dilated loops of small bowel or dilated large bowel, absence of air in the rectum, and multiple air-fluid levels. Kidney stones may be seen, but patients with kidney stones usually do not have a classical "acute abdomen." Findings such as "sentinel loops" may be seen with pancreatitis, but they are not specific and are uncommon.

Ultrasound examinations are most useful for women with potential obstetric or gynecologic problems. Transvaginal ultrasound is likely to reveal gynecologic problems or first trimester complications (see Chapter 14). Occasionally, ultrasound performed on an urgent basis identifies gallstones, but patients who have eaten often demonstrate excessive bowel gas or contraction of the gallbladder. Computed tomography (CT) is useful in identification and management of multiple causes of acute abdominal pain, including small- and large-bowel obstruction, pancreatitis, mesenteric infarction, appendicitis, diverticulitis, intra-abdominal abscess, biliary tract disease, abdominal trauma, and abdominal aortic aneurysm.

Review of Presentation of Some Causes of Acute Abdomen

Appendicitis

Appendicitis is often an illness of young adults, but it may occur at any age. Classically, discomfort or pain starts in the periumbilical area, then moves to the right lower quadrant (McBurney's point) over a few hours. Nausea, general malaise, constipation or diarrhea, and low-grade fever may all accompany appendicitis but are not helpful for the clinician in making or ruling out the diagnosis. Anorexia is commonly present and may be the most reliable symptom. Sometimes after significant early symptoms, the patient temporarily feels improved if he or she lies still. This occurs at the time of appendiceal rupture and the development of peritonitis.

Physical examination performed early is nonspecific, but it gradually becomes more specific. Direct tenderness is present with slight pressure in the right lower quadrant; rebound tenderness localizes to the right lower quadrant, as does referred tenderness. Although rectal examination may demonstrate tenderness, its absence does not reliably rule out appendicitis. The patient may hold the right leg in flexion, and extension is associated with localized pain (psoas sign). The obturator test (rotation of the thigh) is associated with increased pain. A firm tap on the right heel can also elicit tenderness. With further development of peritonitis, rigidity of the abdominal muscle wall develops.

The white blood cell (WBC) count is often mildly elevated, but absence of leukocytosis may be misleading in some patients, particularly the elderly. The urinalysis may demonstrate mild pyuria, but this is not a reliable finding. A pregnancy test should be performed in all premenopausal women and adolescents, and a gynecologic history and appropriate examination should be completed, depending on information suggestive of gynecologic causes. A negative appendectomy has been found to occur more often in women, in patients with complaints of pain disproportionate to objective findings, in the absence of vomiting, and in those with a longer duration of symptoms.[10, 11] On the other hand, other authors have found that the diagnosis of appendicitis is frequently missed in women, with misdiagnoses of pelvic inflammatory disease and urinary tract infection.[12]

Problems in diagnosis also occur when the appendix is not in the classical location, when the symptoms develop slowly or appear recurrently, or in the elderly when signs and symptoms are less specific. In some series, adults over the age of 50 experienced significantly poorer outcomes, mainly resulting from delay in diagnosis. Ultrasound has not been proven to be as useful in adults with suspected appendicitis as CT. CT scans have proven to be both specific and sensitive, allowing safe reduction in negative appendectomy rates.[13] CT provides the additional advantage that alternative diagnoses may be confirmed by this diagnostic study.[14]

In children, confusion sometimes occurs with abdominal lymphadenitis (mesenteric adenitis), usually presenting with symptoms of concurrent viral infection. These children tend to have less classical examination findings. Without rebound tenderness in the right lower quadrant, serial examinations and follow-up may be reasonable. Additionally, ultrasound examination is useful in children when the diagnosis of appendicitis is not clear. Although sensitivity and specificity are good, its greatest value appears to be a decrease in hospitalization and/or surgery with negative ultrasound examination because the negative predictive value is very high (96%).[15] CT has also been used to diagnose appendicitis in children. Children younger than 3 years of age with appendicitis are more likely to experience delay in diagnosis or perforation, and to demonstrate fewer specific findings on examination, such as localized tenderness and rebound, and a greater number of nonspecific findings, such as fever and abdominal distention.[16] Thus, the older and the very young patient with possible appendicitis form high-risk groups that merit special follow-up and/or diagnostic measures.

Gynecologic Causes of Acute Abdominal Pain

Mittelschmerz Syndrome. Mittelschmerz syndrome manifests with the acute onset of sharp, lower abdominal or pelvic pain, usually unilateral in midcycle when ovulation may cause the release of small amounts of fluid and blood into the peritoneal cavity. Patients should have stable vital signs, may demonstrate a minor degree of peritoneal irritation on abdominal examination, and do not give a preceding history of periumbilical diffuse pain (as with appendicitis).

Ovarian Cysts. Ovarian cysts may cause acute abdominal/pelvic pain with leakage of fluid into the peritoneal cavity and/or stretching of the ovarian capsule with growth of the cyst, especially if there is hemorrhage into the cyst. Usually, pain from a nonleaking cyst is mild and may be exacerbated by intercourse or other pressure on pelvic structures.

Adnexal Torsion. Adnexal torsion occurs sporadically, with the vast majority of cases occurring in women who have ovarian cysts, ovarian hyperstimulation, or other ovarian neoplasia,[17] or during pregnancy. Subacute torsion may occur intermittently; acute episodes of torsion are characterized by severe, sharp, unilateral pelvic and lower abdominal pain, which is unremitting. Physical examination findings may be unrevealing except for adnexal tenderness, but may include adnexal mass. Two-dimensional ultrasound findings are variable and include ovarian and other adnexal masses. Diagnosis may be made conclusively with color flow Doppler verification, demonstrating cessation of blood flow to adnexal structures.[18]

Pelvic Inflammatory Disease. Pelvic inflammatory disease presents more commonly in young women and adolescents; onset of symptoms may occur weeks to months following exposure to a sexually transmitted pathogen. Additionally, the spectrum of pelvic inflammatory disease includes endometritis resulting from instrumentation of the uterus. Historical data that should be collected include previous history of pelvic and other sexually transmitted infection, a change in sexual partners in the preceding 2 to 3 months, age younger than 25 years, and the use (or lack of use) of barrier contraceptive methods. Patients may complain of nausea, vomiting, or abnormal uterine bleeding. Usually, nausea and vomiting are seen only in more severe cases, developing after onset of pain. Although abnormal uterine bleeding is common, it is usually not profuse. The clinical onset of symptoms frequently occurs following the menses.

Supportive physical findings for a diagnosis of pelvic inflammatory disease include the following—cervical motion tenderness, mucopurulent cervicitis, bilateral lower quadrant and adnexal tenderness that may be unilaterally more pronounced, and tenderness on palpation of the cul-de-sac. Patients with gonococcal infection usually display fever and leukocytosis, and they may demonstrate mild peritoneal signs. Patients with *Chlamydia* infection usually experience less severe pain, little or no fever, a normal white blood cell count, and less tenderness on examination. Right upper quadrant tenderness with or without liver enzyme elevations coexistent with pelvic inflammatory disease (Fitz-Hugh–Curtis syndrome) is uncommonly seen. A third type of pelvic inflammatory disease has been documented by culture of peritoneal fluid,[19] usually with mixed anaerobic and aerobic Gram-negative bacteria, such as *Bacteroides fragilis* and *Peptostreptococcus*.

The role of mixed anaerobic/aerobic infection and other potential pathogens, such as *Mycoplasma*, remains somewhat difficult to determine because culture of the cervix does not reveal a cause in these cases. Although pelvic inflammatory disease is a common illness, some authors believe the diagnosis is made more frequently than it is supported by evidence from positive cultures[20] or than it meets Centers for Disease Control (CDC) criteria in urgent and emergency settings.[21] Alternatively, it is likely that many episodes of salpingitis are indolent in nature and do not stimulate women to seek emergent medical care. Diagnostic testing that is available on an urgent basis (e.g., complete blood count [CBC], erythrocyte sedimentation rate [ESR], C-reactive protein [CRP], ultrasound) is not sufficiently sensitive, nor is it specific enough, to confirm a diagnosis of pelvic inflammatory disease or to eliminate it as a cause of abdominopelvic pain. Therefore, the diagnosis of pelvic inflammatory disease remains a clinical diagnosis, and clinicians are usually challenged to make disposition without confirmatory information at the time of the encounter.

Patients who should be considered for hospitalization include those with findings of peritonitis, pelvic abscess, and inability to take oral medication or maintain hydration because of nausea and vomiting, as well as those who have failed outpatient management. Laparoscopic studies of the microbiology of severe pelvic inflammatory disease reveal frequent recovery of anaerobic bacteria along with other pathogens, indicating a need for increased antibiotic coverage in this group.[22]

Acute Biliary Tract Disease

Symptomatic *cholelithiasis* may present as recurrent episodes of sharp, cramping, or colicky right upper quadrant or even epigastric pain, accompanied by nausea or vomiting. Patients may or may not complain of classical symptoms of fatty food intolerance or may demonstrate other risk factors such as female sex, multiparity, age over 40, and obesity. Patients with cholelithiasis should be referred for early elective cholecystectomy (usually laparoscopic) because delays in surgery often lead to recurrent emergency treatment and increased morbidity associated with nonelective surgery.[23]

ABDOMINAL PAIN

Cholecystitis, or inflammation of the gallbladder, is most often associated with cholelithiasis. Patients demonstrate signs of inflammation, such as elevated temperature to greater than 38°C and WBC count greater than 10,000; they may also be tender upon palpation of the right upper quadrant (Murphy's sign). Ultrasound performed on an urgent basis may be limited in accuracy, depending on the skill of the examiner and the presence or absence of excessive bowel gas or contraction of the gallbladder in a patient with recent oral intake. Patients with cholecystitis should be admitted for intravenous hydration, enteric antibiotic coverage, and early cholecystectomy (after 24 to 48 hr) because of improved outcomes over delayed surgery.[24] Alternative regimens for patients at poor risk for surgical procedures include percutaneous cholecystotomy, gallbladder aspiration, and endoscopic sphincterotomy.

Patients with *ascending cholangitis* represent, in general, the sickest end of the spectrum of those with biliary tract disease. With obstruction of the common bile duct (usually secondary to stones), bacterial invasion occurs from the intestine or portal venous system with resulting sepsis. These patients are febrile and jaundiced, and they may present with hypotension, shock, and altered mentation. Usually, WBC counts and alkaline phosphatase and bilirubin concentrations are elevated. These patients warrant admission to a facility that can provide endoscopic or percutaneous cholangiography. Additional patients meriting admission include any jaundiced patients (indicating common bile duct obstruction) and those with gallstone pancreatitis.

Pancreatitis

Patients presenting with acute, constant, boring epigastric or periumbilical pain, especially with nausea, vomiting, and tachycardia, may be suspected of having pancreatitis. This diagnosis is more likely in the patient who abuses alcohol or has biliary tract disease, although multiple other causes exist, including hypertriglyceridemia, drug reactions, and viral causes. The examination findings of a patient with pancreatitis may vary from a mildly ill individual with moderate abdominal tenderness and abdominal distention, to a severely ill patient with shock, hypoactive or absent bowel sounds, jaundice, and bluish discoloration of the flanks (Cullen's sign) or periumbilical region (Turner's sign).

Laboratory abnormalities include elevation of amylase, lipase, and (frequently) WBC count. Serum glucose and bilirubin may be elevated, and serum calcium is decreased in one quarter of cases. Serum alkaline phosphatase and transaminases may be transiently elevated. Chest radiograph may reveal pleural effusion, especially on the left side. CT examination may be helpful in the diagnosis of pancreatitis, delineation of its cause (e.g., gallstones), and assessment of its severity. Ultrasound,

ABDOMINAL PAIN

alternatively, may be used to look for gallstones or to identify a pseudocyst. Differential diagnoses include[9] false-positive elevation of amylase with systemic acidemia (such as diabetic ketoacidosis), perforated hollow viscus, mesenteric vascular infarction, abdominal aortic aneurysm, and biliary tract disease.

Perforated Peptic Ulcer

Most patients who have a perforated peptic ulcer have had epigastric pain and often a history of having taken antacids or over-the-counter H_2 blockers for symptomatic relief. However, about one in five has not had symptoms of peptic ulcer before the development of complications (bleeding or perforation).[25] The pain is usually epigastric but may proceed to the lower abdomen as gastric acid spills into the abdominal cavity. There may be pain through to the back or shoulder, which often requires closer questioning because it may not be severe. Patients may writhe in pain early during the event. Fainting or collapsing is common early. There may be a period of temporary easing of symptoms before significant peritonitis occurs, often with vomiting, continued pain, and weakness. Physical examination typically includes findings of muscular rigidity of the abdomen, probably upper abdominal tenderness, and later distention. In this setting, pain with percussion of the epigastrium is highly suggestive of perforated peptic ulcer. Because there is gastric acid throughout the abdomen, tenderness may be noted on pelvic or rectal examination. An upright radiograph or CT scan often reveals air under the diaphragm. For unclear diagnoses, a water-soluble contrast study is likely to reveal the perforation.

Intestinal Obstruction and Strangulated Hernias

Intestinal obstruction is one of the most common causes of acute abdominal pain in the elderly. In strangulated hernia, the intestine is obstructed within a hernia. Both conditions can lead to localized ischemic, necrotic bowel. Thus, there is overlap with the presentation of ischemic bowel, but intestinal obstruction tends to present with more acute pain that is often crampy and is more often accompanied by vomiting. Intestinal obstruction in the elderly is often due to adhesions, hernias, or cancer. Higher obstruction, in the small bowel, tends to be associated with earlier vomiting and less abdominal distention; lower obstruction, in the distal small bowel or colon, causes later vomiting and greater distention. Patients may experience obstipation, but partial obstructions may be accompanied by episodes of watery diarrhea. Physical examination may demonstrate distention, succussion splash, tympany to percussion, generalized tenderness, and rushes of high-pitched or tinkling bowel sounds. Abdominal radiographs may show distended bowel and multiple air-fluid levels. CT scan also shows distended loops and multiple air-fluid levels but can more clearly reveal the source of the obstruction.

Volvulus

Volvulus represents axial rotation of the intestine upon its mesentery. Volvulus of the sigmoid is most common because the mesentery is longest, followed by the cecum, transverse colon, and splenic flexure. Most patients presenting with volvulus are elderly, but constipation and pregnancy (cecal volvulus) may also predispose to this entity. The patient demonstrates rapid abdominal distention accompanied by reports of severe, continuous acute abdominal pain and episodes of colicky pain. The dilated loop of colon may be palpable on examination. A plain-film radiograph demonstrates the dilated colonic segment, running transversely in the case of a sigmoid volvulus with the dilated loop bent upon itself ("bent inner tube effect") and with air-fluid levels in each side of the loop. An additional radiographic finding that has been described is the "northern exposure sign." This finding is described as the appearance of the dilated sigmoid colon cephalad to the transverse colon on supine abdominal films.[26] Closed loop obstruction quickly produces ischemic bowel. Delay in diagnosis increases the mortality rate, and for this reason patients should be referred for immediate attempts at endoscopic decompression or barium enema reduction (cecal volvulus).[27]

Diverticulitis

Diverticulosis is a common condition in the population over the age of 50, but it may be seen in younger patients. The classical presentation of diverticulitis, however, is an older patient who reports left lower quadrant pain and tenderness; diverticulitis may occur at any location in the colon. A WBC count should be obtained. Because elderly, debilitated patients frequently present with fecal impaction and localized tenderness, a flat plate of the abdomen may be helpful in distinguishing patients with a high impaction not palpable on rectal examination.

Care should be taken not to render a diagnosis of diverticulitis in the absence of fever, leukocytosis, or localized findings of inflammation on examination. Patients with mild diverticulitis (low-grade fever, mild leukocytosis, and mild to moderate tenderness) may be managed as outpatients with a liquid diet and broad-spectrum antibiotics (such as a quinolone). Work-up in these patients should be delayed until the resolution of clinical symptoms and may generally consist of colonoscopy or air-contrast barium enema and flexible sigmoidoscopy.

ABDOMINAL PAIN

Patients who should be admitted include those manifesting fever greater than 38°C, marked tenderness, localizing signs of peritoneal inflammation, signs of obstruction, suspected abscess, or an immunocompromised state, and elderly, debilitated patients. CT scan should be obtained emergently; in cases where CT is unavailable or the diagnosis is unclear, contrast enema with water-soluble contrast or barium may be helpful.

Spontaneous Bacterial Peritonitis

Spontaneous bacterial peritonitis (SBP) is seen in approximately 10% of patients with chronic ascites from liver disease, usually when the patient has reached a decompensated state with hypoalbuminemia, jaundice, and prolonged prothrombin time. The patient may present with sudden onset of fever, chills, generalized abdominal pain with rebound tenderness, or hypoactive/absent bowel sounds. Alternatively, the patient may not manifest impressive abdominal findings and may display more generalized systemic findings on encephalopathy. Patients suspected of this diagnosis should undergo paracentesis and should be hospitalized until a diagnosis is established or eliminated.

Ischemic Bowel

Conditions causing intestinal ischemia fall into several major categories, including (1) acute mesenteric ischemia, resulting from arterial embolic or thrombobotic disease, thrombotic venous disorders, low flow states, or other severe systemic illness and (2) colon ischemia. Acute mesenteric ischemia remains a diagnosis with a high associated mortality (as high as 70%); only early surgery can lower the mortality rate. In addition, persistent vasoconstriction, by itself or in conjunction with arterial occlusion, may contribute to ischemia.[28] Because the causes of mesenteric ischemia are manifold, the clinician must consider the possibility of this diagnosis and attempt correction of any contributing factors, such as a low flow state, in addition to procuring rapid involvement of a surgical consultant.

Patients with mesenteric ischemia typically present with pain that is disproportionate to physical findings. No single laboratory test or diagnostic procedure is consistently reliable. A history of other serious medical illness or a personal or familial history of a hypercoagulable state should be obtained. If examination reveals peritoneal findings, immediate surgical intervention is required. If no peritoneal findings are noted, spiral CT may be obtained to pursue a diagnosis of mesenteric thrombosis. Abdominal angiography may also be helpful in diagnosing mesenteric arterial embolus or thrombotic occlusion. Pneumatosis intestinalis (gas in the bowel wall) and portal venous gas, noted on CT or plain film, are suggestive of mesenteric infarction.[29]

Colon ischemia is the most common kind of bowel ischemia; it presents in a variable manner with pain, tenderness, diarrhea, and lower GI bleeding. Colon ischemia may be associated with hypercoagulable states[30] or serious illnesses, resulting in shock; it may occur postoperatively following aortic surgery or in association with colon cancer, cocaine use, sickle cell disease, and oral contraceptives. Usually, diagnosis is made by colonoscopy or barium enema. Patients with peritoneal signs require immediate surgical management.

Pediatric Patients with Abdominal Pain

A thorough discussion of the acute abdomen in infants and toddlers is beyond the scope of this chapter. Congenital abnormalities, such as congenital obstruction of the small bowel, malrotation of the midgut, or annular pancreas, are more common in infancy. Pyloric stenosis occurs in young infants but does not usually present as an abdominal emergency. Intussusception is more common among slightly older infants and toddlers. A small amount of rectal bleeding should particularly increase suspicion for intussusception, and there is frequently a palpable sausage-like mass in the abdomen. By elementary school age, appendicitis becomes a common cause of abdominal emergencies.

Initial Management

Once the patient has been identified as having an acute abdomen (i.e., one probably requiring surgery), he or she should be stabilized and transferred to an emergency department or directly into a hospital where surgical consultation may be obtained immediately. Occasionally, a patient can be sent to a surgeon's office directly, such as when appendicitis is suspected but unclear. All unstable patients should be stabilized with intravenous line insertion and fluid administration, then transported by ambulance. Complex and elderly patients, in particular, should be transported with medical summaries, including a list of known medical problems, allergies, and findings at the primary physician's office.

Clinicians should consider the appropriateness of administration of pain medication to patients with acute abdominal findings, especially if the patient is in severe pain and delay in definitive care is likely. Administration of pain medication has not been found to normalize findings (such as tenderness) of the acute abdomen.[31–33] Patients should not receive medication of sufficient dosage to cloud the sensorium or alter the ability of the patient to interact with the surgeon or anesthesiologist.

ABDOMINAL
PAIN

Summary

Diagnosis of the acute abdomen is largely based on history and physical findings, as well as a clear knowledge of the patient's risk profile for specific illnesses. Every effort should be made to distinguish surgical and nonsurgical causes of abdominal pain, with additional testing used to confirm or eliminate unclear diagnoses. Patients with unstable conditions and those who demonstrate findings of an acute abdomen should be evaluated as quickly as possible, with expeditious referral for definitive treatment. Patients at either end of the age spectrum often present the greatest diagnostic challenge, with patients in the over-50 age range sustaining a much higher percentage of serious illnesses and poor outcomes if care is delayed.

References

1. Adelman A: Abdominal pain in the primary care setting. J Fam Pract 25:27–32, 1987.
2. Adelman A, Metcalf L: Abdominal pain in a university family practice setting. J Fam Pract 16:1107–1111, 1983.
3. Klinkman MS: Episodes of care for abdominal pain in a primary care practice. Arch Fam Med 5:279–285, 1996.
4. de Dombal FT: Acute abdominal pain in the elderly. J Clin Gastroenterol 19:331–335, 1994.
5. Adams ID, Chan M, Clifford PC, et al: Computer-aided diagnosis of abdominal pain: A multi-centre study. BMJ 293:800–804, 1986.
6. Chui DW, Owen RL: AIDS and the gut. J Gastroenterol Hepatol 9:291–303, 1994.
7. Parker JS, Vukov LF, Wollan PC: Abdominal pain in the elderly: Use of temperature and laboratory testing to screen for surgical disease. Fam Med 28:193–197, 1996.
8. Silver BE, Patterson JW, Kulick M, et al: Effect of CBC results on ED management of women with lower abdominal pain. Am J Emerg Med 13:304–306, 1995.
9. Young GP: CBC or not CBC? That is the question. Ann Emerg Med 15:367–371, 1986.
10. Andersson RE, Hugander AP, Ghazi SH, et al: Why does the clinical diagnosis fail in suspected appendicitis? Eur J Surg 166:796–802, 2000.
11. Graff L, Russell J, Seashore J, et al: False-negative and false-positive errors in abdominal pain evaluation: Failure to diagnose acute appendicitis and unnecessary surgery. Acad Emerg Med 7:1244–1255, 2000.
12. Rothrock SG, Green SM, Dobson M, et al: Misdiagnosis of appendicitis in nonpregnant women of childbearing age. J Emerg Med 13:1–8, 1995.
13. Balthazar EJ, Rofsky NM, Zucker R: Appendicitis: The impact of computed tomography imaging on negative appendectomy and perforation rates. Am J Gastroenterol 93:768–771, 1998.
14. Walker S, Haun W, Clark J, et al: The value of limited computed tomography with rectal contrast in the diagnosis of acute appendicitis. Am J Surg 180:450–454, 2000.
15. Dilley A, Wesson D, Munden M, et al: The impact of ultrasound examination on the management of children with suspected appendicitis: A three year analysis. J Pediatr Surg 36:303–308, 2001.
16. Huang CB, Yu HR, Hung GC, et al: Clinical features and outcome of appendicitis in children younger than three years of age. Chang Gung Med J 24:27–33, 2001.
17. Argenta PA, Yeagley TJ, Ott G, Sondheomer SJ: Torsion of the uterine adnexa. Pathologic correlations and current management trends. J Reprod Med 45:831–836, 2000.
18. Tepper R, Zalel Y, Goldberger S, et al: Diagnostic value of transvaginal color Doppler flow in ovarian torsion. Eur J Obstet Gynecol Reprod Biol 68:115–118, 1996.
19. Eschenbach DA, Buchanan TM, Pollock HM, et al: Polymicrobial etiology of acute pelvic inflammatory disease. N Engl J Med 293:166–171, 1975.

20. Parker CA, Topinka MA: The incidence of positive cultures in women suspected of having PID/salpingitis. Acad Emerg Med 7:1170, 2000.
21. Marks C, Tideman RL, Estcourt CS, et al: Diagnosing PID—getting the balance right. Int J STD AIDS 11:545–547, 2000.
22. Heinonen PK, Miettenen A: Laparoscopic study on the microbiology and severity of acute pelvic inflammatory disease. Eur J Obstet Gynecol Reprod Biol 57:85–89, 1994.
23. Rutledge D, Jones D, Rege R: Consequences of delay in surgical treatment of biliary disease. Am J Surg 180:466–469, 2000.
24. Mulagha E, Fromm H: Acute cholecystitis. Curr Treat Opt Gastroenterol 2:144–146, 1999.
25. Pounder R: Silent peptic ulceration: Deadly silence or golden silence? Gastroenterology 96:626–631, 1989.
26. Javors BR, Baker SR, Miller JA: The northern exposure sign: A newly described finding in sigmoid volvulus. Am J Roentgenol 173:571–574, 1999.
27. Grossman EM, Longo WE, Stratton MD, et al: Sigmoid volvulus in the Department of Veterans Affairs Medical Center. Dis Colon Rect 43:414–418, 2000.
28. American Gastroenterological Association Medical Position Statement: Guidelines on Intestinal Ischemia. Gastroenterology 118:951–953, 2000.
29. Ohtsubo K, Okai T, Yamaguchi Y, et al: Pneumatosis intestinalis and hepatic portal venous gas caused by mesenteric ischemia in an aged person. J Gastroenterol 36:338–340, 2001.
30. Koutroubakis IE, Sfiridaki A, Theodorpoulou A, Kouroumalis EA: Role of acquired and hereditary thrombotic factors in colon ischemia of ambulatory patients. Gastroenterology 121:561–565, 2001.
31. Lovecchio F, Oster N, Sturman K, et al: The use of analgesics in patients with acute abdominal pain. J Emerg Med 115:775–779, 1997.
32. Mahadevan M, Graff L: Prospective randomized study of analgesic use for ED patients with right lower quadrant pain. Am J Emerg Med 18:753–756, 2000.
33. Lee JS, Stiell IG, Wells GA, et al: Adverse outcomes and opioid analgesic administration in acute abdominal pain. Acad Emerg Med 7:980–987, 2000.

ABDOMINAL PAIN

Chapter 12
Gastrointestinal Bleeding

David E. Nicklin

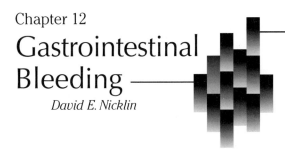

Gastrointestinal (GI) bleeding is a common problem. It is estimated that 125 in 100,000 adults in the United States are affected annually,[1] resulting in 200,000 hospital admissions, as well as total health care costs exceeding $1 billion dollars. GI bleeding may present with chronic low-grade blood loss. Although these patients may have significant anemia, they are hemodynamically stable and are not actively bleeding. With the exception of profound anemia (hemoglobin < 6.0) in patients with comorbidity (such as active coronary artery disease or advanced age), these patients can be safely evaluated in an outpatient setting over days to weeks. Their care does not represent an office emergency and therefore will not be discussed here. This chapter focuses on evaluation and management of patients presenting with moderate to severe active GI bleeding representing an acute, potentially life-threatening emergency.

Office equipment necessary for the evaluation and management of patients presenting with suspected GI bleeding is outlined in Box 12–1.

Box 12–1. *Equipment Required for Evaluation and Treatment of Gastrointestinal Bleeding*

- Guaiac testing slides and developer
- IV catheters (14, 16, 18, 20, and 22 gauge)
- IV solution (normal saline 0.9%, or lactated Ringer's)
- Anoscopes
- Nasogastric tubes (8, 10, and 12 French)
- Normal saline irrigation fluid (iced tap water may also be used)
- Large syringes (60 mL) and large metal basin for lavage

131

CLINICAL RECOGNITION ◄————————

Vital signs, as always, are an essential starting point. Although there is significant variability, postural hypotension alone (a drop in systolic pressure of more than 20 mm Hg, with an increase in heart rate of over 20 beats/min when going from supine to erect) suggests a 20% volume loss; clammy skin, hypotension, and tachycardia while supine suggest 30% to 40% volume loss.[2] If these signs are present, the clinician must start emergency resuscitation, which supersedes all other considerations and is discussed in the section, "Initial Management," later in the chapter.

For patients who are not hypotensive, it is important for the physician to determine how actively they are bleeding. Patients reporting repeated vomiting of "coffee grounds" or of frank blood, or multiple maroon/bloody stools, are likely to have an active, dangerous bleed. Determining the amount of blood in the emesis is useful. Many patients state that they are "vomiting blood," but upon questioning, they reveal that they actually had only a few flecks of blood, or blood streaking of the vomitus. Also, patients (who are understandably frightened) often report a "toilet bowl full of blood." Such statements should be acknowledged but not counted heavily in decision making because as little as 5 mL of blood mixed in the toilet water gives this appearance. Performance of a rectal examination to observe the quality of the stool directly and to confirm the presence of melena or hematochezia is important. Similarly, direct observation of nasogastric aspirate is necessary for confirmation of reported hematemesis. Patients with normal vital signs, who have small amounts of blood in vomitus or stool, may be evaluated by either endoscopy or contrast radiologic studies over the following week.

Upper vs Lower. GI bleeding is classically divided into upper and lower (proximal or distal to the ligament of Treitz, at the duodenal-jejunal junction). This distinction is important and useful because evaluation of risk and rational management differ for upper GI (UGI) versus lower GI (LGI) bleeding. Common causes of UGI and LGI bleeding are given in Box 12-2. The nature of the bleeding often reveals the source. UGI bleeding typically presents with bloody vomitus (either red or black, so-called "coffee grounds") or the passage of melanotic (black, foul-smelling) stool. Melanotic stool is the result of bacterial breakdown of hemoglobin; unlike clotted blood, it does not turn toilet water red.[3] LGI bleeding typically presents with hematochezia, dark red or maroon blood per rectum, often with clots. Blood on the toilet paper or dripping into the toilet water after a bowel movement suggests LGI bleeding from a perianal source. Blood coating a normal stool suggests bleeding in the anal canal. Blood mixed in the stool suggests a source in the descending colon. Maroon stools are generally seen with small-bowel and proximal colon bleeding. Bloody diarrhea suggests inflammatory bowel disease or infectious colitis. At times, however, these clues may be misleading. Up to 20% of patients with a UGI bleed have hematochezia due to active bleeding and rapid transit time.[3] On occasion, a slow bleed in the proximal colon presents as melena, when bacteria in the colon have adequate time to degrade the hemoglobin (Box 12–2).

Box 12–2. *Common Causes of Gastrointestinal Bleeding in Adults*

Upper gastrointestinal bleeding
- Peptic ulcer (gastric or duodenal)
- Gastritis
- Variceal bleeding
- Mallory-Weiss tear
- Neoplasm

Lower gastrointestinal bleeding
   Small intestine (6%)
- Crohn's disease
- Angiodysplasia
- Neoplasm (rare)
- Meckel's diverticulum

   Colon (94%)
- Diverticulosis
- Inflammatory bowel disease
- Ischemia
- Colitis (infectious or radiation)
- Neoplasm
- Anal bleeding (hemorrhoids and anal fissures)
- Arteriovenous malformations

A history of previous GI bleeding should be sought because recurrent bleeding is often from the same site. A history of liver disease or longstanding alcohol abuse suggests possible variceal bleeding. Use of aspirin, nonsteroidal anti-inflammatory drugs (NSAIDs), and alcohol is associated with UGI bleeding caused by peptic ulcers and gastritis. Forceful vomiting of nonbloody emesis, followed by vomiting of blood, is suggestive of a distal esophageal tear (i.e., Mallory-Weiss tear). LGI bleeding most commonly occurs from a vascular source (e.g., angiodysplasia, diverticuli, or hemorrhoids) and is generally painless but may be massive. Some patients have a known history of diverticulosis. Arteriovenous (AV) malformations of the colon are seen more frequently in patients with chronic renal failure and cirrhosis. Their association with aortic stenosis (Heyde's syndrome) has been challenged and is controversial.[4] A history of ulcerative colitis suggests LGI bleeding, although Crohn's disease may be associated with either upper or lower GI bleeding. Previous radiation therapy is associated with radiation colitis, which leads to blood mixed with the stool.

Physical examination provides additional evidence of an upper or lower source of bleeding. Stigmata of liver disease should be sought (e.g., jaundice, increased liver span, cherry hemangiomas, ascites). Tenderness on abdominal examination may suggest peptic ulcer disease, inflammatory bowel disease (IBD), or colitis with localized tenderness in the area of inflammation. Telangiectasias may be seen in Osler-Weber-Rendu syndrome. A rectal examination with anoscopy is essential to check for fissures, hemorrhoids, rectal masses, and any active site of bleeding. Appearance of the stool (black, maroon, or red blood) is important. Stool guaiac testing should be performed to confirm bleeding. Insertion of a nasogastric (NG) tube is required in patients with signs of active bleeding after the physical examination. Bloody (red or dark, guaiac-positive) NG aspirate confirms a UGI bleed. However, up to 16% of patients with a UGI bleed may have negative gastric lavage.[5] Other important findings on physical examination include pale skin and conjunctiva, which suggests subacute or chronic blood loss.

 PHONE TRIAGE ◄———————————————————

During phone triage, determination of the amount of bleeding is important. When a patient reports that he or she is "vomiting blood," he or she must be asked if it is a few flecks of blood, blood streaking of the vomitus, or frank blood with clots. When a patient reports passing a "toilet bowl full of blood," he or she must be asked about the appearance of the stool. If the stool is brown, coated with blood, with blood in the toilet water, it is unlikely that bleeding is severe. When a patient reports dark stools, it is very useful for him or her to bring a stool sample to the office. This is particularly true when a parent reports dark stool (or bloody urine) in an infant in diapers. A variety of foods and medications can result in dark stools. Frequent causes include beets, bismuth-containing compounds (Pepto Bismol), and iron supplements. Guaiac testing of the suspect stool quickly distinguishes these nonmedical causes of dark stools from true GI bleeding.

The passage of bright red blood per rectum is a common complaint, and in younger patients, this is often due to hemorrhoids or anal fissure.

Reassuring history includes young age (younger than 40 years old); a history of hard stools or straining at stool; pain with stooling; recurrent episodes over a period of years; red blood coating the stools, in the toilet water, or on the toilet tissue with wiping; and an absence of systemic signs such as orthostatic dizziness. If these low-risk features are present, the patient may be safely evaluated in the office within several days.

Any patient reporting vomiting blood or coffee ground–appearing material requires immediate evaluation. Patients reporting large quantities of blood and clots per rectum or melanotic stools also should be seen at once. If the patient reports syncope or orthostatic dizziness in combination with active GI bleeding, it may be prudent to send him or her directly to the emergency department.

 ## LABORATORY RECOGNITION ◄———————————

Anemia on laboratory testing is the presenting finding in some patients. This is generally due to chronic slow GI blood loss. It may be systematically evaluated over a period of days to weeks, except when the anemia is severe (hemoglobin below 6 mg/dL) in older patients with comorbidity. In-office hemoglobin and hematocrit testing has a limited role in the evaluation of acute GI bleeding. Unless they are bleeding massively, patients who have suffered significant GI blood loss over a short period (hours) present with signs of volume depletion but with normal or near-normal hemoglobin. Significant anemia in a patient with acute bleeding implies additional chronic blood loss and increases the risk associated with acute bleeding.

Initial Management

In patients presenting with active GI bleeding, the first concern is adequate resuscitation. An algorithm for initial management is shown in Fig. 12–1. After assessment of adequate airway and breathing, circulation should be evaluated. If there is significant hypotension (systolic blood pressure below 100, or a significant decrease from patient's usual blood pressure) with tachycardia (resting pulse over 100), it is critical to begin stabilization of the patient while arranging for transfer and further evaluation. While office staff call for ambulance transport to the hospital, two large-bore (14-gauge, if possible) peripheral intravenous lines should be placed, and 0.9% normal saline or lactated Ringer's solution infused with lines wide open (over 1000 mL/hr). In general, central venous access is not required because longer catheter length results in slower infusion rates. A brief

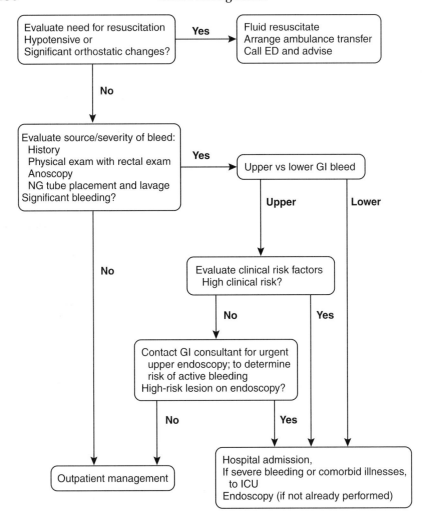

Figure 12–1. Flow chart for management of GI bleeding. (ED, emergency department; GI, gastrointestinal; ICU, intensive care unit; NG, nasogastric)

history and physical examination, as outlined in the "Clinical Recognition" section earlier often distinguishes upper from lower GI bleeding. An NG tube should be inserted, and aspirate tested for blood. The emergency department (ED) receiving the patient should be informed of the patient's presentation and expected time of arrival. In severe cases, the preparation of universal donor (O negative) blood for transfusion on arrival in the ED may be lifesaving. Because emergency endoscopy is required after stabilization, the gastroenterology department should also be informed of the patient's imminent arrival.

In patients who do not require fluid resuscitation and immediate transfer to the ED (vital signs normal, no significant orthostatic changes), the history and physical discussed in "Clinical Recognition" earlier will allow a presumptive diagnosis of either upper or lower bleeding in almost all patients. Decisions regarding management of these two distinct entities are discussed in the following sections.

Upper GI Bleeding. In the past, all patients presenting with active UGI bleeding (grossly bloody NG aspirate or multiple melanotic stools) required hospital admission. With the advent of emergency endoscopy, a significant number of carefully selected patients may be safely treated as outpatients. Because immediate endoscopy has become central to evaluation and management of UGI bleeding, *a physician who can perform endoscopy should become involved in treatment as soon as possible.* Early endoscopy allows evaluation of risk in stable patients, and endoscopic treatment of varices or ulcers in those with continued bleeding. To optimize care, primary physicians should discuss with their consulting endoscopist *in advance* how these urgent referrals can best be handled.

Evaluation of a stable patient in the primary care office includes a complete medical history and physical examination to determine severity and stability of coexisting diseases. In a continuity primary care setting, much of this history will be known to the physician and included in the ambulatory record. A rectal examination, anoscopy, and insertion of an NG tube, along with inspection of the NG aspirate, are required. Observational studies of patients with UGI bleeding have shown remarkable consistency in risk factors for rebleeding and poor outcome.[6-12] Retrospective and prospective studies in more than 3500 patients with active UGI bleeding showed that patients who meet low-risk criteria (Box 12–3) may be safely discharged and treated as outpatients (3% risk of rebleeding requiring admission; one mortality—.03%).[13-15] However, endoscopy is required before discharge so that the bleeding site can be visualized and high-risk findings (e.g., arterial bleeding, ulcer with adherent clot or visible vessel, varices, and portal hypertensive gastropathy) excluded. Although otherwise included as part of a low-risk group, up to 10% of those patients have active rebleeding.[16] Patients not meeting low-risk selection criteria require hospital admission, with intensive care unit (ICU) admission for those with active ongoing bleeding, persistent hypotension, decompensated liver disease, or severe comorbid disease. Admission to the gastroenterology unit may result in shorter hospital stays and should be considered.[17-19] The development of clinical protocols incorporating this approach has recently been shown to reduce admissions and shorten hospital stays.[20]

Lower GI Bleeding. When hemorrhoids and anal fissures are the cause of continuing lower GI bleeding, a complete physical, including rectal examination and anoscopy, will identify a bleeding site and enable the clinician to make the diagnosis. Although patients can have significant

GI BLEEDING

> **Box 12–3. *Guidelines for Selecting Patients for Outpatient Management of Upper Gastrointestinal Bleed***
>
> Absolute: No high-risk endoscopic features, varices, or portal
> hypertensive gastropathy
> Relative: No debilitation
> No orthostatic vital sign change
> No severe liver disease
> No serious concomitant disease (active CHF, COPD,
> coronary disease, etc.)
> No anticoagulation therapy or coagulopathy
> No fresh voluminous hematemesis or multiple episodes
> of melena on the day of evaluation
> No severe anemia (hemoglobin <8.0 g/dL)
> Adequate support at home
>
> Adapted from Longstreth GF, Feiltelberg SP. Outpatient care of selected patients with acute non-variceal upper gastrointestinal haemorrhage. Lancet 345:109, 1995. CHF, congestive heart failure; COPD, chronic obstructive pulmonary disease.

bleeding from hemorrhoids, this is not generally life-threatening because the bleeding is rarely massive and is immediately evident. Therefore, these patients can be safely managed as outpatients with stool softeners, oral iron if anemic, and elective surgical treatment. In patients with active, more proximal LGI bleeding, angiodysplasia and diverticular bleeding account for approximately 85% of cases in which a bleeding site can be identified.[21] Because these problems are largely restricted to older patients, the average age of patients with LGI bleeding is 65 years.

The clinical evaluation of likely cause and stability proceeds as discussed in the section on UGI bleeding; a complete medical history and physical examination are performed to determine the severity and stability of coexisting diseases commonly seen in this elderly population. A rectal examination and anoscopy are required, as is NG tube placement with lavage to exclude hematochezia due to brisk UGI bleeding. Again, early visualization of the bleeding site by colonoscopy is important for diagnosis and prognosis and may allow therapeutic coagulation of bleeding angiodysplasia.[22] Colonoscopy may be impractical in patients with very active bleeding; selective angiography of mesenteric arteries may localize the bleeding site and enable the initiation of therapy with infusion of vasoconstrictors or embolization. Arrangements for urgent consultation with gastroenterology and radiology specialists should be made in advance, and these consultants should be notified early in the evaluation of the patient. A surgeon should also be made aware of the patient's condition because persistent bleeding may require emergent partial colectomy.

GI BLEEDING

Because few patients are potentially eligible, large studies have not been performed of outpatient management of LGI bleeding. Most patients are actively bleeding the day they present, and most are elderly with coexisting morbidities—both of which are contraindications to outpatient care. Further, although bleeding does stop spontaneously in 80% of patients, rebleeding occurs in roughly 25% of these[21]; therefore, they are at higher risk than patients discussed earlier who have peptic ulcers without high-risk features. Patients with active ongoing bleeding, persistent hypotension, or severe comorbid disease are admitted to the ICU; other patients may be admitted to floor beds.

Management of patients with active GI bleeding is summarized in Box 12–4.

Box 12–4. *Summary of Management Steps in Patients Presenting with Active Gastrointestinal Bleeding*

1. Evaluate need for resuscitation. If hypotensive or significant orthostatic changes, provide rapid fluid resuscitation, arrange ambulance transfer to ED, call ED staff to make them aware
2. Evaluation of upper vs lower source of bleed: history and physical, including rectal and anoscopy. Nasogastric tube placement and lavage (all patients with significant bleeding). May do this while awaiting transfer in patients with hypovolemia
3. Contact gastroenterologist and plan emergency EGD (upper bleed) or colonoscopy (lower bleed) for all patients (hypovolemic or not)
4. Patients with upper gastrointestinal bleeding, and clinically at low risk are candidates for outpatient management if EGD shows low risk of recurrent bleeding. Send to endoscopy for evaluation, if feasible
5. Patients with clinical risk factors require admission, as well as urgent endoscopy. Admit to hospital with endoscopy as soon as possible
6. Patients with active ongoing bleeding, persistent hypotension, or severe/decompensated comorbid disease are admitted to intensive care unit, others to floor bed

---

Complications

Potential complications include perforation of peptic ulcer, as well as hepatic encephalopathy in cirrhotic patients with GI bleeding. Peritoneal signs on abdominal examination are atypical and require careful evaluation. Patients with suspected liver disease should be checked for asterixis. Also, the risk of aspiration is significant in patients with massive upper GI bleeding, or those with altered mental status due to hepatic encephalopathy or intoxication with drugs or alcohol. Early placement of an endotracheal tube should be seriously considered in patients at risk.

Pediatrics

In general, evaluation of GI bleeding in children is similar to that in adults, with assessment of severity of bleeding and evaluation of upper versus lower GI sources. However, a different group of causes must be considered. Causes of GI bleeding in children are presented in Box 12–5. Malrotation with midgut volvulus is a potentially catastrophic event and should be considered in newborns with vomiting and bloody stool. Intussusception, most common before the age of 2 years, may also cause bloody stool and vomiting. Esophagitis due to reflux and esophageal bleeding from ingested foreign body may on rare occasions cause upper GI bleeding in infants and toddlers. Ulcer disease is increasingly diagnosed, particularly in adolescents, and may cause bleeding. Those with severe liver disease are at risk for esophageal varices or portal hypertensive gastropathy. Meckel's diverticulum (ectopic gastric mucosa) may cause significant bleeding and may be diagnosed with radionuclide scanning. Children can develop anal fissures, particularly after hard stool and straining. These patients generally present with small amounts of red blood per rectum, with fissures that can be seen on physical examination. Treatment includes reassurance and addition of fiber to the diet.

Box 12–5. *Causes of Gastrointestinal Bleeding in Children*

Upper
- Esophagitis (due to reflux)
- Esophageal foreign body (ingestion)
- Esophageal varices
- Portal hypertensive gastropathy
- Peptic ulcer disease

Lower
- Malrotation with midgut volvulus (newborn period)
- Meckel's diverticulum
- Duplication cysts (causing intussusception)
- Intussusception (more common before age 2)
- Ulcerative colitis and Crohn's disease
- Polyposis syndromes
- Anorectal fissures

References

1. Longstreth GF: Epidemiology of hospitalization for acute upper gastrointestinal hemorrhage; a population-based study. Am J Gastroenterol 90:206–210, 1995.
2. Koziol-McLain J, Lowenstien SR, Fuller B: Orthostatic vital signs in the emergency department. Ann Emerg Med 20:606–610, 1991.
3. DeMarkles MP, Murphy JR: Acute lower gastrointestinal bleeding. Med Clin North Am 77:1085–1100, 1993.
4. Mehta PM, Heinsimer JA, Bryg RJ, et al: Reassessment of the association between gastrointestinal arteriovenous malformations and aortic stenosis. Am J Med 86:275–277, 1989.
5. Lichtenstein DR, Berman MD, Wolfe MM: Approach to the patient with acute upper gastrointestinal hemorrhage. In Taylor MB, Gollan JL, Peppercorn MA, et al (eds): Gastrointestinal Emergencies. Baltimore, Williams & Wilkins, 1992, p 92.
6. Katschinski B, Logan R, Davies J, et al: Prognostic factors in upper gastrointestinal bleeding. Dig Dis Sci 39:706–712, 1994.
7. Zimmerman J, Siguencia J, Tsvang E, et al: Predictors of mortality in patients admitted to hospital for acute upper gastrointestinal hemorrhage. Scand J Gastroenterol 30:327–331, 1995.
8. DeDombal FR, Clarke JR, Clamp SE, et al: Prognostic factors in upper GI bleeding. Endoscopy Suppl 2:6–10, 1986.
9. Rockall TA, Logan RF, Devlin HB, et al: Risk assessment after acute upper gastrointestinal haemorrhage. Gut 38:316–321, 1996.
10. Bordley DR, Mushlin AI, Dolan JG, et al: Early clinical signs identify low-risk patients with acute upper gastrointestinal hemorrhage. JAMA 253:282–285, 1985.
11. Terdiman JP, Ostroff JW: Risk of persistent or recurrent and intractable upper gastrointestinal bleeding in the era of therapeutic endoscopy. Am J Gastroenterol 92:1805–1811, 1997.
12. Silverstein FE, Gilbert DA, Tedesco FJ, et al: The national ASGE survey on upper gastrointestinal bleeding. II. Clinical prognostic factors. Gastrointest Endosc 27:80–93, 1981.
13. Longstreth GF, Feiltelberg SP: Outpatient care of selected patients with acute non-variceal upper gastrointestinal haemorrhage. Lancet 345:108–111, 1995.
14. Rockall TA, Logan FR, Devlin HB, et al: Selection of patients for early discharge or outpatient care after acute upper gastrointestinal haemorrhage. Lancet 347:1138–1140, 1996.
15. Garripoli A, Mondardini A, Turco D, et al: Hospitalization for peptic ulcer bleeding: Evaluation of a risk scoring system in clinical practice. Dig Liver Dis 32:577–582, 2000.
16. Terdiman JP: Update on upper gastrointestinal bleeding. Postgrad Med 103:43–64, 1998.
17. Quirk DM, Barry MJ, Aserkoff B, et al: Physician specialty and variation in the cost of treating patients with acute upper gastrointestinal bleeding. Gastroenterology 113:1443–1448, 1997.
18. Cooper GS, Chak A, Connors AF Jr, et al: The effectiveness of early endoscopy for upper gastrointestinal hemorrhage: A community-based analysis. Med Care 36:462–474, 1998.
19. Nowak A, Belsaguy AF, Yu Z, et al: Upper GI bleeding. Gastrointest Endosc 50:730–733, 1999.
20. Podila PV, Ben-Menachem T, Batra SK, et al: Managing patients with acute, nonvariceal gastrointestinal hemorrhage: Development and effectiveness of a clinical care pathway. Am J Gastroenterol 96:208–219, 2001.
21. Vernava AM, Moore BA, Longo WE, et al: Lower gastrointestinal bleeding. Dis Colon Rect 40:846–858, 1997.
22. Lee JG: Urgent colonoscopy for the diagnosis and treatment of severe diverticular hemorrhage. Gastrointest Endosc 53:261–263, 2001.

Chapter 13
Orthopedic
Urgencies

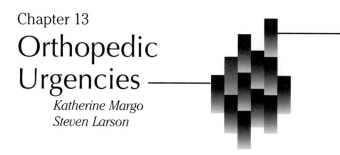

Katherine Margo
Steven Larson

Most orthopedic emergencies are associated with trauma involving a fall or blow. In addition, infection or rheumatologic conditions can present as emergencies with significant pain and swelling in an extremity. Differentiating between these can usually be accomplished after a complete history is obtained.

Fractures

CLINICAL RECOGNITION

Trauma that involves a significant fall or blow to the body puts a patient at risk for a fracture. A simple or closed fracture refers to a fracture with intact skin; an open or "compound" fracture has a break in the skin over the fracture. Comminuted fractures have multiple fragments.

PHONE TRIAGE

The mechanism of the injury should be elicited so that the possibility of significant injury can be assessed. Older patients are at greater risk for fracture, even with relatively minor trauma. After significant trauma, the likelihood of a fracture is increased if a patient is unable to move part of the body or is unable to walk, or if there is a lot of swelling with ecchymoses. The patient should be seen in the office as soon as possible. The patient should be sent immediately to the emergency department if an x-ray facility is not conveniently available, if the patient cannot walk, or if there is an open wound.

If a patient calls and has just been injured and you do not feel immediate emergency room care is warranted, the injured area should be immobilized and ice applied; then, the patient should be brought to the office as soon as possible. If there is intractable severe pain, the patient should come into the office immediately or go to an emergency department.

Signs and Symptoms

In patients with significant fracture, swelling, ecchymosis, and exquisite tenderness with palpation are noted, especially when the involved part is moved. There may also be obvious deformity. This is not always true in more subtle fractures of smaller bones such as those in the wrist or ankle. In addition, because it takes less force to fracture a bone in a geriatric patient, there may be less concomitant soft tissue swelling. Hip and pelvic fractures, which are more common in the geriatric patient, may present only with severe pain on movement. If there is an open wound, a compound fracture must be suspected. All patients with fractures must undergo an evaluation for associated injuries such as damage to nerves, blood vessels, ligaments, tendons, or skin.

Differential diagnoses for suspected fracture include:
1. Sprain, partial or complete tear of ligament
2. Severe contusion
3. Dislocation
4. Cellulitis or septic joint

Initial Management

Initially, the area of possible fracture should be immobilized. If the office physician has the appropriate casting and splinting supplies, many fractures can be treated and followed on site. This can be done with a splinting device or a well-padded plaster splint. An elastic bandage alone should not be used because it does not adequately immobilize the area, and it may compress the already compromised venous and lymphatic systems. The area should be iced and elevated. If the pelvis or hip is involved, the patient should be transported to an emergency department on a board. An open wound near the site of injury introduces the possibility of a compound fracture. This is a more serious injury that will need to be treated as soon as possible by an orthopedic surgeon. All patients should be evaluated for neurovascular compromise that may complicate the fracture. If there is significant malalignment of the involved part with associated neurovascular compromise, gentle traction in the long axis of the limb can be attempted before splinting, although not if there is protruding bone. X-ray facilities should be readily available for full assessment of these injuries.

Shoulder. Most minimally displaced humeral fractures are treated with simple immobilization in a sling. In a fractured humerus with separation of fragments exceeding 1 cm, or angulation greater than 45 degrees, the patient usually needs surgery. The function of the radial nerve needs to be evaluated because it may be injured along the humeral shaft. This evaluation can be done with testing of resisted extension of the wrist. Radial nerve injuries usually recover spontaneously unless they occur after manipulation. Midhumeral fractures are frequently associated with radial nerve and brachial artery injuries, and patients should be referred immediately to an emergency department for evaluation by an orthopedic surgeon.

Elbow. Most elbow fractures are treated with splinting, but if there is significant displacement or a supracondylar fracture of the humerus with comminution, surgery may be indicated.

Forearm. Most forearm fractures are treated with casting unless there is significant malalignment. This can be done easily in the office if the appropriate supplies are available. If both the radius and the ulna are fractured, surgery may be necessary to enable adequate healing and to prevent angulation of the fracture site.

Wrist. Occult fractures are common in wrist trauma, especially in the scaphoid bone. Radiographs may initially be negative; therefore, a patient with tenderness over the scaphoid and pain with radial deviation should be put into a thumb spica splint or cast for 2 weeks before reevaluation occurs. If a fracture is confirmed, the patient should be referred because of the high rate of complications.

Hand. Most finger fractures can be splinted in the office. If a tuft fracture is associated with a subungual hematoma, it should be considered an open fracture and be treated with antibiotics. All flexor tendon avulsion fractures and extensor tendon avulsions greater than 25% of the articular surface should be referred. They should be splinted while orthopedic evaluation is awaited.

Pelvis. Significant trauma often causes this fracture. Because of this, the patient must always be seen in the emergency department to be evaluated for internal bleeding and disruption of the urologic structures. A complete blood count (CBC) and urinalysis (UA) are important for this evaluation. Early radiographs are done to assess the stability of the pelvic ring. If it is fractured in two planes and creates an unstable situation, the patient will need to be admitted. Prolonged recovery will ensue. Adequate pain control and early mobilization are used.

Hip. Early mobilization of the patient after the injury is critical for these fractures, which occur most often in the geriatric population. To enable this, early surgery is usually performed. These patients always need to be evaluated immediately in the emergency department.

A knee radiographic series is only required for knee injury patients with any of these findings:

1. Age 55 years or older
   or
2. Isolated tenderness of patella*
   or
3. Tenderness at head of fibula
   or
4. Inability to flex to 90 degrees
   or
5. Inability to bear weight both immediately and in the emergency department (4 steps) **

* No bone tenderness of knee other than patella.
** Unable to transfer weight twice onto each lower limb regardless of limping.

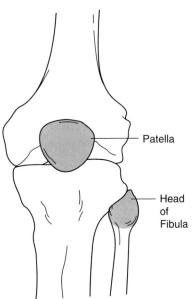

Figure 13–1. Ottawa Knee Rule for use of radiography in acute knee injuries. From JAMA 278:2075–2079, 1997.

Femur. These fractures require more intensive treatment and must be treated by an orthopedic surgeon in the emergency department from the beginning with either traction or surgery.

Knee. The Ottawa Rules for acute knee injuries (Fig. 13–1) say that if any of the following are true, then a radiograph must be obtained: A patient is 55 years old or older, has tenderness at the head of the fibula and isolated tenderness of the patella, is unable to flex to 90 degrees, or has inability to take four steps immediately and in the emergency department.[1] Any displacement of the fracture fragments usually requires surgery. Fracture of the lateral tibial plateau, which is undisplaced, can be treated by a compression dressing and early motion but no weight bearing for 6 to 8 weeks. Displaced fractures of the patella also require surgery, but if nondisplaced, a compression dressing and early mobilization will suffice.

Ankle. Ottawa Rules for the ankle (Fig. 13–2) say that a radiograph is required if there is pain in the malleolar zone with tenderness at the posterior edge of the lateral or medial malleolus, or inability to bear weight both immediately and in the emergency department. Foot radiography is required if there is pain in the midfoot with tenderness at the base of the fifth metatarsal or over the navicular bone, or inability to bear weight both immediately and in the emergency department.[2] Many fractures of the ankle can be simply casted in the office with early mobilization. Bimalleolar fracture and displaced medial malleolar fracture often require surgery.

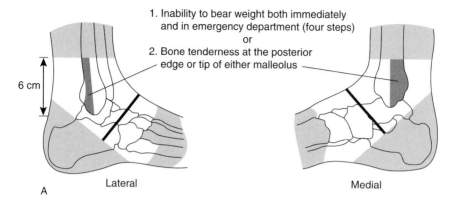

An ankle radiographic series is necessary only if there is pain near the malleoli and any of these findings:

1. Inability to bear weight both immediately and in emergency department (four steps)
or
2. Bone tenderness at the posterior edge or tip of either malleolus

6 cm

A   Lateral   Medial

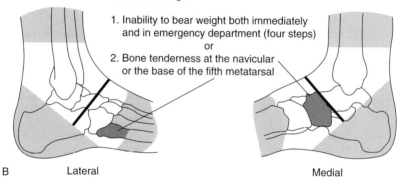

A foot radiographic series is necessary only if there is pain in the midfoot and any of these findings:

1. Inability to bear weight both immediately and in emergency department (four steps)
or
2. Bone tenderness at the navicular or the base of the fifth metatarsal

B   Lateral   Medial

Figure 13–2. A, Refined clinical decision rule for ankle radiographic series in ankle injury patients. B, Refined clinical decision rule for foot radiographic series in ankle injury patients. From JAMA 271:827–832, 1994.

Equipment and Medications

X-ray equipment should be readily available if orthopedic emergencies are to be treated in the office.

Casting and splinting material, either plaster or fiberglass, should be available in several different lengths, 2 to 6 inches in width. Premade splints are available that can be applied to the area with an elastic bandage. Fiberglass supplies must be regularly checked because they are dated and are no longer usable past expiration.

PO and IM pain medications, including narcotics, should be available. Ready-made ice packs can be useful.

Disposition

Patients with intra-articular fractures, both compound and comminuted, should be referred to an orthopedic surgeon immediately because of the risk of long-term problems.

Complications

Volkmann's ischemic contracture, or compartment syndrome, is a feared complication of orthopedic injury that is associated with significant morbidity. Typically occurring in the volar forearm or lower leg, compartment syndrome results when significant trauma increases swelling and pressure in the soft tissue adjacent to bone. As pressure rises, there is a decrease in the perfusion gradient for nutrients, resulting in tissue death. Within 6 hours, vascular compromise results in irreversible tissue injury that particularly affects neurologic and muscular function. The earliest indication of impending compartment syndrome is pain out of proportion to physical findings. Treatment is usually surgical.

Another complication of fractures that is particularly associated with pelvic or femoral injuries is the risk for significant blood loss. Owing to the occult nature of blood loss, patients who sustain such injury may not demonstrate immediate signs of impending vascular compromise. The physician must maintain a heightened awareness of the risks associated with these injuries.

Amputation. Patients with complete or near-complete amputations occasionally appear in a physician's office. The body part should be wrapped in saline-soaked gauze, placed in a plastic bag, and immediately transported on ice to the hospital with the patient.

Pediatrics

Fractures in children are usually less complicated and often do not require surgical intervention. Mild angular deformities usually correct with growth. The closer the fracture is to the end of the bone, and the younger the patient, the greater the amount of angulation that is acceptable. Rotational malalignment persists, however. Fractures that transverse the growth plate vertically can disturb growth and result in angular deformities. These fractures often require surgery. All children who have fractures should be evaluated for the possibility of physical abuse.

Dislocations

A dislocation of an extremity can occur either in traumatic situations, or with significant muscular effort, especially in a patient with past dislocations.

CLINICAL RECOGNITION ◄──────────────────

Patients often recognize their injury as an extremity dislocation. They feel it actually dislocating and can see the deformity. They are usually unable to move it after the dislocation has occurred.

PHONE TRIAGE ◄──────────────────

The patient who has an injury such as a fall, complains of pain, and feels as though something is "out of place" should be told to come into the office immediately, unless there is someone on site with the patient who has experience in assessing and treating dislocations.

Signs and Symptoms

Obvious deformity of the area is usually evident. The patient exhibits reluctance to move the extremity, and there is significant pain in the area. Radiographs should be done to rule out a concomitant fracture.

Initial Management

Shoulder. Fifty percent of all dislocations involve the shoulder. These are usually caused by a fall on an externally rotated, abducted arm. The initial diagnosis of anterior dislocation, the more common type, is usually not difficult. The acromion is usually much more prominent on that side, and the humeral head is not in its usual place. This needs to be reduced as soon as possible, both for pain relief and for protection of the neurovascular structures. Reduction can be achieved by placement of gentle, in-line traction on the arm. If this does not work, Stimson's maneuver can be tried; the patient is placed in a prone position with the affected arm hanging over the side of the table. A 10- to 15-pound weight is tied to the wrist for traction. If this is ineffective, the relocation may need to be performed with the patient under general anesthesia. The shoulder must be immobilized to prevent external rotation for 4 weeks after the initial injury so that recurrences can be avoided. Early referral for physical therapy is essential to avoid a "frozen shoulder."

Elbow. This is usually caused by a fall on the outstretched hand with an extended elbow; 50% of these injuries occur during sports activities. Usually, an obvious deformity results that must be distinguished from a supracondylar fracture. Reduction should be performed as soon as possible. This is accomplished by gentle, steady traction on the wrist with countertraction on the shoulder. The procedure may need to be done with the patient under general anesthesia if the elbow has been dislocated for many hours. The elbow may need to be extended. After reduction, the elbow is immobilized in a splint at 90 degrees for 3 weeks; then, range of motion exercises are performed.

Hip. This usually occurs after severe trauma wherein the knee is struck when the hip and knee are in the flexed position. The hip is usually pushed posteriorly. Early reduction in the emergency department is critical to prevent avascular necrosis. This is accomplished by placing traction on the flexed hip with countertraction on the pelvis. The patient often must be under general anesthesia, is usually admitted for reduction, and does not bear weight for 2 to 3 months.

Equipment

Slings or wraps are needed for upper extremity dislocations.

Pediatrics

Dislocations in children tend to be more easily repositioned. The common nursemaid's elbow can be easily reduced in the office, and congenital hip dislocations require orthopedic referral.

Acute Tendon and Ligament Injuries

Most tendon injuries result from repetitive microinjury. However, particularly on the sports field or in job settings where significant physical effort occurs, an acute injury can occur.

 CLINICAL RECOGNITION ◄————————————

A tendon rupture is suspected when the patient has had an injury after which there is loss of function of a particular motion. A ligament rupture is suspected when a significant injury occurs after which the joint is unstable. In both cases, usually swelling and pain and occasionally ecchymosis are noted at the site. Rapid swelling implies bleeding into a joint, which occurs in large-structure injuries.

PHONE TRIAGE ←

If a patient is unable to move the leg or arm after an injury, particularly if a "pop" is heard, then a tendon or ligament rupture is suspected. The patient should be told to apply ice, immobilize the affected part, and come to the office immediately.

Signs and Symptoms

Swelling, pain, and hypermobility of the joint are noted on examination, as well as reluctance to move the extremity. Alhough ecchymosis is not as common as in fracture situations, in a severe tendon or ligament injury it may occur.

Differential Diagnoses

Differential diagnoses include fracture, acute bursitis, and cellulitis.

Initial Management

Ice and immobilization should be used initially.

Tendon Injuries of the Hand. These often occur with lacerations. A careful functional examination of the whole hand should be performed for all lacerations to evaluate for these injuries. Immediate splinting in extensor tendon injuries may be enough, but flexor tendon injury requires early surgery.

Ligament Injuries to the Knee. This is the most frequent acute injury to the knee and commonly occurs with sports injuries. The mechanism can involve a blow, but the injury may be caused by a twisting, cutting movement. Most common injuries involve the anterior cruciate ligament (ACL), the medial meniscus, and the medial collateral ligament (MCL). In the case of acute trauma with a very swollen knee, it is often difficult to examine and differentiate between the injuries. If rapid swelling occurred, a hemarthrosis is suspected, usually due to an ACL injury. If the joint can be moved but valgus strain is very uncomfortable, an MCL injury is suspected.

Severe Ankle Sprain. Most sprains are easily cared for in the office setting with ice, elevation, and early motion. Complete rupture of the lateral ligaments, injury to the syndesmosis, or concomitant fracture makes more likely the development of long-term complications of an unstable ankle or chronic pain. These injuries should be referred.

Ruptured Achilles Tendon. This injury generally occurs in heavy men who engage in vigorous activity but are not regular athletes. The patient generally hears a "pop" and feels as though something hit from behind. The patient is unable to continue the activity. Many of these injuries require surgery, although there are proponents of nonoperative methods of treatment.

Disposition

Many less disabling tendon and ligament injuries can be managed by the office physician by means of splinting, home care, and physical therapy to treat any continued disability. Complete ligament or tendon rupture requires orthopedic evaluation and timely intervention, which often are delivered in the emergency room setting.

Pediatrics

Children are less likely to experience ligament and tendon injuries because their bones are relatively weak. They are more likely to have a fracture when significant injury occurs.

Swollen Painful Joint Without Obvious Trauma

A swollen joint without trauma may be an orthopedic, rheumatologic, or infectious problem. The differential diagnosis is critical, and testing should be done in an expeditious manner both for comfort of the patient and to prevent devastating consequences, such as those that occur in the case of a septic joint.

 CLINICAL RECOGNITION ←—————————

A patient usually comes into the office complaining of a swollen joint, although he or she still may be able to use the joint. A history of fever, other joint swelling now or in the past, weight loss, and rash should be obtained. The differential diagnoses are listed in Box 13–1.

> **Box 13–1.** *Differential Diagnosis of Swollen Painful Joint Without Obvious Trauma*
>
> Septic joint
> Gout
> Rheumatoid arthritis or other collagen vascular disease associated
>   with arthritis
> Degenerative arthritis
> Cyst such as Baker's cyst of the knee
> Bursitis

 PHONE TRIAGE ◄——————————————

> The patient should be asked how long swelling has been noted and whether pain has been associated with the swelling, or if fever or other joint swelling has occurred. The patient should be seen the same day he or she calls, although not necessarily immediately, unless there is extreme pain or a fever.

Initial Management

If there is any question of trauma, a radiograph should be obtained. If no trauma has occurred, then it usually will not help in management of the injury. Aspiration should be considered in any joint in which there is unexplained swelling, although it may be difficult to perform in small joints such as toes or fingers. It must be determined whether this is a septic joint because the consequences of inadequate early treatment can be severe. Fever, heat, and erythema of the joint with significant limitation of movement greatly increase the likelihood of this diagnosis. If the fluid is cloudy once it has been aspirated, antibiotics should be given pending the results of the analysis.

Equipment and Medications

A large-bore needle with a 10- to 20-mL syringe is adequate for large-joint aspirations. Smaller needles and syringes may suffice for a smaller joint. The laboratory should be called to check which tubes are needed for cell count, culture, crystals, and any other desired test.

Disposition and Transfer

Most swollen knees can be managed by the physician in the office setting. However, it is impossible to determine whether cloudy synovial fluid is the result of infection or crystal disease unless microscopic evaluation is performed to assess for the presence of crystals. Regardless of the patient's history, if aspiration of a hot, acutely swollen joint fails to yield crystals on microscopic examination, the diagnosis of a septic joint must be of primary concern; the patient must be referred for treatment with IV antibiotics.

Pediatrics

Crystal arthropathies are less common in children, but juvenile arthritides must be considered.

References

1. Stiell IG, Greenberg GH, Wells GA, et al: Prospective validation of a decision rule for the use of radiography in acute knee injuries. JAMA 275:611–615, 1996.
2. Stiell IG, McKnight RD, Greenberg GH, et al: Implementation of the Ottawa ankle rules. JAMA 271:827–832, 1994.
3. Wilson FC, Lin PP: General Orthopaedics. New York, McGraw-Hill, 1997.
4. Snider RK (ed): Essentials of Musculoskeletal Care. Rosemont, Ill, American Academy of Orthopaedic Surgeons, 1997.

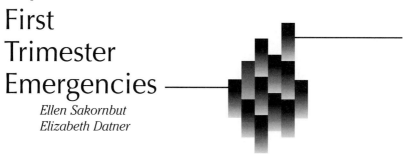
Chapter 14
First Trimester Emergencies

Ellen Sakornbut
Elizabeth Datner

Concerns about early pregnancy commonly cause women to present for urgent medical care. Between 25% and 40% of pregnant women experience bleeding during the first trimester, and about 20% of all pregnancies end in miscarriage. Ectopic pregnancy (EP) occurs at a rate of 1% to 2% of all pregnancies in the United States and remains one of the major reasons for maternal mortality and the leading cause of death in the first trimester.[1] The first trimester of pregnancy is often symptomatic in normal intrauterine pregnancies and a time of increased anxiety. This makes it more likely that women will present whenever they experience symptoms that they perceive to be abnormal.

 PHONE TRIAGE

The nursing and/or front office staff of any physician's office or emergency room must be aware of key complaints associated with pregnancy and with young women who may be pregnant. Patients experiencing pain or bleeding during pregnancy should be evaluated within 24 hours, or more rapidly depending on the severity or progression of symptoms. Often, patients are unsure if they are pregnant, and historical information solicited over the phone may be confusing. Patients presenting without previous confirmation of pregnancy should have a urine pregnancy test (urinary chorionic gonadotropin [UCG]) performed first. Patients with a positive UCG and abdominal pain or vaginal bleeding should be evaluated as urgent or emergent. In addition, the patient with excessive or continued vomiting warrants evaluation within 24 hours. Nursing personnel should be prepared to instruct patients over the phone regarding simple measures to relieve nausea and vomiting.

155

Terminology

Spontaneous abortion (or miscarriage)—passage of products of conception, accompanied by bleeding and, generally, cramping pain before 20 weeks gestation.

Threatened abortion—uterine bleeding before 20 weeks gestational age without dilation of the cervical os or passage of products of conception.

Incomplete abortion—passage of some but not all of the products of conception.

Inevitable abortion—usually embryonic or fetal demise has occurred and the cervical os is open, but tissue has not been passed.

Septic abortion—retained products of conception are present along with signs of infection (tenderness, fever); this may occur with or without instrumentation.

Blighted ovum—implies embryonic demise with fetal resorption and is clearly diagnosable if the gestational sac is 25 mm with no identifiable fetal pole.

Embryonic demise—identified fetal pole without cardiac activity in a fetus measuring 5 to 8 mm as identified by transvaginal ultrasound, or failure to identify cardiac activity in an 8-week-size fetus on transabdominal scanning.

Missed abortion—failure of spontaneous passage of products of conception despite embryonic demise having occurred 4 weeks previously.

Miscarriage

Cause

Examination of the products of conception from first trimester miscarriages reveals genetic abnormalities in a majority of instances. Other identified factors include environmental influences, such as tobacco and other substance exposure, viral and other intrauterine infections, and, occasionally, hormonal problems (luteal phase deficiency). Miscarriages occurring early in the second trimester are more often related to infection, structural abnormalities of the uterus or fetus, or exposures such as crack cocaine.

Evaluation of the Patient with Suspected Miscarriage

History

Embryonic demise often occurs well before the onset of bleeding and/or cramping. The patient may have experienced early symptoms of pregnancy and subsequent cessation of these symptoms. Historical information about menstrual bleeding is important, along with reports of any recently used method of contraception or cessation of hormonal methods of contraception within 90 days before conception. Estimation of gestational age may be less reliable in patients with recent hormonal contraception. Symptoms of recent infection, information on medication usage and other exposures, long-term medical history, previous obstetric and gynecologic history, and review of symptoms such as pain, syncope or near-syncope, bleeding, discharge, or passage of clots or tissue should all be elicited. A history of previous pregnancy failure or poor outcome is helpful because these patients may need extensive long-term follow-up. A history of induced abortion is also relevant, as is information on any instrumentation of the uterus (current or previous); a history of pelvic inflammatory disease, tubal ligation, or infertility treatment; use of an intrauterine device; or treatment for cervical dysplasia (e.g., cryosurgery, cold knife conization, or loop electrosurgical excision of the transition zone). Patients also should be screened for domestic violence.

 ## CLINICAL RECOGNITION ◄

The patient's vital signs, including any tachycardia, hypotension, or orthostatic symptoms, should be recorded. Uterine size may not correlate with gestational age as calculated from the date of the last menstrual period. Fetal heart tones generally can be heard on Doppler at between 10 and 12 weeks, although obesity or a retroverted uterus may make it more difficult for such heart tones to be audible. Gentle elevation of the uterus with one hand in the vagina and the other holding the Doppler directed through the abdominal wall toward the fundus may enable the examining physician to hear heart tones in this instance, or even as early as 9 weeks in a thin patient.

A pelvic examination is necessary for the determination of uterine size and other features characteristic of the pregnancy. Uterine size assessment on bimanual examination may be made more difficult by a retroverted uterus or obesity. Other abnormalities such as fibroids may make the examination inaccurate for the purpose of establishing dates. A uterus that is 4 to 6 weeks in size will not be noticeably larger than a uterus in the nonpregnant state and will not have demonstrated any cervical or lower uterine segment changes. The 6- to 8-week-size uterus is more globular (like an orange), and the cervix and lower uterine segment become softer. By 8 weeks, the cervix has attained a bluish cast that is visible on speculum examination (Chadwick's sign). At 8 to 10 weeks, the uterus is the size of a grapefruit. Bimanual examination during these first weeks may also reveal an enlarged ovary, which can be palpated separately from the uterus. This may represent the corpus luteum cyst of pregnancy.

When the patient complains of bleeding, the presence and quantity of blood in the vaginal vault, bleeding from the cervical os, and friability of the cervical mucosa should be noted. The cervical os should be identified as closed or open. If the external os appears to be open and abortion is inevitable, digital examination of the internal os should be performed. Patients with previous vaginal deliveries may demonstrate mild dilatation of the external os, but the internal os should be closed in normal early pregnancy. A wet preparation and chlamydia and gonorrhea cultures should be obtained during speculum examination and before bimanual examination. Any tissue recovered in the vault should be sent to the pathology department. A "float test" that suspends chorionic tissue in saline demonstrates fronds of villous structures identifiable without microscopy.

Although the patient who is miscarrying often will experience cramping pain, she usually is not very tender on examination. The presence of tenderness and pain in the adnexa must make the examining physician suspicious of an EP. Conversely, the absence of tenderness does not exclude EP. A very tender uterus may result from a septic abortion, with or without a history of instrumentation. Another possible consideration with instrumentation is uterine perforation. Any of these is a potentially dangerous diagnosis, and every effort must be made to differentiate the patient with a common (albeit a possibly distressing) diagnosis from the patient with a life-threatening diagnosis.

 ## LABORATORY RECOGNITION ◄

Laboratory tests that are helpful at this time include a UCG (if one has not already been performed), a hematocrit in the presence of significant bleeding by examination or history, and maternal blood type and Rh testing. The UCG is positive at 50 IU, so a serum quantitative level of human chorionic gonadotropin (hCG) is not necessary in every instance. Serum quantitative hCG is addressed later in the chapter in relation to the patient with a suspected EP. Serum progesterone levels are addressed as well in this later section. Urinalysis should be performed to evaluate for urinary tract infection.

Ultrasound Examination
Patients needing **immediate** ultrasound confirmation of their pregnancy diagnosis include the following: the patient with a tender adnexal mass or

adnexal pain or tenderness without palpable mass; the patient with substantial bleeding in whom operative intervention is being considered; and the patient with findings that indicate instability (e.g., peritoneal signs, unstable vital signs, history of syncope). The patient with unstable vital signs and evidence of shock must be considered as a surgical emergency. Fluid resuscitation should be started while an operatively capable physician is contacted. If diagnostic ultrasound is not immediately available, the emergent consultation should not be delayed for this study. Culdocentesis, along with management of the EP, is discussed later in this chapter.

Patients who present with even small amounts of vaginal spotting in early pregnancy may be concerned. Although the patient whose examination is stable and consistent with menstrual dates need not be scanned immediately, an ultrasound examination performed in an expeditious fashion may provide reassurance or a more immediate disposition. Patients who are stable and pain-free but who present with a nontender adnexal mass warrant ultrasound examination within a few days. Patients with size-date discrepancy and/or vaginal bleeding at less than 20 weeks gestation should also be scanned within a few days or evaluated on a more urgent basis with development or worsening of symptoms.

Ultrasound examination of the first trimester patient is best performed with a combination of transabdominal and transvaginal scanning because some ultrasound findings are better demonstrated on one part of the examination than on another. Although a full bladder facilitates good transabdominal images in the early part of pregnancy, it is not necessary and may displace the uterus when transvaginal scanning is attempted. After the transabdominal part of the examination, the patient should void to empty the bladder. A patient who is suspected of having an acute abdomen must be evaluated rapidly and should be maintained on nothing by mouth (NPO) status. If bladder filling is necessary, this can be accomplished by insertion of an indwelling catheter and instillation of sterile water or saline.

Ultrasound findings that are compatible with a normal pregnancy include the presence of an intrauterine gestational sac, an embryo in the uterus, intrauterine fetal cardiac activity, and a yolk sac in an intrauterine gestational sac. A normal gestational sac is oval or round with a bright echogenic ring, usually located in the fundus. See Figures 14–1 and 14–2 for ultrasound images of early intrauterine pregnancy. Table 14–1 presents further correlation of ultrasound findings with gestational age. If no gestational sac is seen, intrauterine pregnancy is not confirmed. The patient may have an early intrauterine pregnancy, a spontaneous completed miscarriage, or an EP. A quantitative hCG and close follow-up are warranted; see the section on EP later in this chapter.

Clearly abnormal ultrasound findings include a large, sometimes misshapen or irregular gestational sac without an embryo present (blighted

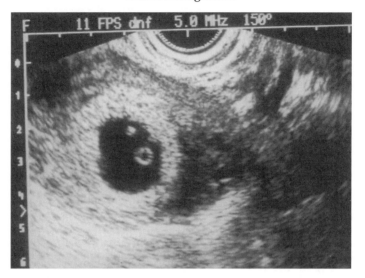

Figure 14–1. Early intrauterine gestational sac (chorionic sac) with small fetal pole and yolk sac.

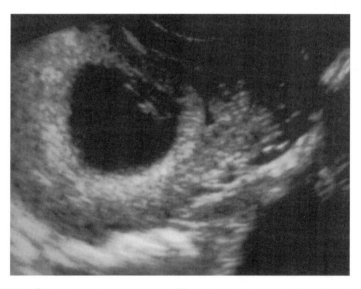

Figure 14–2. First trimester pregnancy: The intrauterine gestational sac is round, with an echogenic "rind," and a live embryo is present.

ovum or embryonic resorption), a gestational sac with irregular echogenic material, an embryo measuring larger than 8 mm without cardiac activity (by transvaginal scan), or irregular echo patterns compatible with retained products of conception. Figure 14–3 demonstrates an abnormal gestational sac with no embryo present. Transabdominal ultrasound that

Table 14–1. Appearance of Structures on Ultrasound According to Gestational Age

Structure	Transvaginal Ultrasound	Transabdominal Ultrasound
Chorionic sac (gestational sac)	35–40 days menstrual age	42 days menstrual age
Yolk sac	42 days	—
Fetal pole	42–45 days	6–7 wk, variable, always by 8 wk, or sac 25 mm
Cardiac activity	7 wk (often earlier)	8 wk

From Ectopic pregnancy—United States. MMWR 44:46–48, 1995.

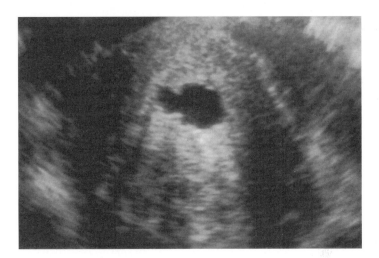

Figure 14–3. An abnormal intrauterine sac is present. The gestational sac is misshapen, and no embryo is present.

demonstrates a gestational sac of 25 mm without an embryo is clearly abnormal. A subchorionic hemorrhage may be seen as a crescent-shaped echolucent area adjacent to the gestational sac. The miscarriage rate with this finding is about 30%.

Specific Diagnoses

1. **Completed spontaneous abortion.** The patient may be able to give a history of passage of tissue or a sac; the uterus will often be small on examination and the cervical os may be closed; bleeding is decreasing. The patient is not particularly tender.
2. **Incomplete or impending spontaneous abortion.** The patient may have passed some tissue or clots and the uterus is still somewhat enlarged. The vaginal examination shows bleeding and/or tissue. The

cervical os is open. No fetal heart tones are heard. The ultrasound demonstrates some intrauterine contents. If no tissue has been passed, this is termed "inevitable" abortion.
3. **Threatened abortion.** The patient has experienced bleeding or pain. The prognosis for continuation of the pregnancy is decreased if she has experienced onset of cramping with the vaginal bleeding. The uterus is enlarged and the os is closed. Fetal heart tones may not be heard, depending on gestational age. Ultrasound examination demonstrates a normal-appearing intrauterine gestational sac or an intrauterine pregnancy with a subchorionic hemorrhage but an apparently viable embryo.
4. **Septic abortion.** The patient has distinct uterine tenderness, possibly accompanied by fever and leukocytosis, and has retained products of conception. These patients generally appear ill.

Management of the Patient with First Trimester Bleeding

The patient who has stable vital signs and no suspicion of EP by history, examination, and ultrasound findings can almost always be managed expectantly. Occasional patients need a suction dilation and extraction or curettage because of heavy bleeding. One study suggests that patients with miscarriage who present with significant intrauterine tissue (gestational sac >10 mm) are more likely to encounter complications of missed abortion, septic abortion, or incomplete abortion, or may require transfusion without uterine curettage.[2] If the patient who presents in such a manner shows postural changes in blood pressure or pulse or is hypotensive or symptomatically orthostatic, she should receive a bolus of crystalloid fluids intravenously while type and crossmatch are processed. The use of blood products must be decided on an individual basis and may be unnecessary after fluid bolus administration. All Rh-negative patients should receive mini–Rh-immune globulin (RhoGAM) (50 µg) within 72 hours for any bleeding episode before 20 weeks gestational age. If mini-RhoGAM is not available, the full-dose version (300 µg) is acceptable. Any tissue passed spontaneously or recovered at curettage should be examined for chorionic villi to substantiate a diagnosis of intrauterine pregnancy.

Septic abortion in spontaneous abortion is accompanied by fatality rates of 0.4 to 0.6 per 100,000. Septic abortion resulting from spontaneous abortion or instrumentation should be managed by admission, tissue cultures, administration of broad-spectrum antibiotics with coverage for anaerobes and gram-negative organisms, and uterine evacuation. Coagulation studies should be monitored because disseminated intravascular coagulation (DIC) is a serious complication.

Miscarriage in the Second Trimester Patient

Late miscarriages (13 to approximately 20 weeks gestational age) are less common than in the first trimester. The patient may present before or after fetal demise has occurred. The uterus may be tender if infection is present or abruption has occurred. Pelvic examination should be performed and cultures obtained for gonorrhea, chlamydia, and group B streptococcus. Examination of the cervix may demonstrate a bulging membrane, cervical dilation, or protruding fetal parts. Ultrasound findings are variable according to the cause of the miscarriage. Management of these patients is complex, and they should be referred to providers with obstetric expertise. If delivery of a second trimester fetus (younger than 20 weeks) is imminent or has occurred, the concerns of the physician and staff should be directed toward the medical stability of the mother and toward the emotional reaction of the patient and her family. Expulsion of the placenta may be delayed or may require surgical curettage. Rh-negative patients should receive full-dose RhoGAM.

Follow-up for Patients with Early Pregnancy Loss

Patients who sustain pregnancy loss at any time may experience significant or complicated grief reactions. They should be followed up for potential emotional and medical issues. These include possible Rh isoimmunization, continued bleeding, infection, contraception, and complications of treatment. Most patients have questions about future pregnancies and require additional discussion about the miscarriage that has occurred. Patients who have experienced repeated pregnancy loss or infertility should have additional consultation if viable pregnancy is a goal.

Evaluation of Suspected Ectopic Pregnancy

Because expectant management is indicated in the majority of women with nonectopic first trimester complications, the crucial question for the clinician becomes, How should emergency diagnostic techniques and consultation be used? Because EP is a serious and commonly encountered condition, it should be considered in any pregnant woman with abdominal or pelvic pain, bleeding, or mass, but some history and/or physical findings make a diagnosis of EP more likely.

History

Historical risk factors include previous EP, infertility, use of an intrauterine device, or tubal ligation; intrauterine exposure to diethylstilbestrol (DES); and previous pelvic inflammatory disease or endometriosis. Physical findings are made more meaningful when correlated with an estimated gestational age. Nonetheless, the date of the last menstrual period can be misleading as a means of dating the gestation owing to the possibility of implantation bleeding in normal pregnancy and the variability of vaginal bleeding in abnormal pregnancy.

 ## CLINICAL RECOGNITION ◄——————————————

A classical history of tubal pregnancy rupture includes symptoms of adnexal pain followed by brief relief of pain, shoulder pain (from peritoneal irritation), and the development of postural instability or fainting. It is fortunate that this presentation is seen less frequently with earlier diagnosis of EP. Usually, vaginal bleeding during EP is not as profuse as that in the patient with miscarriage. The patient may or may not present with pain, but midline cramping should be differentiated from adnexal or lower quadrant pain. Unilateral pain is more likely to represent tubal pregnancy.

The differential diagnosis in patients suspected of ectopic pregnancy includes a normal intrauterine pregnancy, threatened or incomplete abortion, ruptured corpus luteum cyst, acute salpingitis (which may coexist with early pregnancy), torsion of the ovary, acute gastroenterologic conditions such as gastroenteritis, and appendicitis. The clinician should elicit any other pertinent symptoms that may support or eliminate these concerns.

Physical Examination

Tenderness on pelvic examination is usually but not always asymmetrical. A mass may be palpable. The uterus may be slightly enlarged or inconsistent with menstrual dates. Pelvic examination may be normal with a non-enlarged uterus. If peritoneal signs or signs of shock (e.g., hypotension, tachycardia) are present, emergency gynecologic consultation should be obtained simultaneously with the performance of other diagnostic studies.

Diagnostic Testing

The immediate availability of diagnostic testing varies in clinical settings. Physicians in office settings frequently encounter some issues with turnaround time for laboratory tests, and transvaginal ultrasound is not readily available around the clock in a number of settings. Given the variability of resources, an effective and efficient diagnostic process may proceed with different steps. Multiple diagnostic modalities are presented here, along with discussion of their advantages and disadvantages.

Ultrasound Examination

Diagnostic ultrasound provides a definitive, rapid diagnosis in a number of patients presenting with suspected EP. Transvaginal ultrasound is clearly superior to transabdominal ultrasound in the early first trimester owing to its higher resolution and greater capability for detecting findings of pregnancy at an earlier gestational age. Patients with a normal intrauterine pregnancy demonstrated by transvaginal ultrasound may be managed conservatively. Intrauterine pregnancy is best demonstrated by the presence of an echogenic ring surrounding a hypoechoic structure with either a yolk sac and/or a fetal pole demonstrated within the sac (see Figs. 14–1 and 14–2). Care should be taken by the clinician in interpreting a gestational sac because of the phenomenon of a "pseudosac," which is well described in reports of EP. The frequency of coexistence of ectopic and intrauterine pregnancy (heterotopic pregnancy) is about 1 in 10,000, but this diagnosis is seen more frequently among patients treated for infertility. If an intrauterine pregnancy is not identified and there are no other findings suggestive of EP, the patient may be in a very early stage of intrauterine pregnancy. This should be correlated with serum hCG levels.

Transvaginal sonographic findings of EP include an extraovarian round or elongated solid tubal mass or a tubal ring (an extrauterine saclike structure).[3] Free fluid in the cul-de-sac or surrounding other pelvic structures is a nonspecific finding and may represent leakage from a corpus luteum cyst or an EP. The presence of an extrauterine gestational sac with a visible fetal pole (with or without cardiac activity) or a yolk sac in the gestational sac is confirmatory, but occurs less commonly (Fig. 14–4). The size of any mass thought to be an EP should be recorded as useful information for determination of appropriate therapy.

Indeterminate findings on ultrasound include the following: No extrauterine findings of EP are found and no intrauterine fetal pole or yolk sac is identified. Findings include an empty uterus, nonspecific intrauterine fluid, echogenic debris within the endometrial cavity, and an abnormal sac. The likelihood of EP is very low if echogenic debris or a gestational sac is identified within the uterus.[4]

Several studies now demonstrate the effectiveness of physicians in emergency room settings who perform sonographic diagnostic studies for EP.[5, 8] Examiner experience does affect the accuracy of sonographic diagnosis,[6] but negative predictive values in ruling out EP were 100% in a study performed by emergency room physicians in California. This same study found agreement between radiology department interpretation and final diagnosis in 96% of cases.[5]

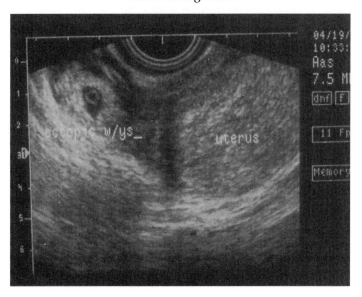

Figure 14–4. An extrauterine gestational sac is present with a yolk sac within the gestational sac.

When ultrasound is not immediately available, the urgency of performing this diagnostic test is increased in patients with unilateral pain and/or a palpable mass and lack of physical findings consistent with developing intrauterine pregnancy. Unstable patients should be evaluated and treated emergently. A more immediate verification of free intraperitoneal blood can be obtained by performance of culdocentesis, accomplished by the aspiration of nonclotting bloody fluid from the posterior fornix (pouch of Douglas) using a spinal needle and aseptic technique. This procedure is rarely performed in recent years but provides ready confirmation of a significant intraperitoneal bleed.

Serum Human Chorionic Gonadotropin Levels

Serum hCG levels rise in a predictable fashion during early pregnancy, with doubling of the hCG every 72 hours or a rise by two thirds every 48 hours until the 10th week of pregnancy. In a patient without ultrasound findings for intrauterine pregnancy, a level lower than 1000 IU/L is most likely an indicator of an early intrauterine pregnancy. Another possible diagnosis is a completed early miscarriage.

Laboratory findings that support the diagnosis of EP include an hCG level greater than 1500 IU/L without transvaginal ultrasound evidence of intrauterine gestation. However, in one recent study, one third of patients with hCG levels higher than 2000 IU/L were later diagnosed with a live, intrauterine pregnancy at follow-up.[7] This suggests that expectant management with close follow-up may be warranted in the stable patient.

Although hCG levels rise in a consistent manner during early normal pregnancy, they do not decrease in a predictable manner in patients who miscarry. Rising hCG levels are more likely to be seen in EP than in spontaneous miscarriage. Falling levels are more likely to be seen in miscarriage than in EP, and levels tend to fall faster in patients with miscarriage. These findings are not sufficiently reliable to provide a means of predicting risk.[8] A retrospective 7-year study of emergency department patients presenting with abdominal pain or bleeding in early pregnancy correlated laboratory findings and outcomes in patients with indeterminate ultrasound findings. Overall, patients with increasing hCG levels were at greater risk for EP than those with decreasing hCG levels ($P < .0001$). Patients with an empty uterus on ultrasound were at greater risk than those with intrauterine contents but no demonstration of a normal pregnancy sac ($P < .0001$). The study identified three high-risk groups: Patients with an empty uterus on ultrasound and hCG values increasing by less than 66% in 48 hours (OR, 24.8); patients with an empty uterus and hCG levels that decreased by less than 50% in 48 hours (OR, 3.7); and patients with an empty uterus and hCG levels increasing by up to 66% in 48 hours (OR, 2.6). Those with levels that decreased by more than 50% in 48 hours were at low risk for EP regardless of ultrasound findings.[9]

Progesterone Levels

Serum progesterone levels in healthy intrauterine pregnancy are usually 25 ng/mL or greater. Levels lower than 11 ng/mL in patients without sonographic evidence of intrauterine pregnancy are highly suggestive of abnormal pregnancy—either ectopic or spontaneous abortion.[10] Many hospitals and urgent care facilities do not have access to rapid serum progesterone levels, limiting their current usefulness for urgent diagnosis of EP. However, in suspected or confirmed EP, the progesterone level may be useful in determining the likelihood of successful medical management of EP, either by expectant management or through the use of intramuscular methotrexate. Patients with serum progesterone levels greater than 7 to 10 are likely to need more than one methotrexate injection or may need surgical treatment.[11, 12] In emergency settings where rapid progesterone levels are available, a serum progesterone of less than 22 ng/mL has a negative predictive value of 100%.[13]

Serum Creatine Phosphokinase Levels

Early investigations of creatine phosphokinase (CPK) elevation in EP were based on the theory that CPK levels would rise with invasion of the smooth muscle of the fallopian tube by the trophoblastic tissue.[14] Serum levels of CPK are lower than normal or are normal in pregnancy until patients go into labor. Initial investigations of CPK for diagnosis of EP produced variable results.[15–18] In the emergency room setting, a case control study comparing women presenting with first trimester bleeding and/or abdominal pain and nonectopic pregnancy with those found to have ectopic pregnancy demonstrated serum CPK elevation in patients with ectopic pregnancy compared with non-EP controls.[19] The mean serum CPK was 118 mIU/dL in the EP group, and 64 mIU/dL in the non-EP group. A CPK greater than 70 mIU/dL was 100% sensitive for detection of EP, with a specificity of 61.9%, a positive predictive value of 72.4%, and a negative predictive value of 100%. Because CPK is also elevated in the presence of damage to skeletal muscle, heart, smooth muscle, and brain, this study excluded women with a recent history of chest pain, trauma, myositis, cocaine use, known renal disease, or intramuscular injection.

The use of CPK in the diagnosis of ectopic pregnancy is limited in the office setting by similar factors to those that limit the use of progesterone levels, although presumably CPK levels are available "stat" in most emergency departments. In addition, CPK is not elevated in ectopic pregnancies in locations where the developing trophoblast does not invade muscle (i.e., abdominal pregnancy). The true positive predictive value of the test is determined by the pretest probability of EP. In an urban emergency department population with a 10% prevalence of EP, the positive predictive value of an elevated CPK would be approximately 23%, with a negative predictive value of 100%. Its use, therefore, appears to be much greater in "ruling out" EP and allowing discharge of patients from the emergency department than in making a certain diagnosis of EP.

The evaluation of a patient with suspected EP is summarized in Table 14–2. In circumstances in which ultrasound is not available on an urgent basis, culdocentesis may be warranted for diagnosis of hemoperitoneum. Culdocentesis is more invasive, less sensitive (100% vs 66%), and less specific (100% vs 80%) for identification of hemoperitoneum than is the detection of echogenic fluid by transvaginal ultrasound.[20]

Treatment of Ectopic Pregnancy

Recent trends in management include the medical treatment of unruptured, early EP. This is not possible without early diagnosis. Delayed diagnosis may be associated with tubal rupture, hemoperitoneum, hypovolemic shock, increased use of blood products, and further sequelae, including death. Admission for EP is sometimes necessary for observation of a patient who is not receiving immediate surgical management and for the surgically treated patient.

Medical Therapy

Methotrexate has been used to treat EP with good efficacy, providing that patient selection is appropriate. Methotrexate is an appropriate

Table 14–2. Diagnostic Scheme for Ectopic Pregnancy in Urgent/ Emergency Care

Perform urinary chorionic gonadotropin (UCG) in patients of child-bearing age with vaginal bleeding and/or abdominal pain. In patients with a positive UCG and a closed cervical os—

If ultrasound is readily available:
Perform transvaginal ultrasound.
- If normal intrauterine pregnancy is seen, manage expectantly
- If findings are indeterminate, draw quantitative human chorionic gonadotropin (hCG) and serum progesterone
- If quantitative hCG is greater than 1500 IU/L, consider consulting obstetrician-gynecologist
- If less than 1500, patients should receive follow-up in 48 hours or earlier if pain increases, or if patients are unstable or experience syncope or near-syncope
- Quantitative hCG should rise at least 66% in 48 hours, or should double in 72 hours. If results are available "stat," consider creatine phosphokinase (CPK) level in patients who have no other medical reason for CPK elevation. If <70 IU/dL, manage as described previously. If >70 IU/dL, consult gynecologist in emergency department If ≥70 IU/dL, consult gynecologist.
- If ectopic pregnancy is demonstrated on ulstrasound, measure size of the mass, determine if there are signs of leakage (e.g., moderate fluid in cul-de-sac, signs of instability), and seek immediate consultation for surgical or medical management. If medical management seems feasible, quantitative hCG and serum progesterone should be drawn

If ultrasound is not readily available:
For all patients with signs or symptoms of instability, tender adnexal mass, or peritoneal signs, obtain immediate gynecologic consult/referral. Consider culdocentesis.
For patients who are stable, schedule ultrasound to be done as soon as possible.
Draw quantitative hCG and progesterone level +/– CPK:
- Patients with progesterone level ≥22 are unlikely to have an ectopic pregnancy and can be managed expectantly
- Patients with CPK <70 are unlikely to have an ectopic pregnancy and can be managed expectantly
- Arrange close follow-up for repeat hCG levels and follow-up of ultrasound results so that a definitive diagnosis may be reached

consideration for any stable patient with an unruptured EP. Methotrexate therapy has been associated with success rates between 64% and 91% based on the following criteria: size of gestational sac or mass less than 3.5 cm, hCG levels lower than 5000 to 10,000 mIU/mL, and serum progesterone levels lower than 7 to 10 ng/mL.[21-23] Methotrexate is usually administered in a dosage of 50 mg/m^2. Levels of hCG are followed weekly, with a second dose adminstered if hCG levels do not decrease. Serious but uncommon complications of methotrexate therapy for EP include methotrexate pneumonitis and neutropenia with subsequent infection.

Surgical Treatment

Surgical treatment of EP remains an appropriate method of treatment for patients who are unstable; those documented with leaking or ruptured EP; and patients with a mass or gestational sac measuring greater than 3.5

to 5 cm. Emergency management in these instances relies on speedy involvement of a consulting gynecologist and operating room staff, as well as adequate fluid resuscitation of the patient with crystalloids and, possibly, blood products.

Other Symptoms or Concerns

Medications

Pregnant patients are generally concerned about whether a prescribed medication is safe for use during pregnancy. The physician must be careful not to provide inaccurate information, particularly if it causes greater anxiety on the part of the patient. Brief exposures to many medications are of minor concern, even if the U.S. Food and Drug Administration (FDA) classification is Class C. If a specific concern cannot be confidently addressed, the patient should be referred to her primary care provider or obstetric care provider.

Hyperemesis Gravidarum

Nausea and vomiting occur in healthy pregnancy on a frequent basis. Urgent treatment should be provided for signs or symptoms of dehydration, ketonuria, or uncontrolled vomiting. The vomiting cycle often abates with simple intravenous hydration provided in the outpatient setting, with or without parenteral antiemetics. Although nonpharmacologic management of this problem is preferable, brief courses of most antiemetic medications (e.g., promethazine, prochlorperazine, ondansetron) are safer than are the effects of dehydration and ketosis. Nonpharmacologic measures include small, frequent, bland meals; separation of dry foods from liquids; and avoidance of smells and tastes that stimulate nausea. Brief admission should be considered if outpatient hydration and antiemetic medication fail to reestablish the patient's ability to ingest small amounts of liquid.

Infectious Diseases

Screening and treatment as indicated are appropriate for all sexually transmitted diseases (STDs). Specific treatments are listed in Table 14–3. A special effort should be made to screen for syphilis in all patients seen for suspected STDs because treatment of other STDs may be ineffective for syphilis. If primary syphilis is diagnosed during the first trimester, this poses a much higher risk situation for the embryo and for continuation of the pregnancy. The patient's obstetric care provider should be notified at once.

Table 14–3. Treatment of Sexually Transmitted Diseases in Pregnancy

Infection	Treatment
Chlamydia	Erythromycin—2 g base or 3200 mg ester/day × 7 days, or 1 g base or 1600 mg ester/day × 14 days **OR** azithromycin 1 g in single dose
Gonorrhea cervicitis	250 mg ceftriaxone IM **OR** cefixime 400 mg PO **OR** azithromycin 2 g in single dose
Syphilis	Penicillin G 2.4 million units benzathine IM for primary or secondary; 2.4 million units × 3 doses 1 wk apart for latent
Trichomonas	Metronidazole 500 mg bid × 5 days **OR** vaginal metronidazole gel hs × 7 days. Treat partner.
Herpes genitalis	Acyclovir 400 mg tid starting at 36 weeks.*

* Acyclovir use in pregnancy has not been associated with teratogenesis. Controversy existed over whether it should be used to prevent recurrent herpes outbreaks and whether this would diminish cesarean sections for this indication. For a discussion of several new studies, see Acyclovir suppression to prevent recurrence at delivery after first-episode genital herpes in pregnancy, an open label trial. In Scott LL, Hollier LM, McIntyre D, et al: Infect Dis Obstet Gynecol 9(2):75–86, 2001.

Varicella exposure is an occasional concern in the first trimester. A nonimmune pregnant woman who has been exposed may be given varicella-zoster immune globulin and should be referred on an urgent basis to her obstetric provider. Most women are immunized against rubella, although titers may not reflect immunity. No effective procedure exists for prevention of maternal infection in the rare event of nonimmune exposure.

Trauma

First trimester trauma patients rarely encounter obstetric complications such as uterine rupture owing to the protected position of the uterus within the bony pelvis. Severe pelvic trauma does pose a threat to the gravid first trimester uterus, but treatment should be directed at maternal stabilization and well-being. Diagnostic or therapeutic procedures that would normally be used, such as radiography, diagnostic peritoneal lavage, computed tomography (CT), or surgical procedures, must be planned based on the needs of the mother. An abdominopelvic CT during the period of organogenesis (days 9–60 conceptual age) is the only single radiologic study that provides enough radiation to the fetus to cause concern about untoward effects. Shielding of the abdomen and pelvis greatly reduces absorption of radiation by the fetus. Fetal heart rate monitoring should be initiated if the fetus is at a viable gestational age to detect signs of distress and allow for emergency cesarean if necessary.

Summary

The diagnosis of EP remains the most worrisome and challenging problem seen during the first trimester of pregnancy by physicians working in urgent and emergency care settings. Use of serum hCG levels and transvaginal ultrasound has allowed improved diagnosis and more timely management for many patients. Patients experiencing symptoms of miscarriage require a diagnostic work-up of their status, but may often need nothing more than expectant management. All patients with first trimester bleeding or trauma during pregnancy should be evaluated for the possible use of RhoGAM. General medical and surgical problems can be diagnosed and treated by usual methods, with the exception of some alteration in medication choices and abdominal shielding when possible during indicated radiographic procedures.

References

1. Ectopic pregnancy—United States, 1990–92. MMWR 44:46–48, 1995.
2. Hurd WW, Whitfield RR, Randolph JF, Kercher ML: Expectant management versus elective curettage for the treatment of spontaneous abortion. Fertil Steril 68:601–606, 1997.
3. Atri M, Leduc C, Gillet P, et al: Role of endovaginal sonography in diagnosis and management of ectopic pregnancy. Radiographics 16:755–774, 1996.
4. Dart R, Howard K: Subclassification of indeterminate pelvic ultrasonograms: Stratifying the risk of ectopic pregnancy. Acad Emerg Med 5:313–319, 1998.
5. Durham B, Lane B, Burbridge L, Balasubramanian S: Pelvic ultrasound performed by emergency physicians for the detection of ectopic pregnancy in complicated first-trimester pregnancies. Ann Emerg Med 29:338–347, 1997.
6. Wojak JC, Clayton MJ, Nolan TE: Outcomes of ultrasound diagnosis of ectopic pregnancy. Dependence on observer experience. Invest Radiol 30:115–117, 1995.
7. Mehta TS, Levine D, Beckwith B: Treatment of ectopic pregnancy: Is a human chorionic gonadotropin level of 2,000 mIU/mL a reasonable threshold? Radiology 205:569–573, 1997.
8. Letterie GC, Hibbert M: Serial serum human chorionic gonadotropin (HCG) levels in ectopic pregnancy and first trimester miscarriage. Arch Gynecol Obstet 263:168–169, 2000.
9. Dart RG, Mitterando J, Dart LM: Rate of change of serial beta-human chorionic gonadotropin values as a predictor of ectopic pregnancy in patients with indeterminate transvaginal ultrasound findings. Ann Emerg Med 34:703–710, 1999.
10. Valley VT, Mateer JR, Aiman EJ, et al: Serum progesterone and endovaginal sonography by emergency physicians in the evaluation of ectopic pregnancy. Acad Emerg Med 5:309–313, 1998.
11. Corasan GH, Karacan M, Qasim S, et al: Identification of hormonal parameters for successful systemic single-dose methotrexate therapy in ectopic pregnancy. Hum Reprod 10:2719–2722, 1995.
12. Ransom MX, Garcia AJ, Bohrer M, et al: Serum progesterone as a predictor of methotrexate success in ectopic pregnancy. Obstet Gynecol 83:1033–1037, 1994.
13. Buckley RG, King KJ, Disney JD, et al: Serum progesterone testing to predict ectopic pregnancy in symptomatic first-trimester patients. Ann Emerg Med 36:95–100, 2000.
14. Lavie O, Beller U, Neuman M, et al: Maternal serum creatine kinase: A possible predictor of tubal pregnancy. Am J Obstet Gynecol 169:1149–1150, 1993
15. Spitzer M, Pinto AB, Dasgupta R, Benjamin F: Early diagnosis of ectopic pregnancy: Can we do it accurately using a biochemical profile? J Women's Health Gend Based Med 9:537–544, 2000.
16. Duncan WC, Sweeting VM, Cawood P, Illingworth PJ: Measurement of creatine kinase activity and diagnosis of ectopic pregnancy. Br J Obstet Gynaecol 102:233–237, 1995.
17. Vandermolen DT, Borzelleca JF: Serum creatine kinase does not predict ectopic pregnancy. Fertil Steril 65:916–921, 1996.

18. Lincoln SR, Dockery JR, Long CA, et al: Maternal serum creatine kinase does not predict tubal pregnancy. J Assist Reprod Genet 13:702–704, 1996.
19. Birkhahn RH, Gaeta TJ, Leo PJ, Bobe J: The utility of maternal creatine kinase in the evaluation of ectopic pregnancy. Am J Emerg Med 18:695–697, 2000.
20. Chen PC, Sickler GK, Dubinsky TJ, et al: Sonographic detection of echogenic fluid and correlation with culdocentesis in the evaluation of ectopic pregnancy. Am J Roentgenol 170:1299–1302, 1998.
21. Stika CS, Anderson L, Frederickson MC: Single-dose methotrexate for the treatment of ectopic pregnancy: Northwestern Memorial Hospital three-year experience. Am J Obstet Gynecol 174:1840–1846, 1996.
22. Perdu M, Camus E, Rozenberg E, et al: Limits of ambulatory medical treatment of ectopic pregnancies by intramuscular methotrexate: Prospective study on 54 patients. Contracept Fertil Sex 26:59–65, 1998.
23. Stovall TG: Medical management should be used routinely as primary therapy for ectopic pregnancy. Clin Obstet Gynecol 38:346–352, 1995.

FIRST
TRIMESTER

Chapter 15
Third Trimester Emergencies

James M. Nicholson

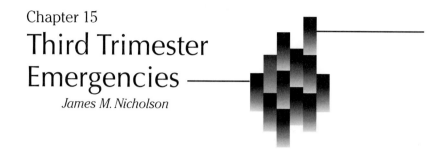

Emergencies that occur during the third trimester of pregnancy represent a unique set of situations in which there are two patients: the mother and the potentially viable fetus. Emergencies can compromise the health and well-being of either or both.

Third Trimester Vaginal Bleeding

Vaginal bleeding during the third trimester of pregnancy is an important symptom, irrespective of the amount of bleeding or the exact gestational age. It complicates about 3% to 4% of all pregnancies, and in half of these cases, the cause is either placental abruption or placenta previa. **Placental abruption** occurs in approximately 1 in 100 to 150 pregnancies and is defined as bleeding that occurs between the placenta and the uterine wall. Gross vaginal bleeding is seen in 80% of cases but is absent in 20% of cases. **Placenta previa** occurs in approximately 1 in 200 pregnancies and is defined as the presence of the placenta completely over, partially over, or very close to the cervical os. Vaginal bleeding from placenta previa can occur at any gestational age but occurs most commonly around 32 to 34 weeks gestation. Both conditions can be life threatening to the mother and the fetus. In the presence of third trimester vaginal bleeding, placental

Table 15–1. Causes of Third Trimester Vaginal Bleeding

	Common	Less Common
Serious:	Placental abruption Placenta previa	Ruptured vase previa Vulvovaginal trauma von Willebrand's disease Leukemia Idiopathic thrombocytopenic purpura
Less serious:	Bloody show Hematuria/UTI	Erosive cervicitis Cervical polyps Hemorrhoidal/GI bleeding

GI, gastrointestinal UTI, urinary tract infection.

abruption and placenta previa should always be ruled out *before other causes are considered.* Table 15–1 lists the common causes of third trimester vaginal bleeding.

CLINICAL RECOGNITION ◄─────────────

Placental abruption is associated with increasing age and parity, with cocaine and cigarette abuse, and with chronic or pregnancy-induced hypertension. It may also be associated with recent abdominal trauma, especially high-velocity accidents. Vaginal bleeding due to placental abruption does not usually start before 20 weeks gestation and is usually associated with lower abdominal or back pain, uterine tenderness, and uterine contractions. It may precipitate preterm labor and delivery, fetal compromise, and maternal coagulopathy. Placenta previa is associated with increasing age and parity, multiple gestations, tobacco abuse, and previous placenta previa. Women with previous cesarean sections and a history of uterine surgery and uterine anomalies are also at greater risk for this disorder. Vaginal bleeding due to placenta previa is usually painless, tends to be intermittent, and typically occurs between 30 and 36 weeks gestation. Unless heavy vaginal bleeding, hemodynamic instability, or fetal distress is present, time should be taken to use two important hospital-based diagnostic tools: pelvic ultrasound and tocodynamometry (uterine contraction monitoring). Ultrasound correctly diagnoses placenta previa in most cases. However, the diagnosis of placental abruption cannot usually be made with ultrasound because pooled retroplacental blood has the same density as placental tissue. Therefore, placental abruption is usually identified through the observation of significant abdominal or back pain, uterine tenderness, vaginal bleeding, and uterine contractions.

Lack of placenta previa on ultrasound and absence of uterine contractions and abdominal pain signal the need to look for other causes of vaginal bleeding (see Table 15–1). A sterile speculum examination (after previa has been ruled out with an ultrasound) can determine the presence of vaginal trauma, cervical polyps, or cervicitis. Vaginal bleeding that begins immediately after rupture of membranes suggests the possibility of ruptured vasa praevia, defined as the presence of fetal blood vessels within the amniotic membranes; rupture of these vessels usually causes severe fetal distress and the risk of exsanguination. Occasionally, patients can mistake bleeding from the urinary or gastrointestinal tract as vaginal bleeding. Hemorrhagic cystitis, bleeding internal hemorrhoids, and rectal fissures are examples of this. Rarely, third trimester vaginal bleeding can be related to a blood dyscrasia such as idiopathic thrombocytopenic purpura (ITP), leukemia, or other coagulopathy.

 PHONE TRIAGE ◀

With the exception of the mild "bloody show" of cervical ripening, any amount of vaginal bleeding in a pregnant patient who is farther than 20 weeks gestation mandates evaluation and treatment in a hospital setting. Basic history should be obtained by phone, including quantity and pattern of bleeding. Have there been any problems with this pregnancy, and has an ultrasound been done? Placenta previa can resolve over the course of a pregnancy, but it almost never develops after the end of the first trimester. Has there been any previous bleeding, recent sexual activity, or abdominal or vaginal trauma? Are there currently symptoms of abdominal or back pain, uterine contractions, decreased or absent fetal movements, or dizziness with standing? Ambulance transfer is usually indicated for anything other than minimal bleeding.

Physical Examination

A patient with active third trimester vaginal bleeding should be approached in a systematic way. Even a gentle digital cervical examination in a patient with placenta previa can precipitate catastrophic hemorrhage. Even a modest delay in diagnosing an active placental abruption can result in serious maternal complications and fetal loss. If the patient is in an outpatient setting, maternal vital signs should be assessed immediately. Systolic blood pressure lower than 95 and/or pulse greater than 120 may suggest possible hypovolemia and impending maternal shock. Heavy bleeding indicates the need for the placement of a large-bore IV tube and rapid volume expansion. The uterus should be displaced at least 15 degrees off the inferior vena cava by a wedge of some kind placed under the right or left pelvis. The health of the mother is always the highest priority, and the best way to support the fetus is to care for the health of the mother.

If maternal vital signs are acceptable, the fetal heart tones (FHTs) should be checked. FHTs greater than 170 or lower than 110 are cause for alarm, and fetal monitoring should be continued along with maternal IV placement, O_2 by mask, and appropriate consultations related to the possible need for emergency delivery by cesarean section. If the FHTs are 120 to 160, a physical examination of the mother *without vaginal examination* should be performed and abnormalities treated appropriately. Excessive uterine tenderness or regular and strong uterine contractions signal possible abruption and the need for emergent referral to a hospital setting. If the maternal examination is benign, an urgent ultrasound should be obtained to rule out placenta previa. If the cause of mild or intermittent bleeding is still not forthcoming following these evaluations, urinalysis via straight catheter placement, rectal examination via digital examination, and coagulation studies should be performed to diagnose other important causes of "vaginal bleeding."

 ## LABORATORY RECOGNITION ◄────────────────────┐

In the setting of third trimester vaginal bleeding, blood counts, coagulation studies, and other more specialized tests are important but are best monitored in a hospital setting. Ultrasound and tocodynamometry are also best applied in a hospital setting.

Initial Management

Third trimester vaginal bleeding usually requires referral to, and evaluation at, a hospital setting; placental and nonplacental causes are not usually amenable to primary office treatment. Therefore, other than the recommendation to rapidly assess, treat, and refer patients to a hospital setting, issues of treatment are beyond the scope of this chapter.

Complications

Complications associated with placenta previa include maternal hemorrhage with risk of shock, fetal distress due to maternal hypovolemia or fetal blood loss, and morbidity associated with preterm delivery. Increased morbidity may also be related to the need for transfusion and/or cesarean section. Placental abruption is associated with a more severe set of complications, including a neonatal mortality rate as high as 30%. Preterm labor and delivery, severe hemorrhage, Couvelaire uterus, consumptive coagulopathy, and multiple end-organ damage from ischemia and the effects of coagulopathy all contribute to morbidity and mortality. A high index of suspicion and a rapid correct diagnosis can significantly reduce maternal and fetal morbidity and mortality.

Disposition and Transfer

A patient who presents to the office with third trimester vaginal bleeding should be urgently transported to a hospital facility with ultrasound, uterine monitoring, and cesarean section capability. Patients with mild self-limited bleeding from placenta previa can be discharged from hospital to home after several hours of fetal monitoring has confirmed maternal and fetal stability, but recurrent episodes of bleeding should always be reevaluated in a hospital setting. Digital vaginal examinations, douching, and sexual activity are absolutely contraindicated until after delivery (which is usually accomplished by a scheduled cesarean section).

Preterm Labor

Preterm labor is the most common emergency affecting women in the third trimester of pregnancy and has been identified as one of the most important modern obstetric health problems. It deserves special attention because of its frequency, its treatability, and its association with preterm delivery, which itself accounts for 10% of all deliveries and more than 75% of all nonanomalous neonatal deaths. Women in the third trimester of pregnancy, but less than 36 weeks gestation, should be evaluated if regular or increasingly strong uterine contractions develop. Bacterial vaginosis, a common, seemingly benign, and treatable condition, has been associated with preterm labor and delivery. Table 15–2 lists the common causes of, and common risk factors for, preterm labor and delivery.

THIRD TRIMESTER

Table 15–2. Causes and Risk Factors for Preterm Labor and Delivery

Causes of Preterm Labor and Delivery	Risk Factors for Preterm Labor and Delivery
Structural Causes	**Past History Factors**
Cervical incompetence	Previous preterm birth
Multiple gestation/hydramnios	More than one midtrimester miscarriage or abortion
Placental abruption	Known uterine anomaly
Uterine anomalies	DES (diethylstilbestrol) exposure
	Incompetent cervix
	History of cone biopsy
Infectious Causes and Exposures	**Current Pregnancy Factors**
Bacterial vaginosis	Preterm cervical dilatation
Urinary tract infection/pyelonephritis	Second or third trimester bleeding
Chorioamnionitis	Extremes of maternal age—<15, >40 y of age
Intra-abdominal infection	Preterm premature rupture of membranes
Abdominal trauma	Cigarette use
Sexually transmitted diseases	Prepregnancy weight <115 lb
Cocaine abuse	
Chronic medical problems	
Chronic social problems	

CLINICAL RECOGNITION ◄————————————————

Preterm labor can be defined in two ways: the presence of regular uterine contractions occurring after 20 weeks gestation but before the start of the 36th week of gestation, associated with either active cervical change over time (dilatation or effacement); or contractions occurring with an initial cervical examination showing dilatation of more than 2 cm or effacement greater than 80%. A list of the symptoms of preterm labor has been developed by Creasy (Box 15–1).

Box 15–1. *Symptoms of Preterm Labor*

- A feeling that the baby is "balling up," which lasts longer than 30 seconds and occurs more than four times per hour
- Contractions of intermittent pain or sensation anywhere between the nipples and knees, lasting longer than 30 seconds and recurring four or more times per hour
- Menstrual-like sensations, occurring intermittently
- Change in vaginal discharge, including bleeding
- Indigestion or diarrhea

Data from Creasy.

PHONE TRIAGE ◄————————————————

A woman in the third trimester of pregnancy, but less than 36 weeks gestation, who contacts a health care facility with the complaint of increasingly severe or frequent lower abdominal or back pain, should be considered to have preterm labor until proved otherwise and should be referred immediately to a hospital for evaluation. In cases in which symptoms seem severe, or if there is a history of premature delivery or rapid delivery, ambulance transfer is indicated. If the symptoms are mild, a brief history should be obtained and recorded. Does she have a history of previous preterm labor? Has she had complications with this pregnancy, a previous urinary tract infection (UTI), or vaginitis? Does she admit to any kind of active infection, dehydration, recent excessive physical activity, or recent sexual activity? All of these factors can stimulate preterm labor. Is there possible rupture of membranes or vaginal bleeding? If symptoms of preterm labor are present, she should be informed that if she does not report to a hospital, she might deliver a premature infant who has an increased chance of respiratory distress, infection, and death. She should be told that effective treatments are available for slowing or stopping most preterm labor if the process is diagnosed and treated in its early stages.

Physical Examination

Mild to moderate uterine contractions before 36 weeks gestation, even without cervical change or uterine bleeding, usually require evaluation. Vaginal examination with laboratory testing should be performed. An oral temperature should be taken. If contractions are regular, treatment with IV fluid should be started pending results of the urinalysis and wet preparation. Moderate to intense uterine contractions might also require the use of hospital-based tocolytic medication and immediate consultation with a specialist. The presence of a maternal fever raises the possibility of chorioamnionitis, pyelonephritis, cholecystitis, or other significant infection. Chorioamnionitis is an indication for delivery.

 ## LABORATORY RECOGNITION ◄————

Laboratory tests can be helpful in the management of preterm labor by identifying important precipitating conditions. UTI, bacterial vaginosis, and cervical group B streptococcal infections are the most common examples. Patients with premature uterine contractions should have a full urinalysis, a vaginal wet preparation for bacterial vaginosis, a group B streptococcal culture, and testing for gonorrhea and chlamydia infections. If excessive uterine contractions have stopped by the time the patient reaches the hospital, these tests still should be performed.

If there is any question about rupture of membranes, a sterile vaginal examination should be done to assess for the presence of amniotic fluid and to perform nitrazine and ferning testing of vaginal fluid. A positive nitrazine test suggests, and a positive ferning test confirms, the presence of ruptured membranes and mandates that all nonessential digital cervical examinations be avoided to reduce the development of chorioamnionitis.

Initial Management

The treatment of premature labor is aimed at uterine relaxation (tocolysis), as well as diagnosis and treatment of possible disorders that

THIRD
TRIMESTER

may lave led to uterine contractions. For preterm labor caused by dehydration and overexertion, successful treatment with bed rest and 1 to 2 liters of IV fluid is usually sufficient. UTIs require hydration and antibiotics.

Preterm labor refractory to rest and hydration may require one of a variety of tocolytic medications. These medications are listed in Table 15–3. More serious conditions such as pyelonephritis require hospital admission with IV antibiotics. Appendicitis or cholecystectomy requires appropriate surgical management. Oral antibiotics for simple UTIs, metronidazole (Flagyl) for bacterial vaginosis, and insistence on adequate hydration, rest, and avoidance of excessive activity are important adjunctive therapies in the treatment of threatened preterm labor. Treatment of current episodes and prevention of future episodes are both important goals.

Table 15–3. Treatment of Preterm Labor

Medication	Initial Treatment	Maintenance Treatment
Sulfate (mg)	4–6 g IV in 100 mL NS over $\frac{1}{2}$–$\frac{3}{4}$ hr	1–2 g/hr IV
Terbutaline	0.25 mg SC q$\frac{1}{2}$–1 h	2.5–5 mg PO
Procardia	10 mg SL q15–20 min	10 mg PO q6h
Indocin	100 mg PR	50 mg PR q8h × 48 hr

Complications

Premature labor can lead to premature delivery. The point of fetal viability is now 22 to 24 weeks gestation, but infants born before 34 weeks usually require prolonged nursery admission, and infants born before 28 weeks may suffer a significantly increased risk of residual physical and developmental problems. Infant morbidity and mortality improve with increasing gestational age until around 36 weeks. It is therefore clear that the aggressive treatment of preterm labor is important in most cases and should occur in a hospital setting. Contraindications to tocolysis include gestational age greater than 36 weeks, known fetal lung maturity, placental abruption, chorioamnionitis, evidence of fetal intolerance of the intrauterine environment, severe preeclampsia, eclampsia, and maternal cardiovascular instability.

In threatened or actual preterm labor in which the gestational age is less than 34 weeks, consideration should be given to promoting fetal lung maturation with corticosteroids. The two common regimens are dexamethasone 6 mg IM every 12 hours for 4 doses and betamethasone 12 mg IM every 24 hours for 2 doses.

THIRD TRIMESTER

Disposition and Transfer

Patients who are diagnosed with preterm labor in an office setting should be transferred to the nearest hospital facility with obstetric expertise. Patients with minimal symptoms and signs of preterm labor may be evaluated in the office setting. If their contractions resolve, they may be discharged to home provided they have not experienced cervical dilatation past 2 to 3 cm, do not have a history of premature delivery, do not live a great distance from the hospital, and do not represent a serious compliance risk. Occasionally, patients are admitted for prolonged bed rest and observation, especially if their fetus is severely preterm (20 to 32 weeks gestation).

Pregnancy-Induced Hypertension

Hypertension in pregnancy has been classified in many ways. The terminology of Hughes is listed in Box 15–2. The syndrome of pregnancy-induced hypertension occurs in at least 6% of pregnancies. Preeclampsia, a syndrome marked by hypertension, proteinuria, and edema, can

THIRD TRIMESTER

Box 15–2. *Hughes Classification of Hypertension in Pregnancy*

A. Pregnancy-induced hypertension: Hypertension that develops as a consequence of pregnancy and regresses post partum
  1. Hypertension without proteinuria or pathologic edema
  2. Preeclampsia—with proteinuria and/or pathologic edema
     a. Mild
     b. Severe
  3. Eclampsia—proteinuria and/or pathologic edema along with convulsions

B. Coincidental hypertension: Chronic underlying hypertension that predated pregnancy or persists post partum

C. Pregnancy-aggravated hypertension: Underlying hypertension worsened by pregnancy
  1. Superimposed preeclampsia
  2. Superimposed eclampsia

D. Transient hypertension: Hypertension that develops after the midtrimester of pregnancy and is characterized by mild elevations in blood pressure that do not compromise the pregnancy. This form of hypertension regresses after delivery but may return in subsequent gestations

Table 15–4. Severity of Preeclampsia

Level of Preeclampsia	Primary Feature	Other Features
Mild–moderate	Systolic BP increase >30 mm Hg Diastolic BP increase >15 mm HG BP>140/90 on two occasions, but <160/110	Proteinuria >1+, but <3–4+ Generalized edema with excessive sudden weight gain
Severe	BP >160/110	Marked proteinuria >3–4+ Oliguria, hepatic dysfunction, cerebrovascular symptoms, scotomata, restlessness, or confusion

BP, blood pressure.

progress to eclampsia, which is distinguished by generalized tonic-clonic seizure activity. Eclampsia occurs in approximately 0.1% of pregnancies but accounts for 15% of maternal deaths in the United States. Mild to moderate preeclampsia and severe preeclampsia are defined in Table 15–4. Severe preeclampsia can be complicated by the HELLP syndrome, a life-threatening multisystem process that includes *h*ypertension, *e*levated *l*iver function tests, and *l*ow *p*latelets. The HELLP syndrome may or may not occur along with eclampsia and has an overall incidence of approximately 0.1%. Any patient past 20 weeks gestation who complains of headache, new generalized edema, visual changes, upper abdominal or epigastric pain, or sudden flulike symptoms should be evaluated for a hypertensive disorder. Although most patients with these symptoms do not have pregnancy-induced hypertension, those that do have this syndrome are at risk for catastrophic outcomes if they do not receive timely diagnosis and treatment. A nonepileptic patient who has a seizure during the third trimester of pregnancy has eclampsia until proved otherwise and requires emergent medical attention.

The cause of pregnancy-induced hypertension is not known. It is more common during the first pregnancy with any given father, with multiple gestations, with extremes of maternal age, in patients with a personal or family history of preeclampsia, and in patients who have other chronic medical problems (e.g., chronic hypertension, diabetes mellitus, renal disease). The timing of progression from mild to severe forms is variable. A particularly severe variant of preeclampsia is seen with the antiphospholipid syndrome. Seizure activity can occur suddenly, at relatively early gestational ages, at early stages of preeclampsia, and before the onset of either proteinuria or severe edema. Chronic hypertension without proteinuria, edema, or other clinical signs or symptoms of preeclampsia does not usually indicate the need for emergency medical contact or intervention but still requires studied attention, especially after the patient has reached term (i.e., >36 weeks gestation).

CLINICAL RECOGNITION

Office recognition of pregnancy-induced hypertension revolves around the finding of significant hypertension (systolic blood pressure greater than 140, diastolic blood pressure greater than 90, or an increase of 30 systolic or 15 diastolic over second trimester baselines). Significant blood pressure elevations are usually associated with sudden excessive weight gain (>4 to 5 lb/wk) and/or proteinuria (>1+). However, the presence of significant *new* hypertension defines by itself a potential clinical emergency. Forty percent of eclamptic patients do not have edema before the onset of their first seizure and 13% do not have proteinuria. The patient with severe preeclampsia may complain of severe headache, visual scotomata, epigastric pain, and shortness of breath, and may demonstrate hyperreflexia, papilledema, tachypnea, and restlessness.

 ## PHONE TRIAGE

A telephone call from a patient complaining of a headache, at a gestational age of more than 20 weeks, should raise concern about possible pregnancy-induced hypertension. Basic historical questions should be asked: Has there been a recent sudden development of pedal or diffuse edema? Has the patient noted visual changes, emotional irritability, severe malaise, or upper abdominal pain? Transport to the office by a responsible adult is acceptable for mild symptoms, but labor floor evaluation is indicated in most cases because of the risk of rapid deterioration with seizures and fetal compromise. Before transportation is provided, the patient should be asked to rest on her side in a quiet, darkened room and with the attendance of a responsible adult. Ambulance transfer to the hospital is indicated for severe symptoms or seizure activity. A patient with suspected pregnancy-induced hypertension should never operate a motor vehicle owing to the potential for compromised driving ability.

 ## LABORATORY RECOGNITION

Patients with suspected pregnancy-induced hypertension should have laboratory testing. Although this testing is usually done within

THIRD TRIMESTER

the hospital setting, outpatient laboratory evaluations are sometimes performed. Severe preeclampsia is associated with uric acid levels greater than 5, a urinary dip protein greater than 1+, and/or elevated serum glutamic oxaloacetic transaminase (SGOT)/serum glutamic pyruvate transaminase (SGPT). A hemoglobin or hematocrit greater than a patient's 28-week gestation levels should be of concern because preeclampsia is associated with hemoconcentration. A platelet count lower than 150,000 may suggest developing thrombocytopenia, which develops in 10% of cases of preeclampsia. Twenty-four-hour urine collection for protein can be measured, and a level of greater than 500 mg/dL is defined as "significant." Normal laboratory tests serve as a baseline for patients with mild or suspected pregnancy-induced hypertension. In patients with moderate to severe preeclampsia, laboratory tests serve to document specific system involvement, as well as the relative severity of involvement. In severe preeclampsia, it is appropriate for serial laboratory tests to be ordered, along with a blood type and crossmatch for at least 2 units of blood and coagulation studies (prothrombin time [PT]/partial thromboplastin time [PTT] and fibrinogen levels) to test for consumptive coagulopathy. These tests can be ordered and samples drawn in an office setting, but the presence of severe preeclampsia mandates transfer to a hospital facility. Lastly, the presence of hypoglycemia may signal acute fatty liver of pregnancy, another rare but serious condition associated with preeclampsia.

Initial Management

Patients with suspected pregnancy-induced hypertension should be evaluated immediately. If blood pressure (BP) is stable, no excess weight gain has occurred, and urine is negative for protein, a follow-up visit in 3 to 4 days is indicated, as well as a discussion of the importance of bed rest and close telephone follow-up if further symptoms of preeclampsia develop. For those patients with mild preeclampsia, hospital admission is recommended for close observation, enforced lateral position bed rest, a no-added-salt diet, and a quiet environment. For patients with new severe hypertension, marked proteinuria, and/or generalized edema, admission to a labor and delivery unit, obstetric consultation, very close observation, and laboratory testing are indicated.

The mainstay of treatment for pregnancy-induced hypertension is admission, treatment with magnesium sulfate, and delivery. Magnesium sulfate is usually given as a 4- to 6-g load IV over 30 to 60 minutes followed by a 1- to 3-g/hr maintenance IV drip. Hydralazine 5 mg IV and labetolol 10 mg IV are effective antihypertensives, but should be given only for severe hypertension and only on an inpatient basis. The intravascular volume in preeclampsia is typically contracted and should be gently replaced. The seizures of eclampsia are best prevented through the regular use of IV magnesium sulfate. In cases in which seizure activity is refractory to treatment with magnesium sulfate alone, adjunctive diazepam IV 5 to 10 mg or pentobarbital IV 125 mg can be given. Repeat dosing may be needed. Refractory seizure activity in the presence of therapeutic magnesium levels and adjunctive medication should raise the possibility of intracerebral disease, including intracerebral hemorrhage, but this complication is rare.

Complications

Preeclampsia can cause decreased uterine perfusion, uteroplacental insufficiency, and fetal distress/demise. Eclampsia occurs in 1% of cases of preeclampsia, or in 1 in 2300 deliveries. Severe preeclampsia usually requires aggressive induction and is associated with increased rates of fetal distress and cesarean section delivery. In its severe forms, pregnancy-induced hypertension can cause multisystem damage with placental abruption, thrombocytopenia, pulmonary edema, acute renal failure, hepatic dysfunction or rupture, adult respiratory distress syndrome (ARDS), and cerebrovascular disease. Hemorrhagic stroke and cortical blindness from parietal ischemia/infarction are rare complications. These complications are ideally prevented by controlling hypertension, preventing seizure activity with $MgSO_4$, and expeditiously promoting delivery. The ultimate cure for pregnancy-induced hypertension is delivery, but seizure activity and the HELLP syndrome have been reported in patients up to 10 days after delivery.

Disposition and Transfer

Patients with labile hypertension that resolves with lateral bed rest and who do not exhibit other signs of preeclampsia can be treated in an outpatient setting with instructions to avoid excessive activity, to follow a no-added-salt diet, and to make frequent office visits for reevaluation. Patients who meet the criteria for having preeclampsia should be admitted for strict bed rest, observation, laboratory testing, and consideration of induction of labor.

Abdominal Trauma in the Third Trimester of Pregnancy

Significant abdominal injury occurs in 7% of women during the third trimester of pregnancy and accounts for 50% of all maternal deaths during pregnancy. Table 15–5 lists the common causes of abdominal trauma in

THIRD
TRIMESTER

Table 15–5. Cause of Third Trimester Abdominal Trauma	
Causes of Abdominal Trauma in Term Pregnancy	**Percentage**
Motor vehicle accidents	50
Domestic abuse and assault	22
Falls	22
Miscellaneous	1

Data from Connolly 1997.

the third trimester of pregnancy. High-speed motor vehicle accidents with multiple traumas have a 50% placental abruption rate; slower-speed accidents with minimal outward injury have a 1% to 6% abruption rate. Almost all patients with abdominal trauma in the third trimester require immediate medical evaluation to document fetal well-being, to help the woman cope emotionally with a threat to her pregnancy, and to evaluate for the presence of the four common major sequelae to abdominal trauma in the third trimester: uterine contusion, placental abruption, uterine rupture, and preterm labor. Description of a mechanism of injury that does not make sense should trigger concern about domestic abuse. Women in the third trimester who have been physically abused should be immediately evaluated, not only to assess for maternal and fetal well-being but also to assess for the likelihood of future abuse.

 ## CLINICAL RECOGNITION ◄─────────────

The diagnosis of trauma is typically identified in the chief complaint. Outward signs of injury may or may not be present. Facial, neck, or arm bruising; an explanation of a cause of injury that does not seem to make sense; or a "hovering partner" (i.e., a husband, boyfriend, or partner who is very interested in staying in the examination room during the interview or examination portion of an evaluation) should raise concerns about the possibility of physical abuse. Firmness, combined with sensitivity and a high level of awareness, can often uncover important historical details. In these situations, it is critical that the health care team find ways to question the woman apart from all other parties.

 ## PHONE TRIAGE ◄─────────────

Serious trauma affecting women in their third trimester usually results in the transfer of the patient from the scene to a hospital without the notification of her primary care office. However, a woman who is past 20 weeks gestation, who has had mild to moderate trauma, and who is not acutely symptomatic may present, in person or by telephone, to a primary care office for evaluation or treatment. These cases should be handled with great care and with a very low threshold for rapid referral to the nearest emergency room.

A brief history is important: What was the date and time of the accident? What, in the caller's words, was the exact mechanism of injury and what was the situation surrounding the accident? Have any obvious symptoms, such as vaginal bleeding, leakage of fluid, abdominal cramps/contractions, or dizziness/orthostasis, developed since the time of the accident? The presence of any of these events dictates the need to have the patient referred directly and quickly to an emergency room. Situations in which the patient's partner initiates the call increase the possibility that physical abuse was involved in the accident.

LABORATORY RECOGNITION ←

Laboratory testing in the setting of third trimester abdominal trauma should occur in a hospital setting. A "normal" office complete blood count (CBC), for example, can be falsely reassuring in the presence of acute intrauterine or intra-abdominal bleeding, and most tests relevant to the diagnosis of pregnancy-related complications (e.g., placental abruption, consumptive coagulopathy, and fetal/maternal transfusion) require hospital laboratory expertise.

Initial Management

Most trauma affecting women during the third trimester requires full evaluation, including basic history, vital signs, physical examination, and at least some form of fetal monitoring. Hospital evaluation is almost always indicated because life-threatening complications can initially be asymptomatic. Patients with only mild trauma, normal monitoring for 4 hours, and lack of vaginal bleeding can generally be discharged to home with instructions to call in the event of abdominal pain, back pain, uterine bleeding, or uterine contractions. If the cause of the trauma was or might have been physical abuse, the woman should be approached confidentially and firmly and with an attitude that projects understanding and interest in helping rather than accusation or prying. Referral to support networks, scheduling of follow-up visits for further discussion, and general support for women who have been victims of abuse are critical pieces of a care plan.

Trauma involving moderate-speed accidents and/or any trauma with residual abdominal or back pain requires a more thorough work-up, including ultrasound evaluation, blood work, and a prolonged hospital stay for observation and prolonged monitoring. Abdominal trauma of any kind associated with increasing abdominal pain, back pain, vaginal bleeding, uterine contractions, or vital sign irregularities requires urgent evaluation. Obstetric and general surgical consultation, an urgent ultrasound, and basic laboratory testing must be obtained, along with continuous fetal monitoring. **In cases involving vaginal bleeding, a vaginal examination should not be done unless an ultrasound has ruled out placenta previa.** Tocolytics should not be given until placental abruption has been ruled out because uterine relaxation in the presence of abruption can dramatically worsen the rate of hemorrhage. Penetrating injuries to the abdomen of a woman during the third trimester always require hospital evaluation and usually the cooperative involvement of obstetricians and general surgeons.

Treatment of mild abdominal trauma generally requires only observation, fetal monitoring, reassurance, and anticipatory guidance. Situations involving potential physical abuse require a high index of suspicion, the ability to confront the pregnant woman in a supportive manner, and a preset plan for referral to support, counseling, and social service agencies. Management of severe abdominal trauma in the third trimester of pregnancy is beyond the scope of this chapter.

Complications

Complications due to trauma in women during the third trimester primarily include placental abruption due to direct placental trauma or shearing forces, onset of premature labor due to placental abruption or uterine wall contusion, or, more rarely, uterine rupture or traumatic rupture of membranes. Undiagnosed placental abruption can cause fetal demise, major life-threatening maternal blood loss, and disseminated intravascular coagulation (DIC). Premature labor and delivery are associated with increased fetal morbidity and mortality. Injuries caused by physical abuse can be a harbinger of more aggressive and potentially lethal abuse in the future; one of the complications of not diagnosing injuries due to physical abuse is the effect that subsequent episodes of abuse can have on the pregnant mother and her fetus.

Disposition and Transfer

Almost all cases of trauma in women during the third trimester require a full evaluation, including fetal monitoring. This theoretically can be done in the office setting in cases of mild trauma. However, for anything more than mild trauma, hospital evaluation is indicated. Nonstress test (NST) evaluation, basic blood testing, and ultrasound assessment of the uterus, fetus, and placenta are important. Stable cases, even those involving mild, stable placental abruption or arrested premature labor, require close observation. Unstable cases are best treated in the hospital setting as the point of initial contact until the pregnant patient is stabilized and/ or delivered. The health and well-being of the mother are almost always given priority over those of the fetus. Emergency cesarean section, irrespective of gestational age, and cesarean hysterectomy are indicated in certain situations to protect the life of the mother.

All undelivered patients with recent abdominal trauma should be strongly cautioned to call and report to a hospital in the event of new significant abdominal or back symptoms, vaginal bleeding, leakage of fluid, or uterine contractions. Victims of suspected physical abuse should be given appropriate phone numbers for future reference. A follow-up visit with the patient's regular provider in 2 to 4 days is advisable from both a medical and a medical-legal perspective.

Bibliography

American Academy of Pediatrics and the American College of Obstetrics and Gynecology: Guidelines for Perinatal Care, 4th ed. Elk Grove Village, IL, The Academy; and Washington, DC, The College; 1997.

Connolly AM et al: Trauma in pregnancy. American Journal of Perinatology 1997:14(6);331-336.

Creasy R et al.: System for predicting spontaneous pre term birth. Obstetrics and Gynecology 1980:55;692.

Queenan JT, Hobbins JC: Protocols for High-Risk Pregnancies. Cambridge, Blackwell Science, 1996.

Niswander KR, Evans AT: Manual of Obstetrics. Boston, Little, Brown, 1996.

Cunningham FG, Williams JW: Williams Obstetrics, 20th ed. Stamford, Conn, Appleton and Lange, 1997.

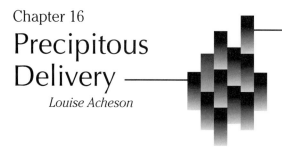

Chapter 16

Precipitous Delivery

Louise Acheson

CLINICAL RECOGNITION

Differential Diagnosis

Usually, it is apparent when a woman is pregnant and in labor. Occasionally, she has denied or concealed the pregnancy and may present with abdominal pain.[1] The fact that she is about to deliver a child becomes evident from an examiner's observation of her gravid abdomen, uterine contractions, and a presenting part in the vagina or a dilated cervix. Rarely, a psychotic woman has delusions that she is pregnant and may act as if she is in labor, but physical signs of pregnancy are not present. Box 16–1 includes the questions that should be asked of a patient who may be in labor.

Box 16–1. *Questions to Ask a Patient Who May Be in Labor*

When a woman calls and may be in labor, answers to the following questions are essential for triage[2]:
- Where is the patient, and who is with her? It is helpful to speak directly with the woman rather than with an intermediary, if at all possible.
- What transportation is available to her? Have emergency and medical services been called? (If it sounds like birth is imminent, have the patient call EMS.)
- How many previous births has she had? Any history of previous uterine surgery (cesarean section)?
- What is gestational age (based on due date, last menstrual period, and/or ultrasound examination)? If she is 1 month or more before her due date and has symptoms of labor, bleeding, or ruptured membranes, advise her to go immediately to a hospital.

Box continued on following page

193

Box 16–1. *Questions to Ask a Patient Who May Be in Labor* (Continued)

- How does she describe the contractions or pains? When did they begin, where does she feel them, how long does each contraction last, what is the time from the beginning of one to the beginning of the next, is this interval regular or variable, can she talk through the contraction or does she have to stop what she is doing? (In active labor, contractions usually last 45 seconds or longer, intensify as labor progresses, occur regularly at intervals of 5 minutes or less, and interrupt conversation. Direct patients experiencing these symptoms to their planned place of delivery.)
- Does she consistently experience an urge to bear down? Does it feel like she needs to move her bowels or like the baby is coming out? Has labor changed, rapidly becoming more intense? These may indicate that she will give birth soon.
- Has she experienced a gush or dribbling of fluid form the vagina? What color? Since when? If there is green or brown fluid, ask her to lie down on her left or right side until the fetus can be checked.
- Does she have vaginal bleeding? How much? If it is more than a usual menstrual period, immediate transport to a hospital is indicated.
- What position was the fetus in (head down or not?) and how dilated was the patient's cervix when last checked?
- Has there been concern for any medical problem or complication during this pregnancy?
- Possibility of injury: Has she been hit or kicked? Is now safe? (Ask this if the pains are premature or seem unlike usual labor pains.)

PRECIPITOUS DELIVERY

Epidemiology

Factors associated with precipitous (i.e., very rapid) labor include:
- Multiparity
- Previous rapid labor(s)
- Premature labor
- Placental abruption with tetanic contractions
- Labor precipitated by acute use of cocaine

Other factors associated with presentation of a patient for care when delivery is imminent include:
- Young teens who conceal pregnancy
- Mentally impaired patients who may deny or not recognize pregnancy/labor
- Delay in the patient's ability to procure transportation
- Rarely: Relatively painless first stage of labor

Initial Assessment

The three assessments most important to make when someone presents in labor are:

1. How imminent is the birth? (Is there time to transfer the patient before delivery?)
2. How far along in pregnancy is the woman?
3. Is this labor abnormal or normal?

Imminence of Birth

To tell how long it is likely to be before the birth, it is helpful for the clinician to know[2, 3]:

1. *How long she has been having painful contractions* (the average labor at term for a first baby is 12 hours and the average labor for subsequent babies is 8 hours, but there is WIDE variation). Usually, labor pains get stronger and more intense as delivery approaches.
2. *Whether the amniotic sac has ruptured* (signified by fluid dripping from the vagina).
3. *How dilated the cervix is.* A trained examiner wearing a sterile glove can perform a digital vaginal examination to assess cervical dilation (Fig. 16–1).

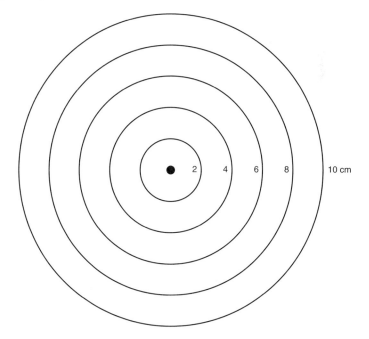

Figure 16–1. Circles of different diameters for cervical examination. 10 cm = complete dilation.

4. *Whether the presenting part of the fetus has moved down into the lower vagina or is showing at the introitus.* If so, there is no time for transport!
5. *What sensations the woman is experiencing*—whether she feels an urge to bear down or rectal pressure. Most women are at least 8 cm dilated when they feel a strong urge to bear down during contractions. *Rectal pressure usually indicates that a presenting part has moved low into the vagina*, and delivery may be imminent.

Birth is imminent if a presenting part of the fetus is distending the perineum or visible in the introitus. Birth may follow within minutes to an hour if strong, painful contractions are occurring and the cervix is dilated almost completely (8 to 9 cm—a rim of cervix 1 to 2 cm wide is palpable around the presenting part) or completely (no rim of cervix is palpable around the presenting part). The woman may exclaim, "The baby is coming!" and she is usually right. If labor has been rapid (especially in a multiparous woman), birth may be imminent if she is contracting strongly, the cervix is at least 6 cm dilated, and the membranes spontaneously rupture (fluid gushes from the vagina). On the other hand, a woman having her first baby may push for 1 or more hours from the time when the cervix is completely dilated until the fetal head descends to the vaginal opening. A judgment must be made about whether there is time to transport the woman to a hospital or childbirth center before she gives birth.[4, 5]

Gestational Age

Gestational age is important to know in an emergency situation for two reasons. First, every effort should be made to transport patients in *preterm* labor (24 to 34 weeks gestation) to a regional perinatal center before delivery. If this is impossible, the most skilled available personnel should prepare to resuscitate and stabilize a premature infant.

Second, if signs of labor are occurring early in pregnancy (*before* 22 weeks), when a premature infant is unlikely to survive, clinicians, patient, and family need to be prepared for a perinatal death, and labor should be managed accordingly. When the gestational age is uncertain, but the fetus may be viable yet premature, preparations should be made for transfer, neonatal resuscitation, and support according to the best judgment of the clinicians.

Term labor occurs 37 to 42 weeks after the first day of the last normal menses (LMP). The estimated due date can be calculated by adding 9 months and 7 days to the date of the LMP. For example, an LMP of January 1 gives an estimated due date of October 8. By convention, weeks of gestation are calculated from the LMP (menstrual date), rather than from the date of conception.

Other indicators of gestational age are listed in Box 16–2.

PRECIPITOUS DELIVERY

Box 16–2. *Indicators of Gestational Age*

- The top of the uterine fundus is at the umbilicus at 20 weeks gestation.
- The mother first perceives fetal movement at 16 to 20 weeks.
- The number of centimeters from the pubic symphysis to the top of the fundus (fundal height) approximately equals the number of weeks gestation between 20 and 36 weeks.
- Ultrasound examination: If done before 30 weeks gestation, the gestational age based on sonographic measurements is likely to be accurate to within 2 weeks. Late in pregnancy, sonographic dating is subject to an error of plus or minus 3 weeks.

Quality of Labor

Abnormal labor is an indication that the patient must be transported to a hospital as rapidly as possible unless delivery is imminent. If transport is not feasible, the most experienced persons available to help should be called.[6, 7]

Presentation

Normally, the top of the fetal head (vertex) presents in the cervix or vagina. Abnormal presenting parts include the feet, buttocks, face, arm, shoulder, and umbilical cord.[8]

Feet or Buttocks (Breech Presentation). Types of breech presentations are footling breech (one or both feet presenting), frank breech (buttocks first with knees extended), and complete breech (buttocks first with knees flexed). Footling breech carries a high risk of umbilical cord prolapse and (if the fetus is viable) should result in an urgent cesarean delivery if facilities are available. Frank or complete breech presentation at term may become evident so late in labor that the only feasible course is vaginal delivery, or the patient and practitioner may choose to attempt a vaginal breech birth in a hospital prepared for cesarean delivery.

Whether delivery occurs by cesarean section or vaginally, breech presentation carries a higher risk of birth injury than vertex presentation. The main danger of a vaginal breech delivery is a trapped fetal head, leading to asphyxia. (See Box 16–3 for appropriate procedure for emergency breech delivery.)

Premature breech delivery is preferably accomplished by cesarean section because of the risk that the smaller fetal head may be trapped by an incompletely dilated cervix if vaginal delivery is attempted.

Face, Arm, or Shoulder. If the face is presenting, vaginal delivery is not an option unless the chin is toward the mother's front. Vaginal delivery

Box 16–3. *Emergency Vaginal Breech Delivery*[8, 15, 26]

As soon as the diagnosis of breech presentation is made, the mother should be transported to a labor and delivery unit with skilled attendants, if at all possible. Any slowing of the progress of labor should alert one to the possibility of a difficult delivery and should prompt further consideration of immediate transport. If labor has been rapid and delivery is imminent with the infant presenting by breech, assisted vaginal breech delivery may be necessary. The following steps describe the process of breech delivery, once the breech is in the mother's lower vagina:

1. Have an assistant ready to help you.
2. The infant's back should always be toward the mother's front, never toward her back.
3. Wait until the cervix is *completely* dilated before instructing the woman to begin to push.
4. She should push gently during contractions until the baby's buttocks and legs emerge spontaneously (be patient; don't try to pull the baby out).
5. When the baby's umbilicus emerges from the vagina, gently pull down a loop of the cord to give it some slack.
6. Support the baby with your two hands on its pelvis: fingers on the anterior iliac crests, thumbs on the sacrum. Never squeeze the baby's abdomen. As the infant's scapula appears, gently rotate the baby's trunk 45 to 90 degrees in one direction. If the uppermost arm does not spontaneously emerge at that point, use the index finger and thumb of one hand to grasp the baby's humerus and sweep it across the anterior chest and down to the baby's side (outside the vagina at the end of this maneuver). Turn the baby's trunk in the opposite direction and perform a symmetrical maneuver to deliver the other arm. The head cannot be delivered until after both arms are out!
7. Throughout the delivery, your assistant should place one hand above the mother's pubis and press gently over the baby's occiput to keep the head **flexed**.
8. Now the baby's back should again be toward the mother's front. Support the baby's abdomen on the volar surface of your forearm while placing your index and middle fingers on the baby's malar areas (cheekbones) to help flex the head. (A towel placed around the baby's abdomen like a sling and held up by your assistant may be helpful.) Place the middle finger of your other hand on the baby's occiput, spreading your index and fourth fingers to rest on the baby's shoulders (or keep all three fingers on the occiput). This hand, too, keeps the head flexed

Box continued on following page

Box 16–3. *Emergency Vaginal Breech Delivery*[8, 15, 26] *(Continued)*
for delivery. The baby's body should always be in the same axis as the head; NEVER hyperextend the neck! 9. During a contraction, ask the mother to push. The baby's body should be level with or somewhat below the plane of the vagina until the chin is visible at the introitus. After the face begins to appear, begin to rotate the baby's trunk in an upward arc. The mouth can be suctioned and an episiotomy cut if necessary. Supporting the baby's body in line with its flexed head, complete the delivery by rotating the baby in a "backward somersault" onto the mother's abdomen. 10. The head is the largest and most difficult part to deliver. If the head is trapped and is compressing the cord, one has 7 to 8 minutes before fetal asphyxia is likely. Fortunately, most precipitous breech deliveries at term do not lead to this complication. Emergency measures include the use of special Piper forceps for breech extraction, Dührssen's incisions (which involve cutting the cervix if it is incompletely dilated [incisions at 11 o'clock and 1 o'clock positions between paired ring forceps]), and (employed in some parts of the world as a last resort) symphysiotomy (with anesthesia) to enlarge the bony birth canal.[21, 22]

also is impossible when an arm or shoulder presents. Infants in this position usually cannot be turned, and cesarean delivery is necessary.

Umbilical Cord Prolapse

If the fetus is still alive, cesarean section should be done urgently. Meanwhile, the mother must assume a hands-and-knees position and an examiner must hold up the presenting part using one hand in the vagina, so that the presenting part does not compress the cord against the cervix or birth canal and cut off circulation to the fetus. This must be maintained *at all times* (including transfer and transport of the mother) until abdominal delivery is accomplished.[6] No attempt should be made to replace the prolapsed cord into the uterus. It should be handled as little as possible because handling it may cause vasospasm. The fetal heart rate is 120 to 160 beats per minute when cord compression is being successfully prevented. Terbutaline 0.5 mg may be injected subcutaneously to decrease contractions during transport. (Intravenous terbutaline 0.25 mg bolus also effectively reduces uterine contractions, but inhaled terbutaline 1 to 2 mg is ineffective.[9]) This dose may be repeated after 15 minutes if necessary.

Fetal Heart Rate

A normal fetal heart rate is 120 to 160 beats per minute (bpm). Fetal heart tones may be heard with a regular stethoscope, a fetal stethoscope, or a hand-held Doppler or ultrasound device. Auscultation of fetal heart rate is not the first priority during a precipitous labor and birth, but as a check of fetal well-being, it is recommended that fetal heart rate be assessed every $^1/_2$ hour during active labor and every 5 to 15 minutes after the cervix has completely dilated.

Fetal demise should be confirmed by several unsuccessful attempts to find a fetal heartbeat using proper equipment, or preferably on ultrasound examination. Heart rates outside the normal range may be signs of fetal distress. Unless delivery is about to occur within 7 to 8 minutes, measures should be taken for "intrauterine resuscitation." These include[7]:

- Positioning the woman on her left side. If the heart rate does not return to normal within 30 to 60 seconds, other positions are worth trying, including the opposite side and on hands-and-knees.
- Administering oxygen to the woman at a rate of 6 liters per minute by mask.
- Rapidly giving a bolus (e.g., 250 mL) of intravenous fluid.
- If a prolonged, tetanic contraction or cord prolapse is causing fetal distress, contractions can be diminished by the administration of terbutaline.

The woman's vital signs should be assessed, the contractions palpated, and a vaginal examination performed to detect abnormal bleeding or cord prolapse. An accelerated fetal heart rate detected when an examiner's finger rubs the fetal scalp is a somewhat reassuring sign. *Persistent* fetal bradycardia less than 100 bpm is an emergency and should result in transport unless delivery is about to occur.

During active labor, contractions normally last 45 to 100 seconds and occur at 1- to 4-minute intervals. An examiner can palpate contractions by keeping a hand on the mother's abdomen above the navel. During late labor, contractions usually become progressively more intense, frequent, and painful, and may be associated with the urge to bear down.

A tumultuous pattern of frequent, long contractions or a tender uterus that stays firm and does not relax between contractions may be a sign of placental abruption, which necessitates emergent delivery and evaluation of the mother for occult retroplacental hemorrhage or consumptive coagulopathy.

Amniotic Fluid

Amniotic fluid is usually clear. If the membranes have ruptured, a pool of fluid may be seen in the vagina during examination with a sterile speculum; the pH is greater than 4, turning nitrazine paper deep blue, and a dried smear of fluid on a glass slide is likely to form a fern pattern.

Green amniotic fluid containing meconium is observed in at least 15% of normal births but may also indicate fetal distress. If meconium is observed, to prevent meconium aspiration, the infant's mouth, then nose should be thoroughly suctioned before delivery of the rest of the body and before the infant's first breath, with the use of a small catheter attached to wall suction or to a suction pump, or a bulb syringe.

Vaginal Bleeding

A small amount of blood mixed with vaginal mucus commonly appears during labor as the cervix dilates ("bloody show"). Bleeding more copious than a normal menstrual flow may be abnormal. Dangerous causes of vaginal bleeding are[7]:

- Placental abruption (separation of the placenta from the uterus before the birth)—often associated with pain, bleeding, an abnormal fetal heart rate, and tetanic contractions.
- Placenta previa (placenta overlying the cervical opening)—in this situation, a digital vaginal examination can cause exsanguination. A gentle speculum examination can be done to evaluate vaginal bleeding during pregnancy, but if the woman is bleeding, a *digital* vaginal examination should NEVER be done until the placenta is known not to be previa!
- Fetal bleeding—for example, from tearing of umbilical vessels crossing the fetal membranes (vasa previa). Blood collected and mixed with sodium hydroxide solution turns brown if it is maternal and cherry red if it is fetal blood (Apt test).

Maternal Vital Signs

Fever often indicates an infection, especially chorioamnionitis, an infection of the fetal membranes and endometrium. An otherwise unexplained maternal fever is an indication for the prompt administration of intravenous antibiotics such as penicillin, ampicillin, ampicillin-sulbactam, or clindamycin and gentamicin.[7, 10]

Group B streptococcus is the most common cause of early neonatal sepsis and postpartum endometritis. Prophylactic administration of penicillin G or ampicillin is recommended at the onset of labor in women known to be colonized with group B streptococcus, in all premature labors, and in labors at term with ruptured membranes longer than 12 hours and fever or tachycardia (maternal or fetal) unless broader-spectrum antibiotic coverage is administered or the patient is allergic to penicillin.[10, 11] (Box 16–4.)

Hypertension: Blood pressures of 140/90 or greater, measured between contractions, should prompt evaluation for preeclampsia. This evaluation includes[7]:

> ## Box 16–4. *Drugs to Administer to the Mother for Premature Labor or Rupture of Membranes between 24 and 34 Weeks Gestation, Unless Delivery Is Imminent**
>
> *Corticosteroids*[13]
> Betamethasone 12 mg intramuscularly q24h × 2 doses
> OR
> Dexamethasone 6 mg intramuscularly q12h × 4 doses
>
> *Antibiotic prophylaxis for group B streptococcus*[11]
> Penicillin G 5 million units IV, followed by 2.5 million units IV q4h
> OR
> Ampicillin 2 g IV, followed by 1 g IV q4h
> If the patient is allergic to penicillin, give clindamycin 300 mg IV q6h
>
> *To stop contractions*[7]
> Terbutaline 0.5 mg subcutaneously or 0.25 mg inravenously. May repeat after 15 min if necessary
> OR
> Magnesium sulfate 2–6 g IV over 20 min, then 1–4 g hr IV infusion for 8–24 hr
>
> ---
> *The same antibiotic regimens are recommended by the Centers for Disease Control and Prevention as intrapartum prophylaxis for group B streptococcal infection in all mothers known to be colonized OR with intrapartum risk factors (e.g., premature labor, rupture of membranes longer than 12 hours and fever or tachycardia, other evidence of chorioamnionitis).[11]

- Frequent blood pressure measurements
- Measurement of proteinuria
- Questioning of the patient about symptoms, including headache, scotomata, and epigastric pain
- Examination for edema, liver tenderness, and hyperreflexia
- Assessment of fetal well-being
- Laboratory studies, including platelet count, hematocrit (for evidence of hemoconcentration), liver and renal function (alanine transaminase [ALT], blood urea nitrogen [BUN], creatinine, and serum uric acid), and possibly tests for coagulopathy

A woman in labor with preeclampsia should receive a bolus of 2 to 4 g of magnesium sulfate intravenously over 20 minutes to prevent eclamptic seizures. This is usually followed by an infusion of 2 g/hr, but it is advisable not to administer an infusion during transport. The drug can be re-bolused on arrival if necessary. Magnesium sulfate 2 g can also be given intramuscularly in preeclampsia if IV infusion is not possible. Should magnesium cause respiratory depression, the antidote is intravenous calcium chloride or calcium gluconate.

Box 16–5 summarizes the key steps for evaluating the woman in labor.

Box 16–5. *Summary of Initial Assessment of the Woman Presenting in Labor*

History

Gestational age estimate:
Add 9 months and 1 week to last menstrual period to obtain
expected date of delivery
Measure centimeters from pubic symphysis to top of uterus =
weeks gestation after 20 weeks. Term pregnancy = 37–42 wk
Symptoms of labor
Group B streptococcal colonization?

Examination

Maternal vital signs (respiratory distress, fever, hypertension
require evaluation and treatment)
Abdomen gravid?
Fetal heartbeat detected?
Fluid or bleeding?
Presenting part? (Vertex. If cord prolapse, arm, foot, breech, face,
get expert help—transport!)
Cervical dilation
Presenting part in lower vagina or distending perineum?
Contraction pattern
Maternal discomfort, cooperation

Disposition and Transfer

Mothers who deliver alone and unattended are likely to suffer emotionally as a result of the experience, even if mother and baby are physically well. Someone should always stay with the woman about to give birth.[12]

When a medical professional is present, it is preferable for the baby to be delivered in the physician's office or the patient's home rather than in a vehicle en route. Usually, if the birth is imminent, transport to a hospital or birth center should be delayed until after delivery and stabilization of the newborn. If the mother has given birth and is not bleeding, it may be elected to transport her before delivery of the placenta.

A woman in premature labor before 34 weeks gestation should if at all possible be transported to a hospital with a level 2 or 3 nursery that is prepared to care for premature infants. Transport of the mother to the perinatal center before the birth is always preferable if it can be accomplished.[4, 5] At between 24 and 34 weeks gestation, a woman with ruptured membranes or whose cervix is changing with contractions should, if possible, immediately receive corticosteroids (see Box 16–4).[13] In addition, magnesium sulfate or terbutaline may be recommended in an attempt to stop contractions. The regional perinatal center should be contacted when premature labor or rupture of membranes is diagnosed. Regional perinatal centers often have transport teams that can be dispatched to stabilize and transport sick or premature infants who have been born elsewhere, in case transfer of the mother before delivery cannot be accomplished.

A complicated labor (with malpresentation, hypertension, bleeding, or thick meconium, for example) is an indication for urgent transport before delivery if feasible, or for enlisting additional professional help if transport is not feasible. Always contact the receiving hospital's obstetrics unit to let them know the patient's condition and the need to prepare for an emergency, especially if an emergency operative delivery may be needed. Any available prenatal records and laboratory results should go with the patient.

When a patient in labor is being transported, she should if possible be accompanied by an attendant trained to perform vaginal deliveries and neonatal resuscitation, and by another person (perhaps a friend or family member) whose role is to provide the mother with comfort measures and emotional support en route and at the receiving facility. A large-bore intravenous line is a wise precaution in case it is needed for administration of fluid and medication for postpartum hemorrhage. Oxygen and equipment for emergency delivery should accompany the laboring woman. In most cases, she can assume any comfortable position except that she should not lie flat on her back. In the supine position, the weight of the uterus on the great vessels may impede venous return and decrease placental blood flow.

If the baby and placenta have already been delivered, and both mother and baby appear stable, then a medically skilled attendant is less necessary during transport, and intravenous access is optional. It is important, however, that the infant be dried and kept warm at all times. Having the baby suckle at the breast may help to keep the infant warm and may cause the uterus to contract, reducing the mother's bleeding. For successful breast-feeding to occur, an attempt to nurse during the first 2 hours after birth is important.

Initial Management: Vertex Vaginal Delivery[3, 6, 14, 15, 17]

If a woman in normal labor appears to be progressing rapidly and will deliver soon, outside the hospital, this section can be a guide to the process. A flow sheet for recording the process, kept with the supplies for delivery, may be helpful.[18]

First, the woman and her support person(s) should be escorted to wherever the birth will occur—in bed, in a treatment room on an examination table, and so forth. She should not lie flat on her back but may deliver in lithotomy position slightly tilted to one side, in a side-lying position with an assistant holding up her uppermost leg, or on hands and knees.

Box 16–6. *Equipment and Medications for Childbirth*

Essentials[2, 14, 15]

- Soap or antibacterial cleanser
- Sterile scissors or razor blade to cut the cord
- Two sterile strings ("umbilical tape" is perfect) or Kelly clamps for the umbilical cord
- Several pieces of clean cloth or 4″ × 4″-gauze: To wash the mother's genitals, to wipe out the baby's eyes and mouth, to clean up afterward
- Warm towels, blanket, or soft cloth to dry and wrap the baby after birth
- Something to put under the mother to contain the fluids and blood from childbirth

Full List of Equipment and Supplies

- Betadine or other cleansing solution
- Sterile speculum, sterile swab, nitrazine paper, glass slide (not necessary if delivery is imminent)
- Protective gown, goggles, sterile gloves for attendants, if feasible
- Instruments for a sterile "delivery pack":
    2 Kelly clamps
    2 pairs of scissors (one for cord, one for mother)
    Suction bulb (e.g., "nasal aspirator")
    2 sterile towels
    Receiving blankets
    Pack of 4″ × 4″-gauze squares
    2 Allis clamps (optional)
    2 small hemostats (optional)
    Umbilical tape or cord clamp (optional)
    Basin for placenta
    Ring forceps (2 or more)
    Needle holder
    Absorbable suture such as 3-0 Vicryl on a long, curved needle
    Skin forceps
    Tubes for collecting umbilical cord blood samples
    Peri-pads or adult diaper for mother's postpartum use
- Doppler or fetal stethoscope
- Large-bore IV
- Newspaper or some sort of absorptive padding and sheet for under mother
- Waterproof cover for bed or surface on which she is delivering
- Source of warmth for infant (blankets warmed in dryer, hot water bottle, 99°F bath, radiant warmer, mother skin-to-skin)

Box continued on following page

PRECIPITOUS
DELIVERY

Box 16–6. *Equipment and Medications for Childbirth (Continued)*

- Receiving blanket/towel/cap for baby
- Suction device, if available
- Bag-valve mask for infant, infant endotracheal tubes of various sizes, laryngoscope
- Bedpan or pelvic examination table (for examination of mother after delivery) (Facilities anticipating frequent out-of-hospital births, if staffed by professionals skilled in operative vaginal delivery, should consider having a hand-held vacuum device [e.g., My-T-Vac] and forceps available for emergency delivery in cases of fetal distress.)

Drugs and Doses[7]

Often needed
- IV fluid, such as lactated Ringer's solution, for rapid volume replacement in case of hemorrhage
- Pitocin: 10 to 40 units (usually 20 U) per liter of IV fluid, after delivery of the placenta OR 10 U IM
- Local anesthetic (e.g., 1% Xylocaine for perineal incision or repair)
- Oxygen with mask and tubing

Rarely needed (may not be feasible to stock in most offices)
- Methergine (methylergonovine) 0.2 mg IM
- Magnesium sulfate, diluent, and antidote: Calcium gluconate $MgSO_4$ 2–4 g IV over 20 min. Can be given IM.
- Terbutaline 0.5 mg for subcutaneous injection OR 0.25-mg intravenous bolus
- Penicillin 5 million units or ampicillin 2 g intravenously over 20 min
- Dexamethasone 6 mg intramuscularly for premature labor or ruptured membranes at 24–34 weeks gestation
- Nitroglycerin spray 200 mcg per spray, 2 sprays into mouth prn (e.g., in case of postpartum uterine inversion to momentarily relax the uterus for manual replacement of the inverted segment)[16]

Equipment and supplies for the birth should be assembled (Box 16–6). If time allows, it is helpful for intravenous access to be established in case fluids and medications are needed to treat postpartum hemorrhage. In more than 80% of cases, however, neither is needed.

Continuous support is valuable for the laboring woman. The woman's partner and/or a laywoman (friend, relative, or office staff member) who has experienced childbirth should remain with her to provide comfort and reassurance. If the woman giving birth has taken childbirth preparation classes or has previously experienced a natural childbirth, she can be reminded of methods for relaxation, controlled breathing, and visualization that may help her to cope with labor pains. If she is inexperienced, it is even more important for someone to communicate in a positive manner that labor is progressing in an expected way, that the pains are a sign of this, that it will not be long until the birth, and that she will be able to get through each contraction, one at a time. Even if the woman is screaming, attendants should speak quietly, face to face, while touching her. A permissive, rather than urgently directive manner often works best, but if it is truly urgent that the woman follow a particular direction, then it is appropriate to state that she needs to do this NOW for the sake of herself and the baby.

Stages of Labor (Box 16–7)

Box 16–7. *Stages of Labor*

First stage
    Contractions that increase in frequency and intensity
    Cervix thins out and dilates
Second stage
    Fetus descends through the birth canal and is born
Third stage
    Delivery of the placenta

First Stage of Labor

As the fetal presenting part descends, most unanesthetized women feel an urge to push during contractions, sometimes continuously. The woman should be urged not to bear down voluntarily until the cervix is completely dilated and she has the urge to do so.

Reassure the woman that the last 2 cm of dilation of the cervix is the hardest part of labor but that it probably will not last long, and that when the cervix is out of the way, it will be a relief for her to push.

Second Stage of Labor

During the second stage of labor, contractions usually come every 2 to 3 minutes and are strong and painful. Rectal pressure similar to the pressure of a bowel movement is associated with an urge to push or bear down. The woman should not be left alone when the pains are strong and coming often. If she appears to be in the second stage of labor, clinicians should prepare for delivery.

Attendants' hands should be washed and gloved. The mother's genitals should be washed. The mother should be told to push when she feels pain, to stop pushing when the contraction stops, and to rest between contractions.

Birth of the Baby's Head

When the baby's head stays visible in the vaginal opening between contractions, delivery is imminent. The mother may feel burning as the skin stretches. Reassure her and ask for her cooperation to ease the widest diameter of the baby's head through the vaginal opening.

Put your hand on the baby's head to stop it from coming out too quickly. Usually the baby's occiput is toward the mother's front. Put your other hand on the perineum below the vagina to support the tissues.

Ask the woman to pant or to push more gently to ease the head out gradually through the vaginal opening. She can do the last few pushes between contractions if she feels like it. It is almost never necessary to cut the perineum (i.e., cut an episiotomy) in a precipitous birth. Sometimes, however, despite attempts to deliver the head slowly, the perineum or labia will tear. Bleeding or large tears must be repaired after labor, but they are usually less extensive than tears occurring after an episiotomy. Local infiltration of 1% lidocaine (Xylocaine; 10 to 30 mL) or 0.25% bupivacaine (Marcaine; 5 to 10 mL) can be used for episiotomy or repair.

As soon as the baby's chin passes through the vaginal opening, ask the mother to stop pushing for a short time. Check for an umbilical cord around the neck. If there is a loose loop of cord, slip it outward over the baby's head before delivering the baby's body. If the cord is tightly around the baby's neck and can't be slipped off, clamp the cord in two places and cut between the clamps; then, unwind the cord.

If the amniotic fluid contains green particles (meconium), suction the baby's nose, then mouth, to remove the meconium before the baby's first breath.

Delivery of the Shoulders

Usually, the baby's head emerges facing the mother's back, but soon it turns sideways to face one of her legs. Do not do anything immediately; wait until you see which way the head is going to turn.

Grasp the sides of the baby's head with two hands, and lower it very gently to help the first shoulder come out. If it is not sliding out, ask the mother to push. As soon as the anterior shoulder appears under the pubis, raise the baby's head to ease the posterior (bottom) shoulder out. After the shoulders have passed through, the rest of the baby will slide out easily. Note the time of birth.

Avoid injuring the baby's brachial plexus: (1) Keep the baby's head lined up with its trunk, not bent far sideways; and (2) do not hook your fingers into the baby's axillae to pull on the shoulders.

Shoulder dystocia[19-22] is present when the infant's head is born but the shoulders are stuck behind the symphysis pubis. NEVER PULL ON THE BABY'S HEAD! If the shoulders do not come easily, first call for assistance. Then (with the mother lying on her back), have her open her legs as wide as possible and hyperflex her hips, while an assistant applies suprapubic (NOT fundal) pressure with the heels of the hands (similar to the position for administering chest compressions in cardiopulmonary resuscitation [CPR], except in a suprapubic location, facing the same direction as the infant). Also, have the mother push. Again, exert gentle downward traction, holding the baby's head in both of your hands, OR have the mother roll to a hands-and-knees position and try delivering the posterior shoulder first by applying gentle downward traction on the baby's head.[21]

If these maneuvers are not successful, put your hand along the baby's back and try to turn the shoulders obliquely to dislodge the anterior shoulder from behind the mother's pubic bone.[19-21] Suprapubic pressure can be continued, and if necessary an episiotomy can be cut posteriorly in the midline to enlarge the vaginal opening. Again, have the mother push.

If attempts to turn the baby's body in either direction are not successful, you may have to deliver the posterior arm.[19] Reach into the mother's vagina along the baby's back, find the scapula that is closest to the mother's back; then, use your fingers to sweep the posterior arm across the baby's chest and face until it is extended beside the baby's head, outside the mother. Usually, the anterior shoulder will then deliver easily.

Each of these steps should be tried for 30 to 60 seconds, and they may be repeated in any order. If the shoulders and body are not delivered within 7 to 8 minutes of the birth of the head, neonatal hypoxia from lack of oxygenated blood flow to the brain is likely.

As a last resort, replacement of the baby's head into the vagina while preparations are made for emergency cesarean section, or, where there are no facilities for cesarean section, symphysiotomy (cutting through the mother's pubic symphysis) has occasionally been successful.[22, 23]

Care of the Baby at Birth[17, 24]

Warmth is essential! Place the baby on the mother's bare abdomen. (If there is thick meconium, ideally the baby should be placed under a warmer, and endotracheal suctioning should be performed by a skilled professional to clear the trachea of meconium.)

Dry the baby's trunk and head. Remove wet cloths and replace with dry ones to keep the baby warm. Position the baby's head with the neck slightly extended to open the airway. Wipe out the baby's mouth with clean gauze, or suction the mouth, then the nose, using a bulb syringe or suction catheter. This will usually stimulate the baby to cry and breathe. (See Box 16–8 for Apgar scoring.)[24]

Box 16–8. *Apgar Scores (Range 0–10)*

This system is commonly used for "scoring" the infant's responses and appearance at 1 and 5 minutes of age:

Observation	0	1	2 points
Heart rate	Absent	<100 bpm	≥100 bpm
Respiratory effort	Apneic	Irregular, gasping	Regular, crying
Response to suctioning	No response	Some response	Facial grimace, sneeze, cough
Muscle tone (arms, legs)	Flaccid	some flexion	Strong flexion
Color	Blue, pale	Body pink, hands and feet blue	Pink

If vigorous stimulation does not result in spontaneous breathing after 30 seconds, follow the steps for neonatal resuscitation. If the baby is breathing, check the heart rate. If it is below 100, follow the steps for neonatal resuscitation (Box 16–9).[24]

Box 16–9. *Neonatal Resuscitation*[24]

If an infant does not breathe immediately, or has only gasping respirations:
1. *Provide tactile stimulation* for about 30 sec
    Vigorously rub the infant's back.
    Slap or flick the soles of his/her feet.
2. *Evaluate respirations:* If not breathing or only gasping:
    Positive pressure ventilation (PPV) with bag and mask, 100% oxygen
        Connect a bag and infant mask to oxygen source (Where there is no equipment available, mouth-to-mouth resuscitation can be considered).
        Position the infant with neck slightly extended (A rolled cloth behind the neck may help).
        Position the mask on the infant's face; check the seal by ventilating and observing for a rise of the chest.
        If no chest movement, reposition and try again.
        If the chest moves, ventilate the infant for 15–30 sec (10–30 breaths at a rate of 40–60 breaths/min, 15–40 cm water pressure).
3. *Check the infant's heart rate:*
    Heart rate >100 beats per min (bpm) and spontaneous respirations

---

Box continued on following page

PRECIPITOUS DELIVERY

Box 16–9. *Neonatal Resuscitation*[24] *(Continued)*

Stop PPV and observe. Give free-flow oxygen if necessary.
Heart rate >100 bpm but no spontaneous respirations
    Continue PPV. Assess every 30 sec.
Heart rate 60–100 bpm and *increasing*
    Continue PPV. Assess every 30 sec.
Heart rate 80–100 bpm and *not increasing*
    Continue PPV and assess adequacy of ventilation: Chest
    motion and oxygen flow.
Heart rate <80 bpm
    Continue PPV and assess its adequacy. Start chest
    compressions.
4. *Perform chest compressions:* This will require a second person—
one to ventilate and one to perform chest compressions
    Make sure that the infant's back is against a firm surface.
    Locate the lower third of the baby's sternum (just below the
    level of the nipples).
    Compress the sternum $^1/_2$ to $^3/_4$ inch, using either
        (a) Both thumbs on the lower sternum, pointing toward
            the baby's head, with your hands encircling the chest
            but not squeezing it OR
        (b) Two fingers of one hand, perpendicular to the baby's
            chest.
    Compress at a rate of 2 per sec, pausing to deliver a breath for
    $^1/_2$ sec after every third chest compression. This will result in
    90 chest compressions and 30 breaths per min.
    After 30 sec (45 chest compressions or 15 cycles of 3
    compressions and one breath), stop for 6 sec to assess heart
    rate and breathing. If the heart rate is >80, stop chest
    compressions and assist respirations as in #3, assessing
    every 30 sec.
5. *Decompress the stomach:* If PPV is needed for longer than 2 min,
insert an orogastric tube to decompress the stomach.
    Use an 8 French feeding tube.
    Measure the length to correspond to the distance from bridge
    of the baby's nose to the ear lobe plus the distance from the
    ear lobe to the tip of the xyphoid process.
    Insert through the mouth.
    Remove gastric contents with a 20-mL syringe, then detach it
    and leave the tube open.
    Tape the tube to the infant's cheek and resume PPV.
6. *Employ endotracheal intubation*
    If PPV is unsuccessful using a bag and mask, or if it needs to be

Box continued on following page

Box 16–9. *Neonatal Resuscitation*[24] *(Continued)*

continued for an extended time, endotracheal intubation of the infant is indicated if equipment and a skilled professional are available. Epinephrine and naloxone can be given by endotracheal tube during resuscitation, as well as through an umbilical vein catheter.

7. *Administer medications:* An endotracheal tube or umbilical vein catheter is needed to administer medications for neonatal resuscitation. These interventions should be employed by professionals trained in their use:

Epinephrine should be considered if the heart rate is 0 or if it is still <80 bpm after 30 sec of chest compressions and PPV. It may be repeated every 3–5 min, if necessary. Use a concentration of 1:10,000. Give 0.1 to 0.3 mL/kg (e.g., 0.5 mL for a 3-kg term infant) rapidly IV or through the endotracheal tube. Dilute it to 1–2 mL with normal saline if giving it endotracheally.

Volume expansion with normal saline or Ringer's lactate should be considered if there is evidence of bleeding or suspicion of hypovolemia. The dose is 10 mL per kg IV over 5–10 min (syringe or drip).

Sodium bicarbonate is used during a prolonged resuscitation and only in conjunction with adequate ventilation. A 0.5-mEq/mL (4.2%) solution comes in 10-mL syringes. The dose is 2 mEq/kg IV, infused slowly over at least 2 min. A term-sized infant will need about 12 mL of the solution.

If the baby is breathing and has a heart rate greater than 100, check skin color. If cyanosis of the lips is noted (central cyanosis), give free-flow 80% to 100% oxygen by mask or from tubing with your hand cupped over the baby's face, until the face is pink. Once the infant becomes pink, oxygen should be gradually withdrawn, until he or she remains pink in room air.

After the baby has begun breathing (or if you need to move the baby for resuscitation), tie or clamp the umbilical cord in two places and cut between them. There is usually no urgency in cutting the cord. Remember that the umbilical cord is directly connected to the infant's circulatory system; the baby's end of it should never be unsecured or allowed to bleed.

Wipe the baby's eyes with clean cloth or gauze. (Administer erythromycin eye ointment, if available, within the first hour of life.) Keep the baby warm (e.g., next to the mother's body, covered with dry blankets or towels). If a clothes dryer is on the premises, it can be used to heat blankets or towels for mother and baby. Put the baby to suckle at the breast within the first 2 hours after birth, if the mother is planning to breast-feed.

Delivery of the Placenta

Do not rush! Do not pull on the cord. Delivery of the placenta may take up to an hour. It may be allowed to occur spontaneously unless the mother is bleeding heavily. Urgent transport to a hospital should be considered if the placenta is retained for longer than a half-hour, or if bleeding occurs without expulsion of the placenta.

The placenta should come out easily. When it does, examine it to see if it is complete. If the placenta looks torn or pieces are missing, strongly consider transport to a hospital for uterine exploration or curettage.

Postpartum Bleeding

As soon as the placenta is delivered, massage the uterus through the abdomen with one hand until the uterus becomes firm and vaginal bleeding stops. The other hand may be placed inside the vagina to compress the uterus from below (as in a bimanual examination but with your whole hand inside the vagina). An assistant may continue to massage the fundus abdominally afterward to keep it firmly contracting so as to minimize blood loss. This should be done at least every 15 minutes for the first 2 hours after birth, and whenever increased bleeding is noticed.

If available, oxytocin (Pitocin) can be given immediately after the placenta delivers, either 10 U IM or 20 to 40 U in 1 L of IV fluid, running at 125 mL/hr (or more rapidly as needed to keep the fundus firm). IM oxytocin may be repeated up to 3 times at 15-minute intervals, if necessary. Other drugs effective for postpartum hemorrhage due to uterine atony are methylergonovine (Methergine), 0.2 mg intramuscularly (causes transient blood pressure elevation and should be avoided if the patient has hypertension or vascular disease) and 15-methyl/prostaglandin F2α (Hemabate), 0.25 mg intramuscularly every 15 minutes for up to three doses.[25] Hemabate is not practical to keep in most physicians' offices, however.

Postpartum Examination of the Mother

When the fundus is firm, the mother's genitals should be examined for lacerations. (This can be done at the hospital if the patient is not bleeding heavily and is about to be transported.) Remember that this examination will be quite uncomfortable for most women. A flashlight, headlamp, or spotlight is essential for adequate visualization. The woman ideally should have her buttocks raised above the bed or be in stirrups as for a pelvic examination. A small gauze square held in a ring forceps can be used to view the vaginal sidewalls to make sure there are no tears. The labia minora and perineum should be examined for deep or bleeding lacerations.

According to the professional attendant's skills and available equipment, lacerations can be repaired with the use of locally infiltrated anesthetic solution (e.g., 1% lidocaine without epinephrine, up to 30 mL total), either at the birth location or at a receiving hospital. If repair will occur after transport, try to achieve hemostasis by applying local pressure to the wound or hemostats to any visible bleeding vessels; then, cover the mother's perineum with clean peri-pads, sterile cloth, or an adult diaper. If repair is not necessary or has been completed, gently wash off all blood with warm water and dry the area before using a pad or diaper. A cold pack to the perineum reduces swelling and discomfort.

Acknowledgments

I gratefully acknowledge the invaluable contributions made by Dr. Frank X. Klamet and Dr. Nancy Samudio to the sections on normal labor and birth. I am indebted to my colleagues at freestanding birth centers in Seattle (especially Cathy Doherty, C.R.N., Linda Harris, R.N., Donna Wahwasuck, R.N., and Stanley Harris, M.D.) and in Ohio (especially Sarah Danner, C.N.M., Al Evans, D.O., and John Tumbush, D.O.) for practical advice and insight from experience with precipitous delivery and birth outside the hospital.

References

1. Miller LJ: Psychotic denial of pregnancy: Phenomenology and clinical management. Hosp Commun Psychiatr 41:1233–1237, 1990.
2. Roberts J, McGowan N: Emergency birth. J Emerg Nurs 11:125–131, 1985.
3. Baldwin R: Normal labor and delivery at home. In Special Delivery: The Complete Guide to Informed Birth. Berkeley, Calif, Celestial Arts, 1979, pp 58–75.
4. Elliott JP, Sipp TL, Balazs KT: Maternal transport of patients with advanced cervical dilatation—To fly or not to fly? Obstet Gynecol 79:380–382, 1992.
5. Low RB, Martin D, Brown C: Emergency air transport of pregnant patients: The national experience. J Emerg Med 6:41–48, 1988.
6. Gianopoulos J: Emergency complications of labor and delivery. Emerg Med Clin North Am 12:201–211, 1994.
7. Brancel M: Obsetetric Urgency/Emergency Guidelines, 1995. [Mark Brancel, M.D., 2263 Commonwealth Ave., St. Paul, MN 55108.]
8. Ratcliffe SD, Baxley EG, Byrd JE, Sakornbut EL (eds): Family Practice Obstetrics, 2nd ed. Philadelphia, Hanley & Belfus, 2001, pp 477–495.
9. Kurup A, Arulkumaran S, Ingemarsson I, Ratnam SS: Can terbutaline be used as a nebuliser instead of intravenous injection for inhibition of uterine activity? Gynecol Obstet Invest 32:84–87, 1991.
10. Ratcliffe SD: Chorioamnionitis. In Ratcliffe SD, Baxley EG, Byrd JE, Sakornbut EL (eds): Family Practice Obstetrics, 2nd ed. Philadelphia, Hanley & Belfus, 2001, pp 448–453.
11. Centers for Disease Control and Prevention: Prevention of perinatal Group B streptococcal disease: A public health perspective. MMWR 45:1–24, 1996.
12. Harper RG, Seaton E, Spinazzola R, Schlessel JS: Unexpected, unattended deliveries. N Y State J Med June:330–331, 1990.
13. NIH Consensus Development Panel on the Effect of Corticosteroids for Fetal Maturation on Perinatal Outcome. Effect of corticosteroids for fetal maturation on perinatal outcomes. JAMA 273:413–418, 1995.
14. Cumbie B, Clement S: Emergency childbirth. Nursing 27:33, 1997.
15. Werner D, Thuman C, Maxwell J: Where There Is No Doctor: A Village Health Care Handbook, 2nd English ed. Palo Alto, Calif, The Hesperion Foundation, 1992, pp 208–220.
16. Hicks JC: Use of nitroglycerin spray in uterine inversion. J Am Board Fam Pract 13:374–375, 2000.

17. Tennyson M: Labor at 20,000 feet. Am J Nursing 100:49–52, 2000.
18. McBee P: ED precipitous labor and delivery flow sheet. J Emerg Nurs 21:326–328, 1995.
19. Carlan SJ, Angel JL, Knuppel RA: Shoulder dystocia. Am Fam Physician 43:1307–1311, 1991.
20. Ramsey PS, Ramin KD, Field CS, Rayburn WF: Shoulder dystocia: Rotational maneuvers revisited. J Reprod Med 45:85–88, 2000.
21. Sanyer O, Gaskin IM: Shoulder dystocia. In Ratcliffe SD, Baxley EG, Byrd JE, Sakornbut EL (eds): Family Practice Obstetrics, 2nd ed. Philadelphia, Hanley & Belfus, 2001, pp 441–448.
22. Wagner RK, Nielsen PE, Gonik B: Shoulder dystocia. Obstet Gynecol Clin North Am 26:371–383, 1999.
23. Cook J, Sankaran B, Wasunna AEO (eds): Surgery at the District Hospital: Obstetrics, Gynaecology, Orthopedics, and Traumatology. Geneva, World Health Organization, 1991, pp 15–48 (pp 34–35 for symphysiotomy).
24. AHA/AAP Neonatal Resuscitation Program Steering Committee: Textbook of Neonatal Resuscitation, 4th ed. Elk Grove Village, Ill, American Academy of Pediatrics and American Heart Association, 2000.
25. Alamia V, Meyer B: Peripartum hemorrhage. Obstet Gynecol Clin North Am 26:385–397, 1999.
26. Eisinger S, Koller WS: Malpresentations, malpositions, and multiple gestation. In Wolkomir M, Parsons GP, Damos JR, Eisinger SH (eds): ALSO Course Syllabus, 3rd ed. Kansas City, Mo, American Academy of Family Practice, 1996, pp 117–135.

Chapter 17
Infectious Emergencies

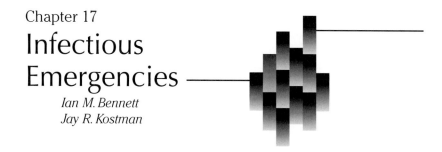

Ian M. Bennett
Jay R. Kostman

Infectious disease emergencies that present in the primary care setting are both interesting and dramatic. Acutely ill, infected patients present with symptoms suggestive of a broad differential diagnosis. This chapter begins with a review of the initial evaluation and management of those with a possible infectious diagnosis (acutely toxic patients). Subsequent sections address several specific diagnoses: bacterial meningitis, pneumonia, cystitis, pyelonephritis, and urosepsis. These were selected for their relative prevalence and/or potential catastrophic consequences. The discussion is limited to the treatment of immunocompetent patients.

The Acutely Toxic Patient

The ability to adequately respond to a severely ill patient in the outpatient setting requires a well-established office procedure for triage and treatment. Figure 17–1 provides a flow diagram for offices, which highlights important areas of response to the acutely toxic patient.

 ## PHONE TRIAGE

Any receptionist or secretary getting phone calls regarding acutely ill patients must be particularly aware of situations that require urgent review. In general, patients with underlying predisposing factors for infectious diseases, including immunosuppression (human immuno-deficiency virus [HIV] infection, chemotherapy, immunosuppressant therapies), extremes of age, or recent surgery, who present with fever either should be seen immediately in the office, or should be directly assessed by a physician by phone to determine the urgency involved. Patients with problems breathing, speaking, staying awake, or walking may need to go immediately to the closest emergency department. A physician or other clinical provider present in the office should be contacted immediately in these cases instead of messages being routed for routine review. If a health care provider in the office cannot

217

immediately review the situation, then the receptionist should direct the patient to contact an emergency response service, for example, by dialing 911. If a physician can review the case, do not let the patient or family member hang up before the provider takes the call.

RECEPTION
Assess risk factors for infectious emergency
  - Fever in age extremes, recent surgery, cancer therapy
Note triggers for expedited care
  - Difficulty staying awake, difficulty breathing or finishing
    sentences, collapsing, vomiting
Initiate expedited care
  - Contact nursing staff or physician directly
  - Bring patient to examination area

NURSING
Implement initial response
  - Room patient and assess severity
  - Lay patient down if there is risk of collapse
  - Contact physician to apprise of potential emergency
  - Prepare materials for placement of 2 18-gauge IV
    catheters and administration of oxygen therapy
Check vital signs
  - Routine vital signs (axillary or rectal temperature for
    patients with severe abnormality or rapid respiration)
  - Pulse oximetry
  - Serum glucose
Monitor patient
  - Ensure that patient is not alone at any time

PHYSICIAN
Implement initial response
  - Assess level of consciousness
  - Review vital signs
  - Obtain brief history, if available
  - Perform rapid physical examination
  - Assess need to activate emergency response system (911)
Begin additional evaluation
  - Order ECG
  - Consider ABG if signs of hypoxia and/or hypotension exist
  - Blood cultures x 2
  - Urinalysis and culture
Initiate therapeutic maneuvers
  - Direct initiation of IV fluids for delirium or hypotension
    (250–500 mL of 0.9 M saline bolus)
  - Initiate oxygen therapy for signs of respiratory distress or
    hypoxia
Determine disposition
  - Reevaluate need to transfer immediately to emergency
    department or ICU
  - Follow disorder-specific treatment plan based on
    differential diagnosis

Figure 17–1. Initial response to an acutely toxic patient. ABG, arterial blood gas; ECG, electrocardiogram; ICU, intensive care unit.

INFECTIOUS EMERGENCIES

CLINICAL RECOGNITION ◄

Classic signs and symptoms of infectious illness include vital sign abnormalities, inability to maintain normal range of body temperature (high or low), chills, abdominal pain, gastrointestinal distress, headache, vision changes, changes in level of sensorium, and dermatologic stigmata. The possible primary causes of an acute infectious disease emergency are broad. Although viral illnesses are the most common infectious diseases to present to the primary care office, it is difficult for the physician to distinguish a viral cause from a more worrisome bacterial infection. Focal abnormalities and symptoms should be identified. For instance, the presence of upper respiratory congestion in a patient with fever and chills makes the diagnosis of a viral syndrome much more likely than in a patient with respiratory distress and fever/chills without symptoms of rhinorrhea or postnasal drip.

Noninfectious illnesses can mimic acute infectious disease emergencies. Primary cardiac syndromes may include many of the physical signs of an infected patient. An electrocardiogram (ECG) should be obtained if the patient has significant risk factors for coronary artery disease (CAD) (e.g., sex, age, hypertension, diabetes mellitus) or a history of acute coronary syndromes. The possibility of a pulmonary embolism must be considered in any patient with dyspnea (associated signs include pleuritic chest pain, tachycardia, and evidence of deep vein thrombosis).

Meningeal signs and delirium may be the results of a vascular intracranial event, or they may reflect metabolic derangements from a variety of causes. Dehydration and metabolic acidosis resulting from a non–central nervous system (CNS) infectious disorder can cause changes in mental status. A computed tomographic (CT) scan of the head to rule out subarachnoid bleed and increased intracranial pressure is prudent before a lumbar puncture is performed in anyone with an abnormal funduscopic examination or focal neurologic symptoms.

Initial Management

Blood and urine cultures should be collected before any antibiotic therapy is begun. In the case of possible CNS involvement (meningitis or encephalitis), a lumbar puncture should be performed promptly for collection of cerebrospinal fluid (CSF) for examination, testing, and culture. In the case of suspected bacterial meningitis (see later), antibiotics should not be delayed for lumbar puncture.

Initial treatments for the acutely toxic patient include volume expansion, blood pressure support, respiratory support, and potential early antibiotic therapy. Patients with less severe illness often improve once mild to moderate dehydration is corrected. Large-gauge IV catheters should be placed during initial evaluation and treatment. Blood draws for laboratory work can be done simultaneously with IV placement (Note: Blood cultures should not be taken from the same site as the IV catheter so that contamination can be avoided). A rapid bolus of 250 to 500 mL of normal saline should be given immediately as it is not likely to cause fluid overload and may provide rapid benefit.

In hemodynamically stable patients, the use of antibiotic therapy should be delayed until a reasonable working diagnosis can be developed that can direct antibiotic choice. The early use of antibiotics can make subsequent definitive diagnosis difficult. Close follow-up for a deteriorating condition is needed for outpatient management.

Equipment and Medications

Materials required for the initial care of patients with infectious emergencies must be kept in primary care offices. The ability to carry out initial evaluation and therapeutic maneuvers can be critical to the final outcome of an infectious disease emergency. Collection of blood and urine cultures, testing for serum electrolytes and complete blood count with differential, and performance of lumbar punctures can be carried out in the primary care office, thereby saving evaluation time. Initiation of therapies such as fluid resuscitation and IV or PO antibiotics can reduce delays in provision of important treatments. Box 17–1 is a checklist of recommended materials with a relatively long shelf life that can be stocked in the office setting.

Box 17–1. *Recommended Supplies for the Primary Care Office for Response to Infectious Emergencies*

Monitoring Equipment
1. Pulse oximeter
2. ECG machine
3. Automatic blood pressure cuff

IV Materials and Fluids	
1. 0.9 M (normal) saline	1-liter bags
2. 18- and 20-gauge IV catheters	
3. IV extension tubing	
Culture Collection	Price per pack in dollars (number of items per pack)
1. Blood culture vials	
a. Aerobic	$227 (50)
b. Anaerobic	$163 (50)

Box continued on following page

> ## Box 17–1. *Recommended Supplies for the Primary Care Office for Response to Infectious Emergencies* (Continued)
>
> 2. Urine culture
>   - Vials (Vacutainer urine C&S) $48 (50)
>   - Midstream collection kit $139 (100)
>   - Pediatric catheterization kit $20 (1)
> 3. Lumbar puncture kit
>   - Adult $22 (1)
>   - Pediatric $22 (1)
> 4. Urine analysis
>   - Urine chemistry dip-stick $71 (100)
> 5. Blood collection materials
>   ABG syringe transporter $60 (24)
>   Blood sample tubes
>   - 4–6 mL evacuated blood collection tubes such as the BD vacutainer system $30–50 (100)
>   - Vacutainer tube holders $11 (100)
>   - Needles $18 (100)
> 6. Gonorrhea/Chlamydia culture swabs $62 (100)
>
> | Medications* | | | |
> |---|---|---|---|
> | 1. Antibiotics | Dose | Cost | (units) |
> | – Ceftriaxone | 250-mg vial | $68 | (10) |
> | – Doxycycline | 100-mg tab | $10 | (100) |
> | – Azithromycin | 250-mg tab | $263 | (50) |
> | – Trimethoprim-sulfamethoxazole | DS tablet | $14 | (100) |
> | 2. Analgesia/antipyretics | | | |
> | – Ibuprofen | 600-mg tab | $4 | (100) |
> | – Acetaminophen | 325-mg tab | $2 | (150) |
> | 3. Other | | | |
> | – Glucose (D_{50}) | IV ampule | $11 | (25) |
>
> BD, Becton Dickinson, Franklin Lakes, NJ; C & S, culture and sensitivity; ECG, electrocardiogram.
> *Shelf life approximately 2 years for antibiotics.

Disposition and Transfer

Disposition must be reviewed in an ongoing manner. In cases of severe distress requiring immediate transfer, initial care includes IV lines/fluids and respiratory support (e.g., oxygen, breathing treatments, and bag-valve-mask respiration); these facilitate care during transport and in the emergency department. Blood cultures should be taken and laboratory samples drawn while the patient awaits transport so that delays in therapy can be reduced.

Most patients do not require immediate transfer, and disposition decisions can be delayed until a better understanding of the illness is established. Initial therapeutic maneuvers may result in significant improvement in the patient's status. The patient may be able to go home with close follow-up in the presence of competent family members who can monitor patient condition and progress.

The indications for hospitalization include the need for close monitoring, inadequate support at home, intravenous medications, pain management, and inability to take nutrition and fluids by mouth. In many health care systems, home health care can address most of these needs outside of the hospital setting. If the patient appears stable but needs IV therapy, home health services should be contacted immediately from the office. Often, the patient can have a short hospital admission with transfer to home care after initial stabilization.

In the case of a patient who is admitted directly to the hospital, a significant portion of the initial evaluation can be completed in the office and a therapeutic plan initiated. Transport to the hospital need not include Advanced Cardiac Life Support (ACLS)-trained providers. In the case of a more urgent need for transfer, the use of an ACLS ambulance service is prudent, and direct transport to a local emergency department for further evaluation should be undertaken. In the case of severe decompensation with need for blood pressure and respiratory support, office personnel should call ahead to an intensive care unit (ICU) to discuss the case and arrange for immediate transfer to that setting.

Epidemiology and Pathophysiology

The number of infectious disease emergencies presenting in the primary care setting is difficult to estimate. Hospital discharge diagnoses for specific diseases in 1993 indicate that 179,000 cases of sepsis (72,000 of which were caused by *Escherichia coli*); 13,000 cases of bacterial meningitis; 29,000 cases of bacterial pneumonia; 108,000 cases of pyelonephritis; and 16,000 cases of gonococcal or chlamydial pelvic inflammatory disease were treated in the inpatient setting for that year.[1] Because these numbers account for hospitalizations only, a much larger number of cases of pneumonia, pyelonephritis, and pelvic inflammatory disease were treated in the outpatient setting.

Acute infectious disorders comprise a spectrum of severity from local disease to sepsis, or the systemic inflammatory response syndrome (SIRS). Limited disease may rapidly progress to SIRS if not initially treated appropriately, or in patients at the extremes of age or with comorbidities.

Pediatrics

The acute care of the toxic pediatric patient is guided largely by age. Infants younger than 60 days of age with a temperature greater than 38°C

(100.4°F) and children from 60 days to 36 months of age with a temperature greater than 39°C (102.2°F) with no focal signs of a specific illness (e.g., congestion, otitis media) should be thoroughly evaluated. A complete birth history, including prematurity, intrapartum antibiotics, prolonged rupture of membranes, maternal infections in pregnancy (chlamydia, herpes simplex virus [HSV], and group B streptococcus [GBS] colonization), and unexplained hyperbilirubinemia, should be elicited from the parents of the infant younger than 60 days of age. Initial evaluation of the patient should include an assessment of the "toxic" appearance of the patient. The playfulness of the child, his or her consolability and interaction with others, and whether he or she smiles appropriately are all significant indicators of severity of illness. Because an infant younger than 60 days of age is difficult to assess in this way, evaluation should include blood culture, urine catheterization, lumbar puncture, and chest radiograph. Admission for 24-hour monitoring is also common, to allow close monitoring of progress.

A febrile child without focal symptoms is at risk for occult bacteremia.[2] Empirical antibiotic treatment in this population is controversial because the overall incidence of adverse events in untreated children is small. Of children from 3 to 36 months of age with a fever of 39°C or higher, only 2% to 3% will have occult bacteremia (90% *Streptococcus pneumoniae*), and 75% of these will resolve spontaneously.[3, 4] One estimate indicates that 414 children would need to be treated to prevent one case of serious bacterial infection.[5] Because of the potential severe consequences for the few children who progress to meningitis (3% of those who have progressive occult bacteremia), practice guidelines have recommended collection of a urine culture, a total white blood cell (WBC) count, and blood culture. When close follow-up is possible, a well-appearing child may have urine cultures alone collected. Children with a toxic appearance and WBC greater than 15×10^9/L warrant antibiotic therapy.[6, 7]

Specific Infectious Disorders

Meningitis

One of the most dramatic and feared infectious emergencies to present to the primary care office is bacterial meningitis. The early identification and treatment of this disorder are the most important factors in decreasing morbidity and mortality. Overall mortality is estimated at 14% with variation based on the causative organism (*Haemophilus influenzae* 6%, *Neisseria meningitidis* 10.3%, and *S. pneumoniae* 26.3%) and with sensorineural hearing loss (10% in children) and learning deficits (30%) manifesting as common sequelae. Overall, the diagnosis is uncommon, with 13,000 cases estimated in 1993 and nearly three times that many patients presenting with aseptic or viral meningitis.[1]

Any patient who presents with signs and symptoms of meningeal irritation (Box 17–2) raises suspicion of meningitis. Infection of the cerebrospinal pia-arachnoid tissues leads to prominent symptoms of headache, meningismus, photophobia, and nausea/vomiting, and often is associated with changes in mental status. These symptoms may be preceded by those of upper respiratory infection (URI). In addition, systemic signs of infection such as fever/sweats and rigors may indicate a

---

Box 17–2. *Cardinal Signs of Meningitis and Initial Laboratory Testing*

Cardinal signs of Meningitis

- Headache
- Meningismus
- Altered mental status
- Photophobia
- Fever
- Preceding URI
- Nausea/Vomiting
- Rigors
- Soaking sweats
- Focal neurologic abnormalities
- Rash (in *Neisseria meningitidis*)

Laboratory Testing in the Evaluation of Possible Meningitis

CSF	*Bacterial Meningitis*
Cell count	1×10^3–1×10^5/μL (usually >500)
Differential	Predominantly PMNs
Protein	>50 mg/dL
CSF/serum glucose ratio	<40%
Gram stain	Positive 65%–95%
Bacterial antigen	*Haemophilus influenzae, Streptococcus pneumoniae, N. meningitidis*

Cultures
Blood (2 sets—aerobic and anaerobic)
CSF
Urine

Additional Laboratory Tests
Serum CBC/differential
Serum electrolytes
Serum glucose (for comparison with CSF)

CBC, complete blood count; CSF, cerebrospinal fluid; PMNs, polymorphonuclear leukocytes; URI, upper respiratory infection.

concurrent bacteremia or sepsis. The differential diagnosis includes any state that can lead to meningeal irritation, including viral meningitis or encephalitis, and subarachnoid hemorrhage.

Figure 17–2 outlines the evaluation and treatment of a patient with

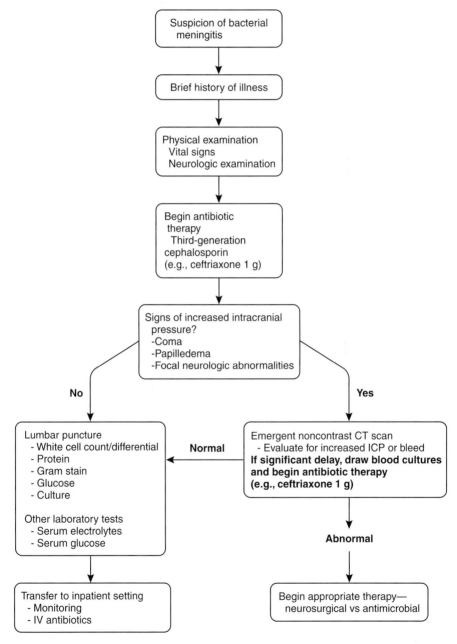

Figure 17–2. Evaluation of a patient with suspected meningitis. CT, computed tomography; ICP, intracranial pressure.

suspected bacterial meningitis. Initial evaluation comprises a brief history of onset of symptoms, predisposing conditions (e.g., immunosuppression, alcoholism, age extremes), and full physical examination, including direct ophthalmoscopy to view the fundus for signs of increased intracranial pressure (papilledema) or intracranial hemorrhage (retinal hemorrhage). Once meningitis is included in the differential, prompt lumbar puncture for collection of CSF should be undertaken. If there is concern for the possibility of increased intracranial pressure (presence of coma, papilledema, or focal neurologic findings), then an immediate CT scan should be undertaken before lumbar puncture is performed. This study provides information regarding intracranial pressure (ICP) and subarachnoid hemorrhage. Despite its potential benefit, it must be kept in mind that this maneuver is a major contributor to delayed initiation of empirical antibiotic therapy,[8] and antibiotics should be started before lumbar puncture is performed if there is a high level of suspicion for bacterial meningitis.

Laboratory evaluation includes CSF for color, WBC count with differential, Gram stain, culture, protein, and glucose (drawing serum glucose also). Opening pressure should be measured with the patient lying on his or her side (>180 mm H_2O suggests meningitis). Blood cultures are positive 70% to 80% of the time in cases of bacterial meningitis. Serum electrolytes help in the evaluation of metabolic derangements. Management includes urgent admission to an ICU setting for monitoring and treatment.

Treatment

Because of the importance of beginning antibiotic therapy promptly in patients with suspected bacterial meningitis, empirical therapy should begin immediately with a third-generation cephalosporin (e.g., cefotaxime or ceftriaxone) to cover *S. pneumoniae* and *N. meningitidis*. Some experts recommend the addition of vancomycin to cover beta-lactam–resistant *S. pneumoniae*. In patients younger than 3 months of age or older than 50, ampicillin is added to cover *Streptococcus agalactiae* and *Listeria monocytogenes*. The use of corticosteroids in adults with meningitis remains controversial owing to an increase in the number of adverse events, particularly gastrointestinal bleeding. Once a specific organism is identified, antibiotic therapy should be changed to cover the specific organism.

Pediatrics

Young patients must be evaluated based on their age. The causative organisms in neonates are generally group B streptococci, *E. coli*, *Enterococcus* species, or *L. monocytogenes*. In infants and children, *H. influenzae* has been the predominant organism, but it appears to be greatly reduced in those who have received the *Haemophilus influenzae* type B (HIB) vaccine series. *S. pneumoniae* and *N. meningitidis* are involved in the bulk of remaining cases. In adults, *S. pneumoniae* and *N. meningitidis* are most commonly followed by other staphylococcal, streptococcal, and *Listeria* species. Possible ports of entry include invasion from the oropharynx or a sinus and bacteremia from a pulmonary or abdominal source. Additional imaging should include chest radiograph if pneumonia is considered. Glucocorticoid therapy has been found to reduce some neurologic sequelae in children and should be given at the time of the first dose of antibiotics at a dose of 0.15 mg/kg of dexamethasone every 6 hours for 4 days.[8]

Community-Acquired Pneumonia

Patients presenting with signs and symptoms of community-acquired pneumonia (CAP) represent an incidence of 1200 per 100,000 population per year. The average U.S. primary care physician is estimated to see two to three patients with CAP per year.[9] Risk factors for hospitalization include age extremes, comorbid illness, and significant physical examination abnormalities (Box 17–3). Cardinal symptoms include cough and fever, pleuritic chest pain, chills, and bloody sputum. Signs include respiratory distress such as tachypnea (with tachycardia or bradycardia) and cyanosis. The patient may also complain of abdominal pain and anorexia. Increasing age (>65 yr) has been shown to be associated with fewer symptoms and contributes to a higher mortality rate among these patients.[10] Atypical agents such as *Mycoplasma pneumoniae* and *Chlamydia pneumoniae* have been shown to account for up to a third of the patients with pneumonia; initial symptoms could not reliably distinguish these from bacterial pathogens such as *S. pneumoniae*.[11]

Box 17–3. *Initial Evaluation for Suspicion of Community-Acquired Pneumonia (CAP)*

Risk factors
Age extremes (<60 days, >50 yr)
Smoking
Comorbidity

Cardinal signs/symptoms
Fever
Chills
Cough
Rusty sputum
Pleuritic chest pain

Risk factors for hospitalization[13]
Age >50 yr
Coexisting illness

Box continued on following page

> ## Box 17–3. *Initial Evaluation for Suspicion of Community-Acquired Pneumonia (CAP)* Continued
>
> Neoplastic disease, congestive heart failure, cerebrovascular
>   disease, renal disease, liver disease
> Physical examination abnormalities
>   Change of mental status
>   Pulse >125 bpm
>   Respiratory rate >30
>   Systolic blood pressure <90 mm Hg
>   Temperature <35°C or >40°C
> Laboratory and radiographic findings
>   Arterial pH <7.35
>   BUN >30
>   Sodium <130
>   Glucose >250
>   Hematocrit <30%
>   Pulse oximetry <90, or SpO_2 <60 mm Hg (room air)
>   Pleural effusion
> *Absence of any of these risk factors is associated with 0.1% mortality and outpatient management is appropriate. The presence of two or more risk factors is associated with increasing mortality, and at least brief inpatient management should be considered.*
>
> **Initial evaluation**
> Full physical examination (vital signs, pulmonary and neurologic
>   work-up)
> Imaging studies
>   Chest radiograph
> Laboratory work
>   CBC with differential
>   Electrolytes
>   Blood cultures (2 sets of aerobic and anaerobic)
>   Arterial blood gas (with signs of hypoxia, including significant
>   respiratory distress)
>
> CBC, complete blood count.

Physical examination of the lungs may reveal signs of parenchymal involvement (e.g., rales, egophony, whispered pectoriloquy) or pleural involvement (e.g., dullness to percussion, friction rub, reduced breath sounds). Auscultation should be carried out in a careful and systematic manner in a quiet area; all lung fields should be listened to, including the axillary areas. Ask patients to take full, deep respirations through an open mouth.

Blood cultures should be collected before initiation of antibiotic therapy. These are positive for the causative organism in 10% to 20% of cases of bacterial pneumonia.[12] Sputum Gram stains that identify gram-positive diplococci or other organisms can be very helpful in determination of initial antibiotic choices. Identification of a definite organism and sensitivities should be used to modify the initial antibiotic choice (see later). However, even if cultures are obtained properly, a causative organism is identified only 50% to 60% of the time. Chest radiographs should be obtained to confirm a diagnosis of pneumonia (including lateral decubitus films if there are signs of pleural involvement). Arterial blood gas measurement should be performed in any patient who is in respiratory distress. A complete blood count with differential should be collected, along with electrolytes, for the evaluation of WBC response, acid-base status, and fluid derangements.

A number of guidelines have been developed to aid in the risk stratification of patients and their initial management and disposition. Fine and associates[13, 14] showed that for adults, a prediction rule based on a scoring system that uses age greater than 50 years, comorbidity, and physical examination findings could accurately identify patients with low risk for death and serious morbidity. Briefly, any adult patient younger than 50 years of age without coexisting illness (e.g., neoplastic disease, congestive heart failure [CHF], cerebrovascular disease, renal disease, liver disease) or specific physical examination abnormalities (e.g., altered mental status, pulse > 125, respirations > 30/min, systolic blood pressure [SBP] < 90 mm Hg, or temperature < 35°C or > 40°C) is in the lowest risk class (class I) with a mortality risk of 0.1 to 0.4 and can be treated as an outpatient unless he or she presents with hypoxemia (pulse oximetry < 90% O_2 saturation at room air or SpO_2 of < 60 mm Hg). Any patient older than age 50 would immediately be placed in a class II level of risk with additional risk variables adding to the class level. Patients in levels II to III who are so classified because of age and a single comorbidity can be considered for outpatient therapy, potentially with home nursing and parenteral antibiotics. Patients with increasing risk variables (class IV to V, with mortality risk of 4% to 10% and >10%, respectively) or who present with hypoxemia should be admitted to the hospital at least briefly for therapy and monitoring.

Treatment

As is summarized in Box 17–4, the initial therapy for CAP includes IV hydration, oxygen supplementation if there are signs of hypoxemia, and the initiation of antibiotic therapy. For outpatient management of adults over the age of 18, azithromycin (500 mg PO × 1, then 250 mg PO qd × 4 days) or clarithromycin (500 mg PO bid × 14 days) is recommended for the coverage of *S. pneumoniae*, *H. influenzae*, *C. pneumoniae*, and *M. pneumoniae*.

Box 17–4. *Initial Treatment of Community-Acquired Pneumonia (CAP)*

Hydration
Oxygen supplementation
Antipyretic
Antibiotic therapy
  Outpatient regimens (>18 yr of age)
  • Azithromycin 500 mg PO × 1, then 250 mg PO qd × 4 days
  • levofloxacin (or other fluoroquinolone with enhanced antipneumococcal activity)
  Inpatient
  • Third-generation cephalosporin (ceftriaxone 500 mg IV or IM qd) + macrolide (erythromycin 15–20 mg/kg/day divided q6hr) OR fluoroquinolone (levofloxacin 500 mg qd)
  • Aqueous penicillin G 6×10^6 units q12h + macrolide
  Pediatric
  • Neonatal (inpatient)—Ampicillin + gentamicin
  • Infant 1–3 mo (inpatient)—Erythromycin 10 mg/kg IV q6h
  • Children 3 mo–5yr (outpatient)—Erythromycin 10 mg/kg PO qid (Inpatient)—Cefuroxime 50 mg/kg IV Q8h + Erythromycin 10 mg/kg IV q6h
  • Patients 5–18 yr (outpatient)—Azithromycin 500 mg × 1, then 250 mg qd

---

Fluoroquinolones with enhanced activity against *S. pneumoniae*, such as levofloxacin and sparfloxacin, also provide adequate coverage. Patients who receive inpatient, non-ICU therapy can be treated with a third-generation cephalosporin (such as ceftriaxone 500 mg) IV or IM with the addition of a macrolide (erythromycin 15 to 20 mg/kg per day divided q6h, or azithromycin 500 mg IV q24h) or a fluoroquinolone with enhanced *S. pneumoniae* activity (levofloxacin 500 mg PO/IV qd). Awareness of local antibiotic resistance patterns, particularly resistance to macrolides, fluoroquinolones, or penicillin in *S. pneumoniae*, helps the physician to determine which regimen may be most effective in specific communities. Immunization of at-risk populations with the appropriate conjugated vaccines is an important part of infection control and should not be neglected.[15]

Pediatrics

From the neonatal period to 3 months of age, all febrile patients require inpatient therapy, and initial evaluation should include blood cultures. Neonatal pneumonia, most likely due to group B streptococcus or *E. coli*, is treated with an initial dose of ampicillin (50 mg) plus an aminoglycoside such as amikacin (10 mg), which may have less ototoxicity than gentamicin. Ongoing treatment schedules depend on the weight and age of the neonate. In patients from age 1 to 3 months, pneumonitis syndrome (usually afebrile) may result from *Chlamydia trachomatis* infection (although RSV is possible), and PO therapy with clarithromycin (7.5 mg/kg bid × 10 to 14 days) or IV therapy with erythromycin (10 mg/kg IV q6h × 10 to 14 days) is indicated. In patients from 3 months to 5 years of age, outpatient therapy can be instituted with erythromycin (10 mg/kg PO qid) or clarithromycin (7.5 mg/kg bid); hospitalized patients should receive cefuroxime plus erythromycin. From ages 5 to 18 years, clarithromycin (500 mg PO bid) or azithromycin (500 mg PO × 1, then 250 mg PO × 4 days) can be used in the outpatient setting.[16] Radiographic imaging plays an important role in the diagnosis and management of patients with pediatric pneumonia and should be employed as needed.[17]

Cystitis, Pyelonephritis, and Urosepsis

Infection of the urinary bladder (cystitis) is common among adult women but is cause for concern among young children and males of any age. Presenting symptoms include urinary urgency, burning on urination, the sense of incomplete bladder emptying, and painful bladder spasm. Diagnosis is made with the combination of clinical symptoms, urine dip positive for leukocyte esterase and nitrites, microscopic examination positive for more than 5 WBCs per high-power field (centrifuged and decanted 10-mL sample in the absence of epithelial cells suggesting inadequate cleaning), and urine culture with more than 1×10^5 colony-forming units of a single organism. Urine samples should be collected with the use of a midstream clean-catch procedure, including cleansing with aseptic wipes.

Infection of the upper urinary tract, or pyelonephritis, is a relatively common complication of simple cystitis in the healthy adult. Risk factors include female sex, pregnancy, history of lower or upper urinary tract infection, and mechanical instrumentation of the lower urinary tract. Cardinal signs/symptoms of pyelonephritis include fever (>38°C), rigors, flank pain on percussion, and evidence of infection on examination and culture of a urine sample. This may advance to urosepsis, particularly in the patient in a debilitated physical state.

Sepsis, or the systemic inflammatory response syndrome (SIRS), is defined by two or more of the following criteria: abnormalities of body temperature (>38°C or <36°C); heart rate greater than 90 beats per minute; respiratory rate greater than 20 breaths per minute or a $PaCO_2 < 32$ mm Hg; total WBC count of more than 12,000 cells/mm^3 or less than 4000 cells/mm^3 or more than 10% band forms on the manual WBC differential count.[18] Risk factors for the development of sepsis include advanced age, debilitated state, dementia, the presence of an indwelling urinary catheter, and recent instrumentation of the bladder for urinary therapy or diagnostic studies.

Initial evaluation should include assessment of illness severity with patients who show signs of sepsis requiring immediate testing and therapy, including a bolus of 250 to 500 mL of normal saline through a large-bore IV catheter; urine and blood cultures; respiratory support through a nasal cannula or mask; and antimicrobial therapy within 30 minutes of evaluation. A pelvic examination should be included in sexually active women with signs of upper urinary tract infection to enable evaluation of possible pelvic inflammatory disease.

Treatment

Treatment regimens for simple cystitis in women of reproductive age include trimethoprim-sulfamethoxazole (TMP-SMX, 1 DS tablet PO bid × 3 days), a fluoroquinolone (ciprofloxacin 250 mg PO bid × 3 days), or nitrofurantoin (100 mg PO bid × 7 to 10 days) in pregnancy. Unless local resistance to sulfa drugs is high among *E. coli* strains or the patient has a sulfa allergy, TMP-SMX is the medication of choice.

Cystitis in men between the ages of 15 and 50 is rare. Short-course treatments have not been studied in men; therefore, a 10- to 14-day course of TMP-SMX, ciprofloxacin, or levofloxacin (250 mg PO every day) is prudent. Follow-up evaluation of a possible mechanical cause of this infection is needed.

For patients presenting in a toxic state, who are unable to take PO fluids and/or who require hospitalization, intramuscular and intravenous antimicrobial treatment may be started in the office setting if supplies are available. As discussed earlier, broad-spectrum antibiotics should be initiated within 30 minutes of evaluation of a patient with possible urosepsis (after blood and urine cultures are collected). Ampicillin or trimethoprim-sulfamethoxazole in combination with an aminoglycoside has excellent coverage for possible urosepsis. Oral therapy with a 7-day course of fluoroquinolones, including ciprofloxacin (500 mg bid) or levofloxacin (500 mg qd), is generally indicated for acute uncomplicated pyelonephritis. Alternatives include amoxicillin/clavulanate (bid × 14 days), or trimethoprim-sulfamethoxazole (DS bid × 14 days). Patients considered for this type of management should be brought back to the office within 72 hours for review of progress.

Criteria for hospitalization include those discussed in the earlier section "The Acutely Toxic Patient," in addition to suspicion of complicated pyelonephritis, including sepsis, renal abscess, or renal failure. Other comorbid conditions such as diabetes or renal insufficiency lower the threshold for hospital admission. Inpatient management of pyelonephritis includes ampicillin in combination with an aminoglycoside, an IV fluoroquinolone, or a third-generation cephalosporin. Therapy should be continued for 14 days, although patients can generally be discharged for home antibiotic therapy within 24 hours of becoming afebrile. Patients with suspected sepsis should be admitted to an ICU setting for continuous monitoring and therapies.

Pediatrics

Pediatric patients require a number of special considerations for the diagnosis and therapy of lower and upper urinary tract infections. The diagnoses of cystitis, pyelonephritis, and urosepsis should be considered in children (boys and girls) with fever lacking localizing signs. In the preschool population, irritability, dysuria, and secondary incontinence (after toilet training is completed) are often associated with urinary tract infection (UTI). In the school-age child, dysuria is a common complaint. Diagnosis in a toilet-trained child can be made from the examination and culture of a properly collected midstream urine sample. Neonates and infants require catheterization or suprapubic aspiration for adequate samples to be collected (external bag collection is not adequate). Samples collected in this manner are considered to have significant bacterial colonization with colony counts of a single organism 1 to 2 logs lower than those collected by clean-catch technique. Evaluation of occult bacteremia in infants includes urinalysis and culture in all children younger than 6 months of age.[19]

Treatment of pyelonephritis in children under the age of 16 should not include the use of fluoroquinolone antibiotics because of the effect that these have on developing cartilage. Most patients with UTIs do not require admission and can be treated with a single injection of ceftriaxone (25 mg/kg) followed by 7 to 10 days of TMP-SMX. Acute pyelonephritis requiring hospitalization should be treated with a 3- to 5-day course of IV antibiotics such as ampicillin with gentamicin, or cefotaxime followed by oral antibiotics such as ampicillin, TMP-SMX, cefadroxil, or cefaclor, for a total of 14 days of therapy.

Because of the high level of permanent renal injury associated with pyelonephritis in children, follow-up evaluation should be carried out; this includes testing for vesicoureteral reflux. Ultrasonography and voiding cystourethrography should be carried out in all children younger than 5 years of age at the time of first febrile UTI (some authors recommend this until the age of 10).

References

1. Graves E: Detailed Diagnoses and Procedures, National Hospitals Discharge Survey for 1993. Hyattsville, Md, National Center for Health Statistics, 1994.
2. Pena BM, Harper MB, Fleisher GR: Occult bacteremia with group B streptococci in an outpatient setting. Pediatrics 102:67–72, 1998.
3. Kuppermann N: Occult bacteremia in young febrile children. Pediatr Clin North Am 46:1073–1090, 1999.
4. Ros SP, Herman BE, Beissel TJ: Occult bacteremia: Is there a standard of care? Pediatr Emerg Care 10:264–267, 1994.

5. Bulloch B, Craig WR, Klassen TP: The use of antibiotics to prevent serious sequelae in children at risk for occult bacteremia: A meta-analysis. Acad Emerg Med 4:679–683, 1997.
6. Gombos MM, Bienkowski RS, Gochman RF, Billett HH: The absolute neutrophil count: Is it the best indicator for occult bacteremia in infants? Am J Clin Pathol 109:221–225, 1998.
7. Yamamoto LG, Worthley RG, Melish ME, Seto DS: A revised decision analysis of strategies in the management of febrile children at risk for occult bacteremia. Am J Emerg Med 16:193–207, 1998.
8. Quagliarello VJ, Scheld M: Treatment of bacterial meningitis. N Engl J Med 336:708–716, 1997.
9. Bartlett JG: Update in infectious diseases. Ann Intern Med 133:285–292, 2000.
10. Metlay JP, Schulz R, Li YH, et al: Influence of age on symptoms at presentation in patients with community-acquired pneumonia. Arch Intern Med 157:1453–1459, 1997.
11. Marrie TJ, Peeling RW, Fine MJ, et al: Ambulatory patients with community-acquired pneumonia: The frequency of atypical agents and clinical course. Am J Med 101:508–515, 1996.
12. Bryan CS: Blood cultures for community-acquired pneumonia: No place to skimp [editorial comment]. Chest 116:1153–1155, 1999.
13. Fine MJ, Auble TE, Yealy DM, et al: A prediction rule to identify low-risk patients with community-acquired pneumonia [see comments]. N Engl J Med 336:243–250, 1997.
14. Fine MJ, Hough LJ, Medsger AR, et al: The hospital admission decision for patients with community-acquired pneumonia. Results from the pneumonia Patient Outcomes Research Team cohort study [see comments]. Arch Intern Med 157:36–44, 1997.
15. Fine MJ, Smith MA, Carson CA, et al: Efficacy of pneumococcal vaccination in adults. A meta-analysis of randomized controlled trials. Arch Intern Med 154:2666–2677, 1994.
16. Schaad UB: Antibiotic therapy of childhood pneumonia. Pediatr Pulmonol Suppl 18:146–149, 1999.
17. Donnelly LF: Maximizing the usefulness of imaging in children with community-acquired pneumonia. AJR Am J Roentgen 172:505–512, 1999.
18. American College of Chest Physicians and Society of Critical Care Medicine Consensus Conference Committee: Definition of sepsis and organ failure and guidelines for the use of innovative therapies in sepsis. Crit Care Med 20:864, 1992.
19. Alpern ER, Alessandrini EA, Bell LM, et al: Occult bacteremia from a pediatric emergency department: Current prevalence, time to detection, and outcome. Pediatrics 106:505–511, 2000.

Chapter 18

Head and Neck Emergencies

Kevin M. Curtis

Ear, Nose, and Throat Emergencies

Foreign Bodies in the Ear

Foreign bodies in the ear are a fairly common problem, particularly in children. In one study of patients who presented to an ear, nose, and throat (ENT) service with foreign bodies in the ear, 12% were younger than 6 years of age, and 48% were between 2 and 3 years of age.[1] Objects commonly found in the ears of children include beads, parts of toys, food, and paper. Adults tend to acquire foreign bodies through self-instrumentation, particularly with pieces of cotton swabs or matchsticks. An unusually troublesome foreign body found in all age groups is the insect, with the most common being cockroaches. Although the large majority of foreign bodies in the external auditory canal are not true emergencies, the resulting symptoms may be very distressing for the patient, and removal is certainly indicated. One exception to the nonemergent nature of these situations is the button battery, which has the potential for erosive perforation of the tympanic membrane.

Patients may present with a clear history of a foreign body and/or with symptoms of pain, fullness, discharge, or decreased hearing. Patients may also be completely asymptomatic and the object detected on routine examination. If possible, it is helpful to ascertain the type of object that is involved, as well as the duration of the problem. Important aspects of the physical examination include identification of the foreign body and, if the tympanic membrane can be visualized, assessment of the presence or absence of perforation.

Because foreign bodies in the ear are generally of no significant danger to the patient, it is imperative that removal does not result in more damage than was caused by the initial insult. Fortunately, most objects are located in the outer two thirds of the external auditory canal. Several methods of removal have been described, including irrigation, suction, and removal under direct visualization.

235

Anesthesia. The external auditory canal is exquisitely sensitive, and foreign body removal is often quite painful. To avoid iatrogenic injury, it is important that the patient remain still during removal. Therefore, although often unnecessary, sedation and local anesthesia should at least be considered. In small children, local anesthesia is usually impractical and sedation is necessary. In some cases, children may require referral to an ENT physician for removal under general anesthesia.

Injections of local anesthesia are given as a four-quadrant block, using a total of 1 to 2 mL of lidocaine (1:100,000) with epinephrine. With a 25- or 27-gauge needle, four subcutaneous injections are administered at the site of entry of the external auditory canal (Fig. 18–1). Adequate visualization with the use of a headlamp or mirror is essential and, if possible, the injections should be given through a large metal ear speculum.

Equipment
  Headlamp or other light source
  Ear speculum (large metal type preferable)

For Irrigation Technique
  10- to 20-mL syringe
  Butterfly catheter or 18-gauge Teflon IV catheter
  Normal saline (room temperature)

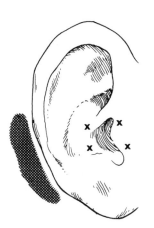

X Points of injection for
     local anesthesia of external
     auditory canal.

  Area of injection for
     local anesthesia of pinna.

Figure 18–1. Sites of injection for anesthesia of the external auditory meatus. (From Stair T: Practical Management of Eye, Ear, Nose, Mouth, and Throat Emergencies. Rockville, Md, Aspen Systems Corporation, 1986, p 42.)

For Suction Technique
  No. 5 Frazier suction tip (or modified IV tubing)

For Direct Visualization Removal
  Alligator forceps
  Right-angle hook
  Earwax wire loop or curette

For Insects
  Mineral oil (microscope immersion oil) or 2% lidocaine
  Equipment for irrigation or direct visualization removal, as listed
  previously

Removal

The choice of removal technique is based on familiarity, equipment availability, and the type of foreign body. Irrigation is easy and fairly effective for most objects. It should not be used, however, for organic or absorbent objects that swell when wet (i.e., food/vegetative matter, paper). Irrigation should also be avoided when there is a known tympanic membrane perforation. Suction is useful for smooth objects that are difficult to grab. Direct visualization removal is appropriate for objects that are uniquely amenable to the use of specific instruments (see later), or when less invasive techniques are unsuccessful.

Irrigation. The goal of irrigation is to direct fluid around the object so that back-pressure develops and forces the foreign body out. The catheter should be inserted only into the outer cartilaginous canal, however. A kidney basin is held under the ear to collect the fluid. Room temperature normal saline is used to avoid caloric stimulation of the inner ear.

1. If a butterfly needle is used, the metal needle and plastic butterfly are cut off and the tubing cut to 2 to 3 cm.
2. Attach the IV catheter or butterfly catheter to a 10- or 20-mL syringe, filled with saline.
3. Place the catheter into the external canal, aimed along the superior wall, and irrigate.

Suction. An alternative to the Frazier suction tip, with less risk of canal trauma, is a section of IV tubing.[1] The end of the tubing needs to be modified to a flange, however, and the literature recommends the use of a "preheated metal atomizer tip" to accomplish this.

Direct Visualization. The right-angle hook is ideal for hard, spherical objects such as beads. The correct approach is to pass the hook beyond the object, turn it 90 degrees, and then withdraw. The loop and curette are better for softer objects that can be scooped out, and the alligator forceps should be considered for irregularly shaped foreign bodies that can be grasped. The mouth of the alligator forceps should not be opened until the tool is in the vicinity of the object.

Insects. The presence of an insect in the ear can cause a great degree of patient discomfort, not only aesthetically, but also from movement of the insect in the canal and against the tympanic membrane. In these cases, the first step is to kill the insect. This can be accomplished with either 2% lidocaine or mineral oil.[2] Once this has been done, either irrigation or removal by direct visualization can be performed.

Disposition

It is important that the clinician repeat the ear examination after the foreign body has been removed. This ensures that removal has been successful; it also allows better examination of the tympanic membrane and provides an opportunity for evaluation of any damage incurred as a result of the procedure. Minimal lacerations of the external auditory canal can be treated with observation alone or with topical antibiotics. Antipyrine/benzocaine (Auralgan) should be offered as needed for several days. Oral antibiotics are indicated only for associated infection.

Most patients who have undergone successful removal of a foreign body from the ear do not require ENT referral. Exceptions include those with tympanic membrane perforation, persistent symptoms of hearing loss or vertigo, or more than minimal trauma to the canal. These patients, in addition to those for whom removal was unsuccessful, should be seen by an ENT physician within 24 hours. Patients with persistence of a button battery or insect require emergent referral.

Cerumen Impaction

Cerumen impaction is most often an incidental finding that obscures visualization of the tympanic membrane. If the blockage is complete, hearing loss may occur. Although cotton-tipped applicators may remove peripheral wax, they often cause deeper impaction. Removal of the cerumen may be accomplished by irrigating with saline or by using an ear curette or wire loop (see "Foreign Bodies in the Ear" earlier in this chapter). It may be beneficial to apply carbamide peroxide (Debrox) to soften the cerumen before definitive removal is undertaken.

Foreign Bodies in the Nose

Foreign bodies are the most common cause of nasal obstruction in children. Because of the underlying anatomy, objects are most often located below the inferior turbinate (on the nasal floor), or they are found anterior to the middle turbinate. Common objects include erasers, paper, pebbles, beads, buttons, food, and parts of toys.

Clinical Presentation

The history may be a witnessed episode of placement of the object into the nose, or it may include symptoms of nasal obstruction or persistent discharge. Pain is not a characteristic symptom of nasal foreign bodies. Initially, the discharge is usually mucoid, but it may progress to a muco-purulent form. In a child presenting with a purulent, unilateral nasal discharge, a nasal foreign body must be considered.

Equipment

Needed in All Cases
Headlamp (or mirror with an indirect light source)
Nasal speculum

Needed in Some Cases
Combination local anesthetic/topical vasoconstrictor (4% lidocaine/phenylephrine)
Long bayonet forceps or alligator forceps
Suction with No. 5 Frazier tip
Right-angle hook
Wire loop

Removal

In cases in which any intranasal manipulation is planned and/or in which it can be easily accomplished, the nasal mucosa should be prepared with a combination local anesthetic/vasoconstrictor. A good option is a 1:1 combination of 0.5% (or 1%) phenylephrine and 4% lidocaine, applied as a spray or as drops. Sedation may be needed in a minority of cases; occasionally, general anesthesia is required. One of the drawbacks of sedation is the increased risk for aspiration of the foreign body if it should be inhaled or forced posteriorly.

An initial attempt should be made to force the foreign body out through exhalation. Those patients who are old enough should be instructed to take a deep breath in, then to exhale with the mouth shut and the un-involved naris occluded, with the index finger placed alongside the nose. For the young child, the procedure is as follows[3]:

Procedure—Removal by "Mouth-to-Mouth" Approach
1. Have the child lie supine on the parent's lap.
2. With one hand, the parent should stabilize the child's chin while holding the mouth open.
3. With the thumb of the other hand, the unobstructed naris is gently occluded.

4. The parent then makes a firm "mouth-to-mouth" seal and delivers a short, sharp puff of air.

If this technique is unsuccessful, either suction or removal through direct visualization should be attempted. With both procedures, adequate visualization (provided by a headlamp, or a mirror and light source) and the use of a nasal speculum are essential. Blind probing or repeated unsuccessful attempts should be discouraged because they may force the object farther posteriorly and result in either aspiration or a more difficult removal. The patient should be seated upright, leaning slightly forward in the "sniffing" position. Insertion of the nasal speculum is accomplished with the handle horizontal and the lower blade along the floor of the nasal cavity.

Examination of the intranasal object may provide an indication of the best technique for removal. For irregular or smaller objects such as cloth or paper, the bayonet forceps work well. For foreign bodies that are more difficult to grasp, including round objects such as beads or pebbles, suction, curved hooks, or wire loops should be considered. Unlike with foreign bodies in the ear, irrigation should not be performed.

It is essential that a repeat examination be performed after removal of the foreign body to ensure complete removal, to look for a second object, and to examine for any trauma or epistaxis.

Disposition

Patients with a button battery that cannot be removed need emergent ENT referral owing to the risk of erosive injury. In addition, anyone with a persistent foreign body who is thought to be at high risk for aspiration should be referred emergently. For other patients who have undergone unsuccessful removal of a nasal foreign body, or for those with a strongly suspected but not visualized object, referral to an ENT physician within 24 hours is appropriate.

Epistaxis

Nosebleeds are a common problem that can often be managed with the use of minimally invasive techniques. The blood supply to the nasal mucosa is provided via both the external and internal carotid arteries through multiple anastomoses. For the purpose of determining cause and providing treatment, epistaxis is classified as anterior or posterior. Approximately 90% of all nosebleeds are of the anterior type, with most occurring in Kiesselbach's plexus on the anterior septum (Fig. 18–2). The majority of these can be managed in an office setting. Posterior nosebleeds should be addressed by an otolaryngologist.

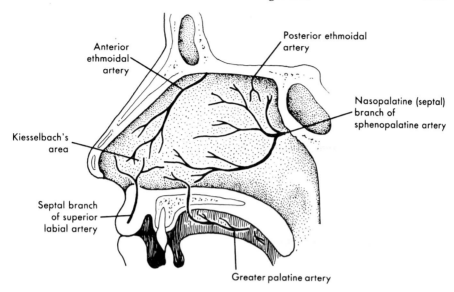

Figure 18–2. Kiesselbach's plexus. (From Rosen P [ed]: Emergency Medicine Concepts and Clinical Practice, 4th ed. St. Louis, Mosby, 1998, p 2726.)

The most common causes of epistaxis are upper respiratory infection and trauma (including nose picking).[3] Many cases of epistaxis have no clear underlying cause, however. The history should include questions on the use of aspirin or anticoagulants; the use of intranasal cocaine; any previous blood dyscrasias; history of liver disease; renal failure; or the use of immunosuppressive medications. Although hypertension does not appear to play a role in the initiation of epistaxis, it may contribute to the persistence of bleeding. More commonly, elevated blood pressure associated with epistaxis may be a reflection of apprehension rather than indicating an underlying medical condition. A history of trauma should be noted so the clinician can consider the presence of other injuries and the possibility of a septal hematoma. Measures used by the patient before presentation may indicate the likelihood of success of direct pressure alone. Finally, in the case of apparent bilateral epistaxis, it is often helpful for the clinician to determine the nostril from which the bleeding began because it is most often the only naris that requires treatment.

Most patients with nosebleeds do not need any laboratory tests. Exceptions may include those on anticoagulants as well as patients with a history that suggests a bleeding disorder.

Equipment

All necessary equipment should be assembled before the examination is begun.

Frequently Needed Instruments
Headlamp (or other light source)
Suction with No. 5 Frazier tip
Nasal speculum
Cotton-tipped applicators
Bayonet forceps
Topical anesthetic/vasoconstrictor
Silver nitrate sticks
Merocel (Medtronic Xomed, Jacksonville, Florida) nasal tampon (5 cm)
Cotton balls
Kidney basin
Towels
Petroleum-jelly–impregnated gauze ($\frac{1}{2}$″ × 72″) (optional)

Additional Items for Posterior Epistaxis
Merocel (Medtronic Xomed, Jacksonville, Florida) nasal tampon (10 cm) or
Nasostat (Sparta, Pleasanton, Calif) balloon with lidocaine (Xylocaine)
  jelly or 10, 12, or 14 Fr Foley catheter with a 30-mL balloon, along
  with a hemostat or umbilical clamp
Lidocaine jelly

Management
The first step in the management of epistaxis is to apply direct pressure. First, the patient should forcibly evacuate the nose of all blood and clots and then apply continuous pressure for 10 minutes (Fig. 18–3). The patient should be encouraged to watch the clock during this period and should be discouraged from stopping periodically to check for persistent bleeding. This latter step can be done while equipment is being gathered.

For a proper physical examination, the patient should be seated upright, leaning slightly forward in the "sniffing" position. If appropriate, the patient should reevacuate the nose of any blood. A combination topical anesthetic and vasoconstrictor should be applied. A good option is a 1:1 combination of 4% lidocaine and 0.5% (or 1%) phenylephrine. The maximum dose of 4% lidocaine is 4 mL in adults and 3 mg/kg in children.[4] The anesthetic can be administered by spraying or by wetting a cotton ball with the solution and inserting it into the nose. The patient should be instructed to hold the cotton ball in place, in the region of the bleeding, by applying pressure with the index finger on the outside of the nose. After 5 minutes, a complete examination should be possible.

Anterior Epistaxis. In all cases, a good light source and a nasal speculum are necessary. The nasal speculum is inserted with the handle horizontal and the lower blade along the floor of the nasal cavity. If there is considerable blood or clots in the nose, attempts should be made to remove them by blowing or providing suction. The examination should

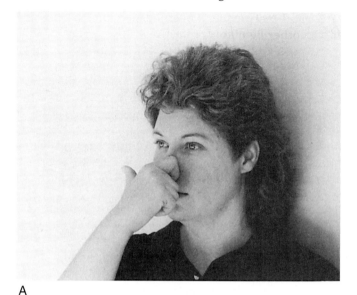

A

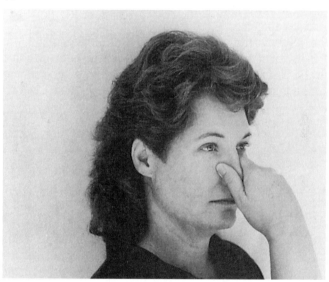

B

Figure 18–3. Direct pressure for control of epistaxis. (From Titanelli JE [ed]: Emergency Medicine: A Comprehensive Style Guide, 4th ed. New York, McGraw Hill, 1996, p 1084.)

begin with inspection of the area of Kiesselbach's plexus. At any point, if an area of recent bleeding is noted, chemical cautery is applied with a silver nitrate stick. Although there have been reports of septal perforation from overaggressive cautery, it is important that silver nitrate be applied continuously for 10 to 15 seconds while the stick is rotated. Silver nitrate is not effective in the presence of ongoing bleeding; in this case, an alternative approach must be employed. Sites with very slow bleeding may be suctioned or dabbed with a cotton-tipped applicator; silver nitrate administration should follow immediately.

If no active bleeding is noted and the previous bleeding source cannot be identified, one of two approaches should be taken. First, the clinician can attempt to induce bleeding by rubbing the mucosa in the area of Kiesselbach's plexus with a cotton-tipped applicator. The alternative is simple application of an antibiotic ointment in the region. The advantage of attempting to induce bleeding from the most likely site is that subsequent directed cautery may decrease the incidence of delayed rebleeding.

If bleeding is not controlled with use of the above measures, packing is indicated. This can be accomplished most easily with a 5-cm Merocel nasal tampon (Fig. 18–4). The tampon is made of compressed cellulose, an absorbable material that swells when wet. When the tampon is used for epistaxis, the moist nasal mucosa and blood cause it to fill the nasal cavity and tamponade the bleeding. It can be held with a bayonet forceps or a gloved hand. Antibiotic ointment can be added before placement to help prevent infection and to ease insertion. For effective use, it is important that the tampon be inserted quickly, both to minimize discomfort and to prevent it from swelling before full insertion has been accomplished. It also should be inserted until all of the tampon has been placed into the nose. Although insertion of the nasal tampon may cause discomfort, once

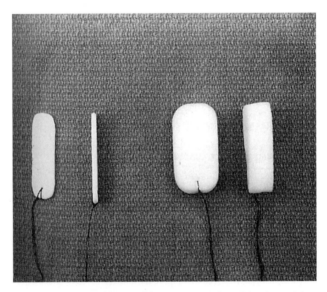

Figure 18–4. A Merocel nasal tampon in desiccated and hydrated forms. (From Titanelli JE [ed]: Emergency Medicine: A Comprehensive Style Guide, 4th ed. New York, McGraw Hill, 1996, p 1085.)

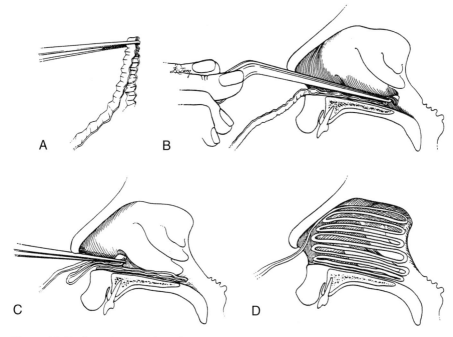

Figure 18–5. Anterior nasal packing with a gauze strip. (From Roberts JR, Hedges JR: Clinical Procedures in Emergency Medicine, 2nd ed. Philadelphia, WB Saunders, 1991, p 1034.)

in place, it is generally well tolerated. If additional expansion of the tampon is needed after insertion, the end can be irrigated with saline.

If nasal tampons are unavailable and less invasive measures have been unsuccessful, gauze packing should be considered. With the use of the nasal speculum and the bayonet forceps, Vaseline gauze is placed in layers from inferior to superior in an "accordion fashion" (Fig. 18–5). Each layer should begin as far posteriorly as possible. Good visualization is essential and blind packing is discouraged. Although the packing should not be forced tightly, 72" of gauze should be able to fit easily into the nose. A tail from the end of the gauze should be left outside of the nose for use in future removal. Only one side of the nose should be packed.

If anterior packing does not control the bleeding, or if it results in continued bleeding down the back of the throat, the source of epistaxis may be located posteriorly. This requires emergent ENT referral. If the bleeding is significant enough that temporizing measures must be done while the patient awaits ambulance transport, posterior packing should be performed.

Posterior Epistaxis. Options for treatment of posterior epistaxis include a 10-cm Merocel nasal tampon, a Nasostat balloon, or a Foley catheter. Use of the nasal tampon is similar to that described earlier, but requires

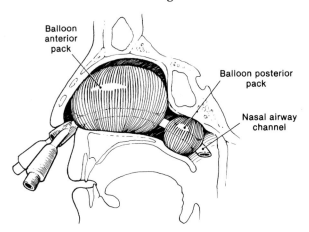

Figure 18–6. Nasostat balloon. (From Stair T: Practical Management of Eye, Ear, Nose, Mouth, and Throat Emergencies. Rockville, Md, Aspen Systems Corporation, 1986, p 92.)

the larger size. It is important that the majority of the 10 centimeters be inserted into the nares. Advantages of this option are the ease of technique as well as the fact that it also serves as an anterior pack.

The Nasostat is a double-balloon device for treatment of posterior epistaxis that is designed to also tamponade anterior bleeding (Fig. 18–6). After the balloons are checked, lidocaine jelly should be applied to the Nasostat. The device is inserted along the floor of the nose and is advanced into the nasopharynx. The posterior balloon is inflated with 4 to 8 mL of water and is gently pulled forward. The anterior balloon is inflated with 10 to 25 mL of air or water, as tolerated.

If neither of the previously mentioned items is available, a 10-, 12-, or 14-gauge Foley catheter can be used to treat posterior epistaxis. The catheter is inserted in a fashion similar to the Nasostat and is advanced until it can be seen in the nasopharynx. The balloon is slowly inflated with 5 to 15 mL of saline as guided by bleeding, pain, and resistance. Once inflated, the catheter is pulled forward and clamped at the nose with an umbilical clamp or a hemostat. An anterior pack is also required; either Merocel or Vaseline gauze can be used.

Disposition

All patients in whom bleeding resolves in the office, spontaneously or by treatment, should be observed for 30 minutes for recurrence. Instructions should be given on the proper technique for applying direct pressure. Patients should be instructed that if the problem recurs, they should apply direct pressure for one or two 10-minute sessions before seeking medical care. For those patients without packing, Vaseline or bacitracin ointment can be used three times a day. Other recommendations should instruct the patient (1) to avoid use of fingers or tissues in the area, and (2) to open the mouth when sneezing.

All patients who are treated with nasal packing require antibiotics. Because the pack occludes the sinus ostia, patients are at increased risk for sinusitis. In addition, the presence of a foreign body may introduce a risk for toxic shock syndrome. Appropriate oral antibiotics include cephalexin or amoxicillin-clavulanate. Patients with anterior packing should leave the packing in place and follow up with an ENT physician within 24 to 48 hours. Patients with posterior packing require hospital admission because of the need for sedation and the risk for hypoxia and hypercarbia. For these patients, as well as for those with persistent uncontrolled epistaxis, ENT involvement should be immediate.

Temporomandibular Joint Dislocation

Mandibular dislocation occurs as a result of trauma or during wide opening of the mouth such as occurs with yawning or laughing. The dislocation can be unilateral or bilateral and results from the condyle(s) becoming locked anterior to the articular eminence. Muscle spasm and inflammation can impede spontaneous relocation.

Clinical Presentation

Patients with temporomandibular joint (TMJ) dislocation generally present with the mouth locked open and with variable degrees of pain. It is important that the clinician ask about trauma because its presence introduces the possibility of a fracture, which warrants radiologic evaluation and/or direct referral.

Procedure for Treatment

In most cases, pretreatment with an IV benzodiazepine such as midazolam is necessary for anxiolysis and muscle relaxation. Medication alone may result in spontaneous reduction. If not, the procedure for reduction is as follows:

1. The patient should be seated with the back supported.
2. The examiner wraps gauze around the thumbs of his or her gloved hands.
3. While the examiner stands and faces the patient, the thumbs are placed inside the mouth on the occlusal surfaces of the lower, posterior teeth.
4. At the same time, the fingers grasp both sides of the mandible near the angle (Fig. 18–7).
5. A downward force is applied to the mandible to free it from the articular eminence.

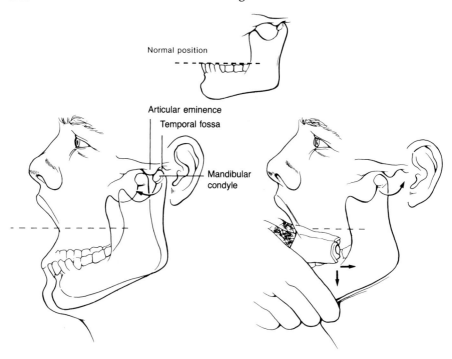

Figure 18–7. Reduction of a TMJ dislocation. (From Harwood-Nuss A [ed]: The Clinical Practice of Emergency Medicine, 2nd ed. Philadelphia, Lippincott-Raven, 1996, p 72.)

6. Once it is felt to be clear, gentle posterior pressure is applied. This step may be unnecessary because once the mandible is brought inferiorly, it often snaps back into place. (This is why it is essential to have the thumbs protected.)

Disposition

Postreduction radiographs should be considered in first-time dislocations. Traumatic cases, patients with an associated fracture, and those who have undergone unsuccessful reductions all require emergent referral to an ENT physician or for oral maxillofacial surgery. Patient instructions include a soft diet for 1 week, avoidance of wide mouth opening, use of nonsteroidal anti-inflammatory drugs (NSAIDs), and follow-up with the provider named in the referral.

Peritonsillar Abscess

Peritonsillar abscess (PTA) is the most frequent abscess of the head and neck in adults.[5] Patients are typically adolescents and young adults;

PTA is rare in those younger than 10 years of age. The palatine tonsils lie in the tonsillar fossa between the anterior and posterior pillars, with the internal carotid artery 2 to 2.5 cm posterior and lateral.[6] PTA is a complication of tonsillitis in which the infection spreads into the peritonsillar tissues, including the space between the tonsil and the superior constrictor. Infections are generally polymicrobial, with group A streptococcus being most common; they include other Gram-positive organisms, Gram-negative organisms, and anaerobes. Potential complications of PTA include airway obstruction, deep neck abscesses, mediastinitis, extension into and hemorrhage of the internal carotid artery, and septic thrombophlebitis of the internal jugular vein.

Clinical Presentation

The classic presentation of a patient with PTA follows several days of fever and sore throat, which then becomes unilateral and increasingly painful. Patients may demonstrate a muffled voice, trismus, drooling, and otalgia. Physical examination may be difficult owing to the inability of the patient to open the mouth adequately. The earliest findings are those of cellulitis with erythematous tonsils and marked unilateral erythema of the adjacent anterior tonsillar pillar and soft palate. As the infection progresses to an abscess, the palate bulges with inferior displacement of the tonsil and eventual deviation of the uvula to the unaffected side (Fig. 18–8).

Equipment

Headlamp (or other light source)
Cetacaine spray
1% lidocaine with epinephrine (1:100,000)
25- to 27-gauge needle on a 3-mL syringe
20-gauge needle on a 10-mL syringe
Scalpel with a No. 15 blade
Suction with a Frazier tip

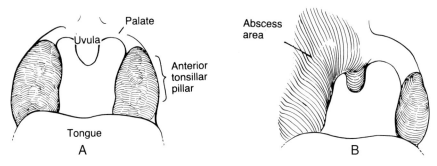

Figure 18–8. Peritonsillar abscess. (From Roberts JR, Hedges JR: Clinical Procedures in Emergency Medicine, 2nd ed. Philadelphia, WB Saunders, 1991, p 1044.)

Procedure

Drainage of a peritonsillar abscess is a procedure for the ENT surgeon. Complications of the procedure include significant bleeding, aspiration, and carotid artery laceration. Aspiration or incision in any other setting should be considered only when there is no possible ENT referral and the patient is at imminent risk for a serious complication.

A PTA can be drained by needle aspiration or by incision and drainage. In either case, the procedure should be directed toward the area of the soft palate with the most notable bulge or fluctuance. To minimize the extent of penetration and therefore the risk of internal carotid puncture, all needles and blades should be "guarded." For needles, a guard can be made by cutting the distal 0.5 cm off the plastic needle cover and placing it back over the needle. The cover is then taped to the syringe to prevent intraoral dislodgement. For the scalpel blade, tape is wrapped generously around the proximal aspect of the blade, leaving 0.5 cm exposed.

1. Have the patient seated in a chair with a headrest.
2. Apply Cetacaine spray to the general area of the abscess.
3. Locally anesthetize the area for drainage using 1% lidocaine with epinephrine via a 25- to 27-gauge needle with guard.

Aspiration

4a. Aspirate using the 20-gauge needle with guard and a 10-mL syringe.
4b. If no pus is obtained at the first site, consider repeating the procedure 1 cm caudal.

Incision and Drainage

4c. Make a gentle stab incision using the scalpel and a No. 15 blade with guard.
5. Suction as necessary.
6. Have the patient rinse with water, saline, or half-strength hydrogen peroxide.

Disposition

All patients with a possible peritonsillar abscess should be referred emergently to an ENT physician for drainage and consideration for admission and IV antibiotics. For those patients who are drained in the office and who demonstrate marked improvement in symptoms, treatment consists of oral antibiotics, analgesics, and follow-up in 24 hours. Similar outpatient treatment is appropriate for those patients diagnosed by an ENT physician with peritonsillar cellulitis as long as the patient is nontoxic, is able to tolerate fluids, and has no respiratory difficulty. An appropriate choice of antibiotics includes amoxicillin/clavulanate or clindamycin.

Ophthalmologic Emergencies

Acute Angle Closure Glaucoma

The iris divides the eye into anterior and posterior chambers. Aqueous humor, which is formed by the ciliary body, fills the posterior chamber and passes through the pupillary opening into the anterior chamber. From there, it is reabsorbed by the trabecular meshwork (Fig. 18–9). The aqueous humor provides nutrition to the lens and cornea, removes metabolic waste products, and gives the eye structural support. Intraocular pressure (IOP) is determined using the balance of production and reabsorption of aqueous humor; it is normally 10 to 21 mm Hg. The iris should contact the lens only at its posterior margin. In a patient with an underlying acute angle, sudden pupillary dilation can cause the iris to become closely

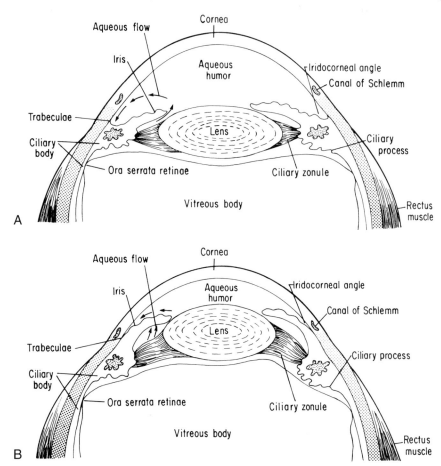

Figure 18–9. Acute angle closure glaucoma. *A,* Normal aqueous humor flow. *B,* obstructed aqueous humor flow due to acute angle closure. (From Yanofsky NN: The acute painful eye. Emerg Clin North Am 6:26, 1988.)

apposed with the trabecular meshwork, thereby obstructing the flow of aqueous humor. The result is acute angle closure glaucoma.

Acute angle closure is estimated to account for less than 5% of all cases of glaucoma,[6] but it is an ophthalmologic emergency. It is more common among hyperopic (farsighted) patients who have naturally narrower angles, in older persons, and in the presence of sudden pupillary dilation, such as occurs in a dark environment or following the use of anticholinergic or sympathomimetic agents. Many patients with acute angle closure have no obvious precipitating event, however.

The most significant complication of acute angle closure glaucoma is permanent visual loss due to ischemia of the optic nerve and retina caused by high intraocular pressure.

Clinical Presentation

The predominant symptoms of acute angle closure glaucoma include a unilateral painful eye and sudden blurred and decreased vision. Patients often have nausea and/or vomiting, and they may see halos around lights. A precipitating event that caused pupillary dilation may be elicited.

On examination, a marked decrease in visual acuity is noted. The eye is injected, most markedly in the perilimbic region. The pupil is at mid-position and is minimally or completely unresponsive to light. The cornea appears hazy and edematous. If the closed eyelid is gently palpated, the underlying globe may feel firm in comparison with that in the unaffected eye. Pathognomonic findings include an increased IOP, usually greater than 50 mm Hg.

Diagnosis

Definitive diagnosis of acute angle glaucoma is made through measurement of elevated intraocular pressure in an appropriate clinical setting. Instruments for determining IOP that may be available in the office include the Schiøtz tonometer or the tonometer pen (see following sections). In the absence of equipment to measure IOP, the "oblique flashlight" test can be used as a less accurate, qualitative assessment of the angle.[7]

Oblique Flashlight Test (Fig. 18–10)
1. Hold a penlight on the temporal side of the affected eye, perpendicular to the visual axis.
2. Gradually bring the light from posterior to anterior until the light illuminates just the lateral aspect of the iris.
3. In an eye with a normal angle, a light in this position also illuminates the nasal side of the iris.
4. In an eye with a narrow angle, a shadow is cast on the nasal side.

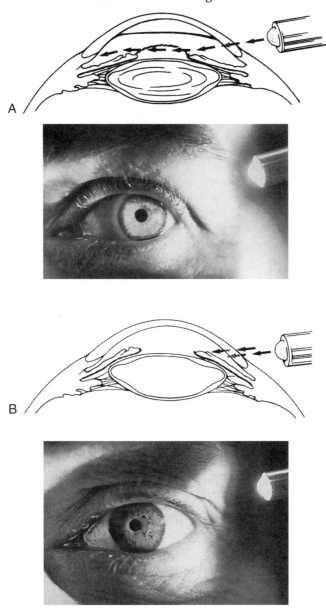

Figure 18–10. The oblique flashlight test. *A*, Normal angle. *B*, narrow angle (From Harwood-Nuss A [ed]: The Clinical Practice of Emergency Medicine, 2nd ed. Philadelphia, Lippincott-Raven, 1996, p 58.)

Although this can be a useful test, in a patient with suspected acute angle closure glaucoma, an apparently normal oblique flashlight test should not preclude emergent referral.

Tonometry

Schiøtz Tonometer. Schiøtz tonometry measures IOP by determining the degree of corneal indentation produced with a known weight. The result is expressed in units that can be directly converted to mm Hg through the use of the table provided with the tonometer. Importantly, low Schiøtz readings correspond to high IOPs.

1. Before using the tonometer, ensure that the lowest weight (5.5 g) is attached.
2. Check the Schiøtz with the convex test button provided. When placed on the test button, the plunger apparatus should move smoothly and the gauge should read zero.
3. Have the patient in a supine position.
4. Instill a drop of a topical anesthetic (proparacaine 0.5%).
5. Instruct the patient to focus on a fixed point straight ahead.
6. Hold the eyelids apart. (However, it is essential that while the eye is held open, pressure should be applied only to the bony supraorbital and infraorbital rims, not to the globe; otherwise, the resulting pressure reading will be affected.)
7. Holding the tonometer with the side handles, lower it gently onto the midpoint of the eye.
8. Note the reading on the scale and remove the tonometer.

It is generally recommended that when a low scale reading is obtained (e.g., <4 units), the measurement should be repeated with a heavier weight to determine the definitive IOP. This is usually unnecessary in the office setting, however, because a qualitatively high IOP in the clinical setting of acute angle closure glaucoma requires treatment and emergent referral.

Tonometer Pens. Tonometer pens are battery-operated devices that are also based on the principle of indentation tonometry. The eye is anesthetized in the same manner as for the Schiøtz. The IOP is provided as a digital readout in mm Hg with no conversion required. A sterile rubber cover should be used and discarded after each measurement. Although the accompanying directions make the use of the tonometer pen relatively easy, some familiarity with the calibration process is helpful.

Indentation tonometry is contraindicated in penetrating eye injury, and it is discouraged in patients with known eye infection that could be transmitted by the instrument.

Treatment

The immediate goal of treatment of acute angle closure glaucoma is to decrease the intraocular pressure by constricting the pupil and pulling the iris away from the trabecular meshwork. In many cases, the necessary medications may not be immediately available, and emergent transfer to an ophthalmologist or emergency department to obtain the medications should not be delayed. If medications are available, initial interventions include:

1. Timolol ophthalmic drops: 1 drop to the affected eye.
2. Pilocarpine 1% or 2%: 1 drop to the affected eye.
3. Antiemetic as needed.
4. Acetazolamide 500 mg PO or IV in consultation with the ophthalmologist.

Disposition

All patients with a suspected diagnosis of acute angle closure glaucoma require emergent evaluation by an ophthalmologist or in the emergency department.

Acute Chemical Exposures

Acute chemical exposures to the eye are a true ophthalmologic emergency. The identification of the chemical as an acid or alkali has some physiologic and prognostic implications; however, in essentially all cases, the most important initial intervention is irrigation, and the sooner initiated, the better the outcome.

The extent of damage to the eye from exposure to chemicals is a function of the volume, concentration, pH, and time to irrigation. Acids cause injury through coagulation necrosis, which tends to limit the extent of penetration. As a result, it is uncommon for acid exposures to cause damage deeper than the cornea. Acids can, however, cause significant corneal injury. Alkali burns to the eye tend to be more serious, causing injury by liquefaction necrosis, with the potential for deep injury within a short time.

Long-term complications of chemical exposure include chronic iritis, adhesions between the lens and iris, cataracts, secondary glaucoma, and visual loss.

Clinical Presentation

Patients who have experienced a chemical exposure to the eye often present with pain, tearing, and possible visual loss. Examination may reveal evidence of facial and periorbital burns or erythema. Examination of the eye often reveals diffuse injection. The extent of injury may vary, ranging from simple epithelial injury, corneal edema, corneal abrasion, and ulceration to, in the most severe cases, an opaque, marbled cornea.

Management

When a patient or family member calls the office after a chemical exposure, instructions should be given to start irrigation immediately, before the substance is definitively identified, and before transport has occurred. In a work setting in which an eyewash station is available, it should be used. Any source of water is acceptable, however. Irrigation should be continued for 5 to 15 minutes; if there is any concern about a serious chemical injury, transport by ambulance to the nearest emergency department should be arranged.

When a patient arrives in the office after a chemical exposure, irrigation should be started even if it has already been performed. If the substance is known, the local poison center should be called for further information and recommendations. Arrangements should be made for transport to an emergency department while irrigation continues.

If the irrigation is complete before the arrival of the ambulance, the pH of the conjunctival fornices can be checked to evaluate the efficacy of treatment. The easiest instrument is a urine dipstick cut just past the pH segment. (If the patient has brought the chemical along, it can also be checked for pH.) Normal tear film pH is 7.4. If the initial postirrigation pH is normal, it must be rechecked in 10 to 20 minutes because the initial reading may be more of a measurement of the pH of the irrigating solution. Any abnormal pH warrants continued irrigation.

Procedure: Irrigation of the Eye
Equipment Needed
    Topical anesthetic (e.g., proparacaine 0.5%)
    1-L normal saline IV bag
    Sterile IV tubing
    Basin to catch fluid
    4″ × 4″ gauze pads

Procedure
1. Anesthetize the eye with 1 drop of proparacaine 0.5%.
2. Have an assistant hold the lids apart using gauze pads.
3. Irrigate the eye using the normal saline and tubing and aiming the stream tangentially at the conjunctiva so that the fluid flows over the entire eye (Fig. 18–11).
4. A minimum of 1 liter for acids and 2 liters for alkalis should be used while the patient awaits ambulance transport.[8]

Corneal Foreign Body

History
Patients with corneal foreign bodies usually present with sudden pain or foreign body sensation. They may or may not know or suspect that something flew into their eye. Of particular concern is a history of possible corneal foreign body in a person who was working with metal on metal, such as with hammering, chiseling, grinding, or drilling. This can result in globe penetration that may not be obvious on physical examination.

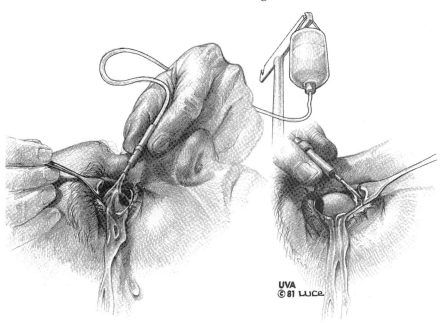

UVA
© 81 LUCE

Figure 18–11. Irrigation of the eye. (From Haddad LM, Winchester JF [ed]: Clinical Management of Poisoning and Drug Overdose, 2nd ed. Philadelphia, WB Saunders, 1990, p 373.)

Physical Examination

It may be necessary to administer a drop of a topical anesthetic before performing any significant examination of the eye. Proparacaine 0.5% works well, with a half-life of 15 minutes.

Eyelid Eversion (Fig. 18–12). Once the anesthetic has taken effect, the first step is to evert the upper eyelid with a cotton-tipped applicator. Grasp the upper eyelashes with one hand and place the tip of the cotton-tipped applicator horizontally against the midtarsal plate. Pull outward and up-ward on the lashes, while holding the applicator in place. If a foreign body is seen under the lid, it can simply be brushed away with the cotton swab. The lid is returned to its normal position by pulling outward and downward on the lashes.[9]

Corneal Examination. The next step in the examination is evaluation of the cornea, which should be done with magnification and with a cobalt blue light source. The cornea is initially examined with simple magnification. If no foreign body is seen, or if an object is identified and removed, it is important that a subsequent examination with fluorescein be performed. Fluorescein fluoresces in the alkaline environment found just below the corneal epithelium, but not in the neutral lacrimal fluid. Therefore, fluorescence occurs in the presence of a breech in the epithelium.

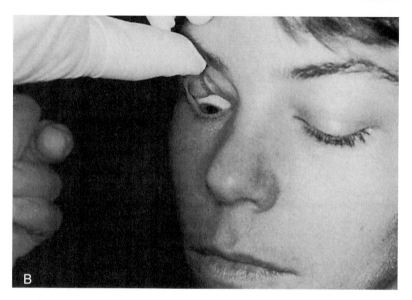

Figure 18–12. Eversion of the eyelid. (From Scott JL, Ghezzi KT: Emerg Med Clin North Am 13:682, 1995.)

Fluorescein is administered by moistening a strip with 1 drop of saline or topical anesthetic and holding it gently against the lower conjunctival sac for 3 to 5 seconds. The eye is then reexamined with a cobalt blue light. Areas of increased uptake may indicate an object not previously seen, or they may reflect an underlying corneal abrasion. If several vertical abrasions are seen, the lids should be reexamined because this pattern is classic for repeated trauma from a foreign body under the upper lid. The conjunctiva can be difficult to evaluate with fluorescein because mucus causes increased uptake.

Treatment

Corneal foreign bodies can be removed with a cotton-tipped applicator or by irrigation. If a cotton swab is used, it should be sterile and moistened with normal saline. Irrigation can be done with the use of an eyewash if available, or as described in the section on "Acute Chemical Exposures." Once the foreign body is removed, the eye should be reexamined with fluorescein.

Special Considerations

Iron or metallic objects pose potential problems for two reasons. One is that iron particles often leave a surrounding rust ring that must be removed. If the foreign body has been removed but the rust ring remains, the patient should be treated with antibiotic ointment, patching, and follow-up with an ophthalmologist in 24 hours for definitive removal.

The other important issue with metallic objects is the potential for penetration of the globe (see "Ruptured Globe and Penetrating Eye Injury."). This is an area of concern, especially when there is a history of metal on metal. In some cases, the eye examination may appear normal because the globe may close around a penetrating object. In others, there may be gross evidence of perforation or a "positive Siedel test." A positive Siedel test is revealed by the streaming of blue or green fluid from a point on the globe that is visualized by the cobalt blue light after fluorescein administration. Because it may require a large amount of fluorescein, it is not a particularly sensitive test for a perforated globe. A positive result, however, must be regarded as indicative of a penetrating eye injury; management and referral should proceed as outlined in the section on "Ruptured Globe and Penetrating Eye Injury." If the clinician suspects a deep metallic foreign body, a plain radiograph should be done. Because plain films do not detect all foreign bodies, however, if they are negative in the presence of a high index of suspicion, the patient should be emergently referred to ophthalmology for possible computed tomography (CT).

Disposition

For those patients in whom foreign body removal is unsuccessful, referral should be made to an ophthalmologist or an emergency department for slit-lamp examination and possible removal with a needle or spud. Those patients with an underlying corneal abrasion should be treated with topical antibiotics with or without a patch (see "Corneal Abrasion"), followed by ophthalmologic care in 24 hours.

Corneal Abrasion

Clinical Presentation

The corneal epithelium is well innervated and highly sensitive to pain. Typical symptoms of corneal abrasion include the sudden development of a foreign body sensation, pain, tearing, and sometimes photophobia. Initial examination reveals injection, often with blepharospasm, interfering with eye opening.

It is frequently necessary to administer a drop of a topical anesthetic, such as proparacaine 0.5%, before any significant examination of the eye is performed. This can be not only therapeutic, but also diagnostic, in that significant relief from the pain supports a corneal source of pain.

Although large abrasions may be seen by the naked eye, most require magnification. If no abrasion is seen with initial magnification, the examination should be repeated with a cobalt blue light after administration of fluorescein (see "Corneal Foreign Body"). Examination of the everted lid should also be performed as part of the search for a causative foreign body. If a foreign body is identified, or a rust ring is noted, management should follow guidelines provided in the section on "Corneal Foreign Body."

Treatment

Because of the loss of the corneal epithelial barrier, abrasions predispose to subsequent infection. Therefore, these patients should be treated with prophylactic topical antibiotics. Many patients will need analgesics— either NSAIDs or oral narcotics. Topical anesthetics should not be prescribed owing to associated delayed healing and secondary keratitis. In general, eye patching is no longer recommended. Eye patching is contraindicated in contact lens wearers with corneal abrasions and when the abrasion was caused by vegetative matter because of the risk of *Pseudomonas* infection.

Patients with significant photophobia should be evaluated for evidence of iritis. A simple test for acute iritis is consensual photophobia, in which illumination of the nonaffected eye elicits pain in the affected eye. If present, a drop of a cycloplegic agent such as cyclopentolate 0.5% should be given and the case should be discussed with an ophthalmologist.

Disposition

Patients treated with cycloplegics should be instructed not to drive because of loss of depth perception. A repeat examination should be performed in 24 to 48 hours, preferably by an ophthalmologist.

Ruptured Globe and Penetrating Eye Injury

Clinical Presentation

A ruptured globe is the result of blunt trauma and should be suspected when the patient reports symptoms of post-traumatic pain and visual impairment. Examination of the eye may reveal a large subconjunctival hemorrhage, hyphema, limitation in extraocular movements, and, less commonly, extrusion of intraocular contents.

Patients with penetrating ocular injury may present with a clear history of intentional trauma or, more subtly, in association with an eyelid laceration. It must also be suspected in all cases of eye trauma resulting from metal on metal, such as occurs with grinding, drilling, or hammering. Physical examination may be normal, even when there is a retained foreign body. The most characteristic finding is an irregular, "tear-shaped" pupil caused by prolapse of the iris.

Physical Examination

If either a ruptured globe or a penetrating ocular injury is suspected, the patient should be initially treated presumptively regardless of a cursory examination that appears unremarkable, or when the eye cannot be adequately examined. When an eye examination is done in this setting, it must be performed without any pressure applied directly to the globe. If the patient cannot open the eye spontaneously, an attempt can be made to assist. This must be done, however, with the pressure of the examiner's hand applied only to the orbital ridge, not to the globe itself.

Treatment
1. The patient should be supine, with the head of the bed at 30 degrees.
2. No drops or ointment is applied to the eye.
3. Keep the patient NPO.
4. Apply a Fox shield or taped paper cup to the eye, if available.
   • Do not use an eye patch or pressure dressing of any kind.
5. Administer an antiemetic, if needed (prochlorperazine [Compazine] IM or IV).
6. Arrange emergent transport to the hospital.

Dental Emergencies

Periapical Abscess

Periapical abscesses typically occur in association with other intraoral infections or from occlusion of a gingival pocket by food.

Clinical Presentation

Patients present with pain and swelling. Examination reveals gingival erythema and an area of fluctuance. If there is evidence of extensive involvement of the surrounding tissues, referral should be made to an ENT or oral and maxillofacial surgeon. Otherwise, incision and drainage is appropriate.

Equipment
  2% lidocaine with epinephrine or Cetacaine spray
  Scalpel with No. 11 blade
  3-mL syringe and 25- or 27-gauge needle
  10- or 20-mL syringe for irrigation
  Normal saline
  Suction (optional)
  Mosquito hemostats (optional)

Procedure
1. Anesthetize the area of maximal fluctuance with 0.5 to 1.0 mL of 2% lidocaine with epinephrine. (If this is not available or is not tolerated by the patient, Cetacaine can be used.)
2. Make a single stab incision.
3. If the abscess does not drain spontaneously, gentle, blunt dissection with mosquito hemostats may be necessary.
4. Irrigate well with saline.

Disposition
  Patients should be treated with oral antibiotics (either penicillin or clindamycin) and analgesics, and should be instructed to perform warm saline or chlorhexidine gluconate (Peridex) rinses four times daily. Dental follow-up should be arranged in 1 to 2 days.

Fractured Teeth

The treatment of dental trauma is a function of the age of the patient and the involvement of the pulp. Dental fractures are described by the Ellis system based on the extent of injury.

Ellis Class I Injuries
  Ellis class I fractures involve only the outer enamel of the tooth. Examination reveals a chipped area of enamel with no exposed dentin or pulp (see later). Patients have no pain from the injury and no sensitivity to hot or cold. Treatment is elective referral to a dentist.

Ellis Class II Injuries
  Class II fractures involve both the enamel and the dentin, but not the pulp. Exposed dentin is ivory/yellow or very light pink, and is surrounded by white enamel. No drops of blood are seen. Patients have pain and sensitivity to heat and cold. Treatment involves covering the exposed dentin

to (1) decrease pain, (2) minimize the risk of infection, and (3) promote repair.

Equipment

Calcium hydroxide paste (Dycal, Dentsply, Germany)
Dental foil or dental wax
$4'' \times 4''$ gauze pads
Saline

Procedure

1. Clean the area with warm saline.
2. Dab the region with gauze to check for drops of blood consistent with an Ellis III injury.
3. Dry the application site well with gauze. (Dycal will not adhere to a wet surface.)
4. Apply a thin layer of calcium hydroxide paste.
5. Cover with dental wax or foil.

These patients should be given an oral analgesic as necessary and should be referred to a dentist within 24 hours.

Ellis Class III Injuries

Class III fractures involve exposure of the pulp. Diagnosis is made by evidence of red dentin or drops of blood on the tooth. Patients usually have pain and sensitivity to hot and cold but occasionally are anesthetic. These injuries are dental emergencies and treatment is emergent referral. Although application of calcium hydroxide paste may be temporarily useful, it is generally impractical owing to the moisture of the tooth surface. If available and tolerated, the tooth can be temporarily covered with aluminum foil or dental foil.

Subluxed and Avulsed Teeth

Subluxed teeth that are minimally mobile (<2 mm) and have no displacement from their original positions can be treated with a soft diet, analgesics, and dental follow-up in several days. Significantly subluxed teeth require correct alignment and subsequent stabilization as soon as possible.

Avulsed primary teeth should not be replaced in the socket because of the risk of alveolar osteitis. These children need referral only. Avulsed permanent teeth, on the other hand, are a dental emergency, with viability directly related to the time to treatment. A 1% chance of successful re-implantation is lost with every minute that the tooth is outside its socket. However, placement into the socket can be difficult. If this is the case, the best transport/holding medium is Hank's solution ("Save-a-Tooth"), a balanced pH cell culture medium. It may allow viability for 12 to 24 hours.[8] The next best option is probably milk, with normal saline being an acceptable alternative. The worst option is to let the tooth dry.

Equipment
    Saline
    10-mL syringe
    18-gauge Teflon IV catheter
    4″ × 4″ gauze pads
    Suction (optional)
    Dental mirror (optional)

Procedure
1. Hold the avulsed tooth by the crown only (not by the root because this may cause damage to the periodontal ligament).
2. Rinse the tooth with normal saline (no scrubbing).
3. Inspect the socket. Using the syringe, saline, and angiocatheter, irrigate away any blood clots or debris. (Gently suction, if needed.)
4. Hold the tooth with gauze and return it to its position using finger pressure.
5. If the tooth cannot be placed completely into the socket, leave it in place and have the patient hold it there by biting on gauze.
6. Refer the patient to a dentist immediately.

References

1. Jensen JH: Technique for removing a spherical foreign body from the nose or ear. Ear Nose Throat J 55:270–271, 1976.
2. Leffler S, Cheney P, Tandberg D: Chemical immobilization and killing of intra-aural roaches: An in vitro comparative study. Ann Emerg Med 93:1795–1798, 1993.
3. Backlin SA: Positive-pressure technique for nasal foreign body removal in children. Ann Emerg Med 25:554–555, 1995.
4. Rosen P (ed): Emergency Medicine Concepts and Clinical Practice, 4th ed. St. Louis, Mosby, 1998.
5. Roberts JR, Hedges JR: Clinical Procedures in Emergency Medicine, 2nd ed. Philadelphia, WB Saunders, 1991.
6. Stair T: Practical Management of Eye, Ear, Nose, Mouth, and Throat Emergencies. Rockville, Md, Aspen Systems Corporation, 1986.
7. Harwood-Nuss A (ed): The Clinical Practice of Emergency Medicine, 2nd ed. Philadelphia, Lippincott-Raven, 1996.
8. Haddad LM, Winchester JF (eds): Clinical Management of Poisoning and Drug Overdose, 2nd ed. Philadelphia, WB Saunders, 1990.
9. Scott JL, Ghezzi KT (eds): Emerg Med Clin North Am 13:681–701, 1995.

Chapter 19

Spinal Injury

William H. Shoff
Elizabeth M. Datner
Suzanne Moore Shepherd

Early recognition of a spinal cord injury (SCI), or an unstable spinal injury that has the potential to produce neurologic injury, is an opportunity to avert a catastrophe or, perhaps, minimize it. Spinal cord injuries are devastating to the individual both emotionally and physically, to the involved family emotionally, and often, to both financially. The total financial cost, ranging from $1 million to $5 million, derives from hospitalization after the initial injury, rehabilitation of the patient, and loss of earning potential due to disability.[1] Approximately 10,000 to 14,000 new spinal cord injuries occur in the United States annually, representing 2.6% of incidents of major trauma.[2, 3] A bimodal distribution of patients present with SCI. The group most commonly involved includes men between 15 and 24 years of age; a second peak occurs in patients older than 55 years of age.[4, 21] Mortality associated with spinal cord injury is estimated to occur at a rate of 17% among all patient groups, with a lesser rate of 6.9% in those experiencing isolated SCI.[2] Fortunately, more than one half of SCI patients experience incomplete injury and retain some degree of motor and/or sensory function.[12] SCI may result from motor vehicle collisions, missile wounds or other penetrating injuries, falls, assaults, athletic activities, infection, diving, boating, and decompression illness or, less frequently, from high-energy percussive injuries such as those caused by blasts or lightning strikes.[2, 4–7]

The spinal cord, roots, and cauda equina are normally afforded stability and protection by the intact spinal column and its associated ligaments and muscles. Spinal stability has been defined as "the ability of the spine, under physiologic loads, to maintain the relationships between vertebrae such as there is neither damage nor irritation to the spinal cord or roots, nor incapacitating deformity or pain due to structural changes."[8] Injuries such as ischemia, laceration, crush, penetration, stretch, and infection, along with inflammation, can directly injure the cord or convert the normal stabilizing effect of the spine into a potential danger to cord integrity. Relatively mobile areas of the spine, such as the cervicothoracic and lumbosacral junctions, expose adjacent areas of the spine to an increased risk of injury. When injury is severe enough to produce displaced fracture of relatively protected spinal segments, such as the thoracic spine or the sacral spine, devastating cord injury can occur. The thoracic cord is also at increased risk of potential injury owing to its watershed circulation and relatively narrow medullary canal.[9, 10]

The primary care physician must be prepared to assess, immobilize, stabilize, and manage patients with potentially devastating spinal injuries, often in combination with other multisystem injury. Interventions must be instituted as expeditiously as possible, bearing in mind that both animal and human studies suggest an approximately 8-hour window of opportunity for pharmacologic or mechanical intervention to prevent both direct and secondary cord injury. Direct cord injury results from a bony fragment, a dislocated segment(s), a herniated disc, a laceration, or any combination of these. Secondary cord injury occurs as a result of progressive injury-related edema and vasospastic and thrombosis-related ischemia.

Primary care physicians often work in settings that are remote from tertiary trauma care and where they are the closest or only medical care initially available to the patient who has sustained an injury. The purpose of this chapter is to provide them with the knowledge and skills needed to exclude or to recognize and initially manage the patient with a spinal injury in a field setting such as the office or urgent care center, and then to initiate appropriate early transfer to a trauma center.

 ## CLINICAL RECOGNITION ◀—————————————

Patients with spinal cord injury may present with a widely varying clinical picture. Injury may range from transient to ongoing symptoms—pain or tenderness solely at the injury level, or the subjective sensation of paresthesia distal to the injury. Conversely, patients may exhibit significant grossly obvious paralysis. Patients may have neurologic injury alone or neurologic injury in the setting of multisystem trauma. Even without concomitant airway, pulmonary, chest wall, or cardiac injury, neurologic injury may interfere with ventilation, oxygenation, and circulation. Injury to the cervical cord may result in obvious or subtle respiratory compromise, which ultimately may place the patient at risk of death. Patients with cervical or high thoracic cord injury in *spinal neurogenic shock* may present with warm, dry skin and hypotension secondary to decreased sympathetic tone and vagally mediated bradycardia.[56] This syndrome can persist for months after injury. A systolic blood pressure of 80 to 90 mm Hg is rarely produced by SCI alone. The physician must carefully exclude hemorrhage, cardiac injury, and other sources of hypotension before concluding that the patient is exhibiting spinal neurogenic shock.[11, 21]

Although most patients who present to the primary care physician's office with the complaint of neck or back pain and tenderness are found to have ligamentous sprain or muscular injury and no associated cord injury, evaluation of potential neurologic injury includes meticulous testing of motor, sensory, and reflex function. The motor examination tests key muscles (Table 19–1)[9] and is graded on the well-established scale of 0 (no function) to 5 (full normal strength). The sensory examination carefully tests 28 dermatomes (Fig. 19–1), with sensation graded from 0 (absent) to 2 (normal). Paired reflexes are specifically keyed to nerve root levels (see Table 19–1) and are also graded on a 0 to 2 scale. The presence of fecal incontinence, urinary retention or loss of continence, or priapism should be documented. Careful mapping of sensory and motor loss defines the neurologic level of injury, which represents the most caudal spinal cord segment on both sides of the body with normal motor and sensory function, and allows the physician to appropriately focus radiologic testing.[12]

The severity of injury may qualify as *spinal cord concussion*—incomplete sensory loss/paralysis (partial cord injuries discussed in the following section) or *paraplegia/tetraplegia*—complete sensory loss/paralysis. The American Spinal Injury Association (ASIA) impairment scale is the currently accepted grading system for spinal injury (Table 19–2).[13] Patients with spinal cord concussion (intra-axonal injury) exhibit transient paralysis and/or sensory dysfunction appropriate to the level of injury, which typically resolves within 48 to 72 hours of injury.[14–16] Note that the amount of damage to the cord is much less than that seen with spinal neurogenic shock, which is discussed later. Partial cord injuries exhibit partial motor and/or partial sensory function distal to the neurologic level of injury, and *sacral sparing* may be evident.[58] Sacral sparing, demonstrated by intact perineal reflexes (i.e., anal wink, bulbocavernosus reflex), is a very important finding in a paralyzed patient with sensory loss or paralysis because it prognosticates a chance of recovery. The anal wink is elicited by

Table 19–1. Motor and Reflex Tests by Nerve Root Levels

Nerve Root Level	Motor	Reflex
C4	Diaphragm	—
C5	Deltoid, biceps	Biceps
C6	Extensor carpi radialis	Brachioradialis
C7	Triceps, wrist flexors, finger extensors	Triceps
C8	Finger flexors	—
T1	Hand intrinsics	—
T4	Intercostals	—
T10	Abdominals	—
L1, L2	Iliopsoas	—
L3, L4	Quadriceps	Quadriceps
L5	Extensor hallucis longus	—
S1	Gastrocsoleus, flexor hallucis longus	Achilles tendon
S2, S3, S4	Anal sphincter, bladder	Bulbocavernosus, anal wink

Adapted from Trafton PG: Spinal cord injuries. Surg Clin North Am 62:64, 1982.

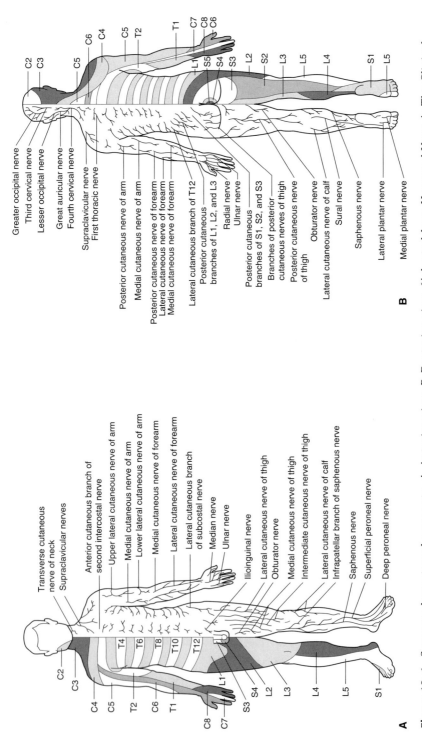

Figure 19–1. Sensory dermatomal segments. *A,* Anterior view. *B,* Posterior view. (Adapted from Harwood-Nuss A: The Clinical Practice of Emergency Medicine, 3rd ed. Philadelphia, Lippincott Williams & Wilkins, 2001, p 497.)

Greater occipital nerve
Third cervical nerve
Lesser occipital nerve
Great auricular nerve
Fourth cervical nerve
Supraclavicular nerve
First thoracic nerve
Posterior cutaneous nerve of arm
Medial cutaneous nerve of arm
Posterior cutaneous nerve of forearm
Lateral cutaneous nerve of forearm
Medial cutaneous nerve of forearm
Lateral cutaneous branch of T12
Posterior cutaneous branches of L1, L2, and L3
Radial nerve
Ulnar nerve
Posterior cutaneous branches of S1, S2, and S3
Branches of posterior cutaneous nerves of thigh
Posterior cutaneous nerve of thigh
Obturator nerve
Lateral cutaneous nerve of calf
Sural nerve
Saphenous nerve
Lateral plantar nerve
Medial plantar nerve

B

Transverse cutaneous nerve of neck
Supraclavicular nerves
Anterior cutaneous branch of second intercostal nerve
Upper lateral cutaneous nerve of arm
Medial cutaneous nerve of arm
Lower lateral cutaneous nerve of arm
Medial cutaneous nerve of forearm
Lateral cutaneous nerve of forearm
Lateral cutaneous branch of subcostal nerve
Median nerve
Ulnar nerve
Ilioinguinal nerve
Lateral cutaneous nerve of thigh
Obturator nerve
Medial cutaneous nerve of thigh
Intermediate cutaneous nerve of thigh
Lateral cutaneous nerve of calf
Infrapatellar branch of saphenous nerve
Saphenous nerve
Superficial peroneal nerve
Deep peroneal nerve

A

268

Table 19–2. American Spinal Injury Association (ASIA) Impairment Scale

Grade of Injury	Type of Impairment
A	Motor and sensory loss complete below level of injury
B	Motor complete, sensory incomplete below level of injury
C	Partially preserved motor function: Majority of key muscles below level with less than grade 3 strength
D	Partially preserved motor function: Majority of key muscle groups below level with ≥3 strength
E	Normal sensory and motor function

Adapted from Ditunno JF, Young W, Donovan WH, et al:The international standards booklet for neurological and functional classification of spinal cord injury. Paraplegia 32:70–80, 1994.

stimulating the anus tactilely and observing contraction of the anus. The bulbocavernosus reflex is elicited by tugging on, or squeezing, the glans penis or pushing on the clitoris, or by tugging on an inserted Foley; when intact, this reflex causes reflexive anal sphincter contraction.

Several important partial cord injury syndromes can occur (Fig. 19–2).[17] Determination of a partial cord syndrome may be difficult owing to the patchy nature of sensory and motor loss. *Central cord syndrome* (CCS) is perhaps the most commonly seen. It usually presents in patients with a narrowed spinal canal caused by congenital stenosis or degenerative spine disease. The most common mechanism for acute injury is forced hyperextension of the neck (e.g., from a fall or motor vehicle crash), which results in more significant injury to the central portion of the cord. The central portion of the cord contains the lateral corticospinal tract. There may be preferential loss of upper extremity strength compared with that of the lower extremities.[18] Sensory loss is variable and many patients exhibit urinary retention.[19] This injury, which is usually managed non-operatively, bears a relatively good prognosis for recovery of at least partial function. Approximately three fourths of patients are able to walk 1 year after the injury. Resolution is heralded by caudocephalic return of function. The *burning hands syndrome*, a variant of the CCS probably produced by contusion of the spinothalamic tract, is exhibited by patients who complain of "burning" dysesthesias of the hands.[20]

The *Brown-Séquard syndrome* is a hemicord injury caused by penetrating injuries, disc disease, and tumor. This syndrome, which represents approximately 2% to 4% of all spinal injuries, classically presents as ipsilateral dorsal column dysfunction and motor deficit, along with contralateral loss of temperature and pain sensation.[57] On occasion, ipsilateral hyperesthesia may be present distal to the level of injury.[21] More commonly, patients present with *Brown-Séquard-Plus syndromes*: Asymmetric paraplegia is seen, with hypalgesia more significant on the side with less motor weakness.[23] These syndromes usually have favorable outcomes, with return of bladder and bowel continence and ambulation.[22] Those due to penetrating injury may fare less well.[23]

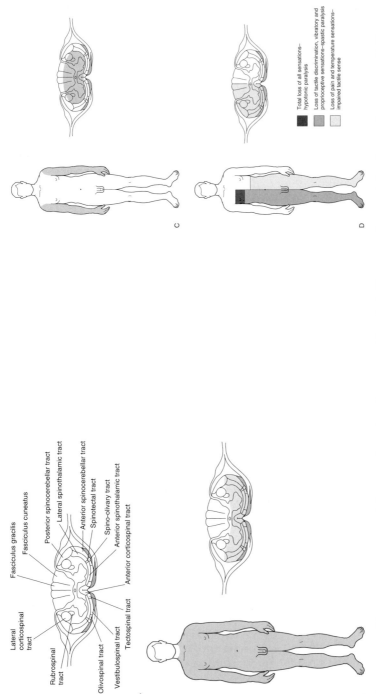

Figure 19–2. Transverse section of the spinal cord at the cervical level. *A,* The ascending and the descending tracts. *B,* Tracts that may be damaged in the anterior spinal artery syndrome. *C,* Tracts that may be damaged in the central cord syndrome. *D,* Involved tracts and the superimposed areas of deficit from an injury at T4 (resulting in the Brown-Séquard syndrome). (Adapted from Harwood-Nuss A: The Clinical Practice of Emergency Medicine, 3rd ed. Philadelphia, Lippincott Williams & Wilkins, 2001, p 498.)

The *anterior spinal cord syndrome*, a relatively uncommon injury, may be produced by thoracic aortic injury, resultant disruption of the blood supply, and ischemia of the anterior cord; direct compression of the anterior spinal artery; or direct blunt injury to the cord by displaced bone fragments, hematoma, or a herniated disc. Flexion "teardrop" fractures are frequently seen in conjunction with this lesion. The patient exhibits loss of temperature and pain sensation and motor function below the level of injury; however, the dorsal column functions of vibration, light touch, and proprioception are preserved.[13, 24] The prognosis for recovery with this injury is unfavorable.

The *posterior cord syndrome* is rare. Injury to the dorsal columns in this syndrome produces disruption of vibration, light touch, and proprioception, as well as resultant difficulty with ambulation.[21]

In rare instances, trauma, such as disc herniation, may injure the cauda equina. The patient may complain of unilateral or bilateral sciatica, bilateral lower extremity weakness, anogenital saddle hypesthesia or analgesia, and bowel and/or bladder incontinence. This situation is a true surgical emergency: Decompression of the injury within 24 to 48 hours of injury produces a significantly better outcome than does late intervention, which may result in permanent bladder or rectal dysfunction.[25–27]

Total loss of spinal cord function below the level of injury carries a poor, but not hopeless, prognosis for recovery. Complete spinal cord injury may be very difficult to accurately diagnose at the time of initial examination owing to the presence of associated *spinal neurogenic shock*. This is seen in the setting of near- or complete physiologic or anatomic transection of the spinal cord, usually at T6 or above. The patient exhibits absence of reflexes, absence of bladder tone, flaccid paralysis, hypotension, hypothermia, and ileus for a period of 24 hours (most commonly) to days to weeks after injury.[21, 22] Over time, spastic paralysis may develop. Spinal shock is also known as warm shock because of the peripheral vasodilatation. Up to 30% of patients require pressors. Resolution of spinal shock is signaled by the return of segmental reflexes and often by the return of anal wink or the bulbocavernosus reflex *(vide supra)*.[21, 56]

PHONE TRIAGE ◄————————————————————————

During phone triage, recognition of potential spinal injury is essential. Patients with potential spinal injury may call the office complaining of a fall/motor vehicle injury/dive or other trauma mechanism that could produce spinal injury. A family member, friend, coach, or bystander at the injury site may call for the patient. The receptionist should not ask that the patient come to the phone but should first obtain the phone number of the caller, the address, and the name of the caller, in that order. Next, the receptionist should turn the call over to a physician in the office; if a physician is not available, then a nurse should take over the call. If the receptionist is alone, he or she should advise the caller to hang up and call 911 or the closest emergency department, in that order. The patient should be evaluated as soon as possible by a physician trained to recognize and manage spinal injuries because the lack of specific neurologic symptoms or the ability of a patient to ambulate after an accident does not rule out SCI. If the caller says that the injury has just occurred, it is important to elicit some assessment of the airway, breathing, and circulation (ABCs) and information on whether the patient can or cannot move. If there is any question of spinal injury and the patient is not in a dangerous location or in need of cardiopulmonary resuscitation (CPR), he or she should not be moved; emergency medical services should be dispatched to the scene immediately. If time and circumstances permit, the following information can be gathered by phone, while emergency medical assistance is in route: Identity of injured body part(s), associated local findings (pain, swelling, and deformity), the timing of events, change in mental status, presence of paresthesias or incontinence (bowel or bladder), and any respiratory difficulty.

Initial Management

A careful initial history and physical examination of the patient with suspected SCI begins with a focused history, assessment of the vital signs, and an appropriate survey of the ABCDEs[28]; this approach enables the clinician to recognize and stabilize life- and limb-threatening injuries. If available, details of the event should be ascertained. Any history of preexisting disease that may increase the risk of cord injury, such as rheumatoid arthritis or disc disease, should be elicited. The physician should inquire about medications, alcohol, and other substances that might interfere with the patient's ability to give an appropriate history or mask clinical signs and symptoms. The initial examining physician may be the only one to speak to an individual with coincidental head injury who is later unable to describe events, the individuals actually at the accident scene, or the initial transporting Emergency Medical Services (EMS) personnel. An initial full neurologic examination should be performed as soon as possible. It will serve as the basis for the patient's initial evaluation and management and ongoing comparative evaluation. It will also provide a frame of reference, if the patient requires transfer to a higher level of care, for the emergency physician, general trauma surgeon, and/or neurosurgeon at the trauma center. It is often helpful to pictorially document the motor, sensory, and reflex findings on the patient's chart.

The clinician should examine the patient for other related injuries, bearing in mind that loss of sensation due to SCI may mask these.

All patients with potential cord injury require spinal immobilization during their initial evaluation and stabilization. Simultaneous resuscitation may be required in the significantly injured patient; this potentially involves delivery of high-flow oxygen, airway management in the semiconscious or intoxicated patient unable to control his/her airway, a nasal or orogastric tube, large-bore intravenous access, serial vital sign monitoring, removal of wet/cold clothing and use of a warmed blanket, and a Foley catheter. Traction should not be applied to the patient's spine until lesions are carefully defined because distraction of the injured cord or roots may cause severe neurologic injury. If a patient with spinal injury needs to vomit, log-rolling and suctioning the patient will produce the least amount of spinal motion.[29] Equipment and medications needed in the office setting for the initial management of SCI are listed in Table 19–3.

It should not be assumed that hypotension in an SCI patient is due to spinal shock. All patients with SCI and hypotension warrant further evaluation for hemorrhage into the thorax and abdominal and pelvic cavities. Pressor support is required in 20% to 30% of patients with spinal shock, most commonly with dopamine.[1] Unfortunately, the optimal blood pressure to be maintained has not been demonstrated, but some authors suggest a mean arterial pressure of greater than 85 mm Hg.[30]

Table 19–3. Office Equipment and Medications Needed to Manage Spinal Injury

Cervical spine immobilization collars (pediatric, small, medium, large)
Blankets
Backboard
Gurney capable of holding immobilized patient and being taken to X-ray facilities
Tape and binding to secure patient to backboard
Intravenous tubing
Intravenous normal saline or Ringer's lactate
Intravenous catheters (14, 16, 18, 20, 22, 24 [size dependent on age and acuity])
Oxygen source and tubing
Nasal prongs, ventimasks, non-rebreather mask, bag-valve mask
Airway management/code cart
Electrocardiographic (ECG) monitor
Pulse oximetry
Wall suction
Nasogastric tubing
Toomey syringe to check nasogastric tube placement
Foley catheters
Tetanus toxoid (store in refrigerator)
Second- or third-generation cephalosporin for intravenous administration
Narcotic pain medication
Nonsteroidal anti-inflammatory agent
Methylprednisolone for intravenous administration
Dopamine

After the ABCDEs are completed, the patient is stabilized, and a meticulous, but expeditious, history and physical examination has identified a potential SCI, further evaluation of the injured spine is warranted. Plain films of the spine are the initial modality used to further characterize the injury(ies). The clinician must decide who does or does not require them. Through careful physical examination, this decision can be facilitated by the distinction of whether the patient is experiencing midline cervical, thoracic, or lumbar tenderness versus paravertebral muscle tenderness. Regarding cervical spine injury, 10 published series (>30,000 cases) have led to the development of criteria for appropriate ordering of cervical spine plain films.[31] These criteria were prospectively assessed in the National Emergency X-Radiography Utilization Study (NEXUS),[32, 33] which included 27,389 patients; researchers concluded that any of the following clinical criteria mandates cervical plain films:

- Altered mental status (brain injury, drug and alcohol, medication, metabolic shock, etc.)
- Posterior midline cervical spine tenderness
- Neurologic deficit (motor or sensory, including distal paresthesias)
- Distracting injury (any other injury that could potentially draw the patient's attention away from the neck injury)

According to these criteria, 15 fractures were missed and only one of these necessitated surgical intervention in this study. None of the missed fractures was unstable. Although thoracolumbar spine (TLS) injuries have not been as thoroughly studied, there have been at least two small-scale studies[34, 35] on TLS injuries similar to the NEXUS study that resulted in a similar conclusion. The total case series for when to order plain films for potential TLS injury, however, included fewer than 600 patients. In one study involving children, TLS plain films were found to be better than computed tomography (CT) for detecting spinal fracture in children.[36] Current criteria for obtaining TLS plain films for the injured patient include:

- Fall from higher than 10 feet
- Ejection from a car or off a motorcycle traveling at a speed greater than 50 mph
- Back tenderness or pain
- Glasgow Coma Scale score lower than 8
- Neurologic deficit (motor or sensory, including distal paresthesias)[37]

Obtaining plain films or other studies for the critically ill patient should not interfere with transferring the patient to an appropriate facility for definitive care.

The initial plain films, if feasible, may provide valuable information about potential SCI. Plain radiographic evaluation of the cervical spine involves three views: true lateral, open-mouthed odontoid, and anteroposterior (AP). A true lateral projection of the cervical spine identifies approximately 90% of significant ligamentous and bony injuries. The family or emergency physician must not accept inadequate imaging. All seven cervical vertebral bodies and the top of T1 should be visualized. A swimmer's view may be required to visualize the cervicothoracic junction in the patient with large shoulders. The open-mouthed odontoid view identifies most of the remaining 10% of injuries. The AP view rarely identifies injury that is not already suspected from the clinical examination.[38–41] Plain radiographic evaluation of the TLS involves two views—lateral and AP. Additional oblique views may be obtained of any portion of the spine to better image the lamina, pedicles, and neural foramina when radicular symptoms are present.[36] In treatment of the patient with significant pain and normal initial films, careful use of flexion-extension views adds additional information regarding potential ligamentous injury and spinal column stability. Interpretation of plain cervical spine films involves several considerations[22, 31]:

- Evaluate the vertebral column alignment on the lateral view by observing imaginary lines connecting four respective anatomic elements—anterior vertebral bodies (C1–T1), posterior vertebral bodies (C1–T1), the spinolaminar line, and tips of the spinous processes. Step-off of greater than 2 mm is abnormal and must be accounted for. It may be secondary to degenerative arthritis, muscle spasm, positioning of the patient, or trauma (previous or acute).
- The soft tissue plane on the lateral view anterior to the vertebral column from C1–C4 should measure no greater than 5 mm, and from C5–T1 no greater that 21 mm in the adult (see later for pediatrics). Any increase in this measurement raises the question of free air, foreign body, hemorrhage, infection, tumor, and vertebral body fracture.
- Flattening of the normal lordotic curve on the lateral view may be secondary to fracture, muscle spasm, or normal variation.
- Anterior displacement of one vertebral body on another on the lateral view represents a double-facet dislocation if the displacement is 50% or more of the width of the body (unstable injury); a single-facet dislocation if the displacement is 25% (stable injury); if less than 25%, displacement may be of no consequence.
- Note that the spaces between the spinous processes on the lateral view are normally equivalent, and that imaginary lines extrapolated from the tip of each process converge. Any divergence from this pattern suggests a disruption of the posterior spinous ligament.
- When the posterior height of the vertebral body on the lateral view is decreased by 25% or more upon comparison with the anterior height, a fracture of the vertebral body should be suspected.
- Examine the elements of each vertebra for signs of disruption of the bony integrity indicating fracture, until proven otherwise.
- Evaluate the vertebral bodies on the lateral film for teardrop fractures, which are displacements of bony fragments from the anteroinferior corner of the body. These are considered unstable fractures until proven otherwise.

- Compare all the disc spaces for relative narrowing on the lateral view, which may be secondary to congenital anomaly, degenerative processes, disc herniation, surgery, or other disease processes. Any relative increase in the spacing suggests annulus fibrosus rupture or longitudinal ligament disruption.
- Evaluate the space between the interior surface of the anterior aspect of the ring of C1 and the anterior surface of the dens (predental space) on the lateral view for widening greater than 5 mm in the adult and greater than 8 mm in the child, suggesting C1 fracture, dens fracture, or disruption of the ligaments that hold the dens in position.
- On the AP view, evaluate for straight alignment of the spinous processes, breaks/step-offs in the cortical surfaces, and evenness of the joint spaces. Any abnormality must be accounted for.
- On the odontoid view, evaluate for symmetry—between the vertical dens and the surfaces of the C1 ring and between the positions of lateral bodies of the C1 ring and the position of the dens in the middle of the ring space. Note the integrity of the dens, being aware that overlying structures radiographically sometimes create a false appearance of fracture. A 5-degree tilt of the dens off the vertical axis is a fracture of the dens until proven otherwise.
- On flexion-extension views, displacement of greater than 2 mm of one vertebral body on another and angulation of 16 degrees or more of one group of vertebral bodies on another are considered abnormal; further studies are indicated.[42, 42a]
- The pediatric spine in comparison with the adult spine has facets that slide more easily, contains more laxity in the ligaments, supports a proportionally heavier head, and has unfused physes. These properties lead to difficulties in interpretation of pediatric cervical spine films, resulting in the observation of pseudosubluxation of up to 3 mm (C2–3 or C3–4; present age < 12 years), anterior wedging (usually C3 or C4), avulsions (actually secondary ossification centers), and more lateral displacement of the lateral masses of C1 than expected (odontoid view).

Interpretation of TLS films involves the following considerations[31]:
- Evaluate for alignment, disc spaces, flattening of the lordotic curve, teardrop fractures, and vertebral body height on the lateral views, as with cervical spine films.
- Flattening of normal lordotic curve on the lateral view may be secondary to fracture, muscle spasm, or normal variation.
- Evaluate for bony integrity on the lateral and AP views, and pay additional attention to the transverse processes and the spinous processes.
- Evaluate anterior displacement of one vertebral body, as with cervical spine films.
- Evaluate for teardrop fractures, as with cervical spine films.

- Evaluate for widening of the paraspinous stripe on the AP film, which suggests fracture.

Additional information may be obtained with CT scanning and magnetic resonance imaging (MRI). CT is indicated: to better delineate bony detail when fracture is present, when neurologic injury is present, when instability is suspected based on plain film findings, and when better delineation of questionable plain film findings is necessary. Furthermore, CT adds information on associated soft tissue injury and may demonstrate additional fractures not suspected on plain films. MRI is used to demonstrate soft tissue injury. It is currently considered the definitive method for delineating spinal cord injury. MRI is less effective at defining bony detail.[42, 43] Both studies are often necessary for best definition of the injury.

With acute blunt cord injury, high-dose methylprednisolone is given early in treatment to reduce secondary cord injury. This recommendation is based on the results of the second National Acute Spinal Cord Injury Study (NASCIS II), a randomized, double-blind, placebo-controlled multicenter trial that evaluated methylprednisolone and naloxone.[44] Patients who received methylprednisolone within 8 hours of injury in this study demonstrated improved motor and sensory function in both the short-term and through-6-month follow-up. Although the original investigators published further follow-up on these patients after 1 year,[45] no well-controlled follow-up studies have been performed to validate these data. Penetrating injuries were excluded from the NASCIS II study. NASCIS III, a third randomized, multicenter trial that investigated methylprednisolone plus/minus a lipid peroxidation inhibitor in all SCI patients, found similar efficacy for methylprednisolone in blunt trauma.[46] The currently accepted dosing of methylprednisolone within 3 hours of blunt injury is a loading dose of 30 mg/kg over 15 minutes, followed by an infusion of 5.4 mg/kg/hr (230 mL D_5W at 10 mL/hr) over 23 hours. The dosing from 3 to 8 hours after blunt injury is the same initially, but the continuous drip is maintained for 48 hours.[21, 43–45] Patients on this 48-hour protocol have developed more significant pneumonias and sepsis.[17]

In patients with penetrating injury, or associated open bony fracture, antibiotics should be administered. The usual choice is a second- or third-generation cephalosporin, initially administered intravenously.[4, 47] Check the patient's tetanus immunization status, and update as necessary.

Disposition and Transfer

Patients who are found not to have evidence of SCI may be treated appropriately for their injuries and discharged home. Rest, ice, and analgesia may be warranted for muscular injury. The patient should be supplied with appropriate follow-up instructions, including signs/symptoms that should promote his/her return earlier than scheduled. Physical therapy/

back exercises may be appropriate once the acute injury has been addressed.

If the patient is found to have SCI, if a concern exists regarding SCI that cannot be addressed in the office setting, or if other significant injury is noted, the primary health care worker should expedite safe patient transfer to a tertiary care facility. The office-based physician should contact the accepting physician and discuss the case because further care may be warranted before transfer. Safe patient transfer is the responsibility of both the transferring physician and the accepting physician. The patient should be appropriately immobilized and stabilized for transfer. The most appropriate mode of transportation should be determined based on local availability and access to the trauma center/hospital. An individual capable of administering fluids, dopamine, and intravenous methylprednisolone, and who is capable of providing appropriate airway support should accompany the patient. Records documenting the patient's history and physical examination, pertinent medical and surgical histories, medications, allergies, and current evaluation and management, as well as copies of any appropriate tests, must accompany the patient. These arrangements, including the accepting physician's name and the plan of action, should be accurately documented.

Pediatric Considerations

SCI occurs much less frequently in children than in adults. The reported annual rate is approximately 18 cases/million.[48] The leading causes in this age group include motor vehicle crashes, especially a motor vehicle striking a pedestrian, followed by falls and sports-related injuries, particularly diving.[48, 49] In general, aspects of the head and neck anatomy of young children predispose them to a greater number of injuries in the C1–4 levels than adults—a relatively larger head, poorly developed neck musculature, and horizontal orientation of the facet joints of the upper cervical vertebral bodies. In children up to 8 years of age, the most common area for cervical spine injury is the occiput to C2. The alanto-occipital dislocation, typically a fatal injury, has been survived. It can be diagnosed by the X-line method: Draw a line from the tip of the basion to the midspinolaminal line of C2; this line should intersect tangentially the edge of the odontoid. Another line drawn from the tip of the opisthion to the posteroinferior corner of the body of C2 should intersect the spinolaminal line tangentially.[50] Upper spinal cord injury results in apnea, cardiac arrest, and significant hypotension, but fewer survivors are left with hypoxic brain injury compared with outcomes seen in adolescent and adult populations.[51-53] Patients with partial cord syndromes, such as Brown-Séquard and central cord lesions, often recover well.

SCIWORA syndrome (spinal cord injury without radiologic abnormality) is described in approximately 4% to 67% of childhood SCI.[54] A spectrum of injury from complete paralysis to transient symptomatology is seen; this may be due in part to spinal cord ischemia and infarction.[54] Owing to the relative elasticity of their spinal cords, the relative weakness of the neck musculature, and the other anatomic differences noted previously, this syndrome is seen most commonly in children younger than 8 years of age. Children with complete injuries and increasingly severe findings on MRI have a significantly poorer prognosis.[55]

The use of methylprednisolone in *SCIWORA syndrome* is recommended by some.

References

1. Bracken MB: Pharmacological treatment of acute spinal cord injury: Current treatment and future projects. J Emerg Med 11 (suppl 1):43–48, 1993.
2. Burney RE, Mario RF, Maynard F, et al: Incidence, characteristics, and outcomes of spinal cord injury at trauma centers in North America. Arch Surg 128:596–599, 1993.
3. Kraus JF, Franti CE, Riggins RS, et al: Incidence of traumatic spinal cord lesions. J Chron Dis 28:471–475, 1975.
4. Jallo GI: Neurosurgical management of penetrating spinal injury. Surg Neurol 47:328–330, 1997.
5. Knopp R: Near drowning. J Am Coll Emerg Phys 7:249–254, 1978.
6. National Center for Injury Prevention and Control: Ten Leading Causes of Death Tables, 1994. Atlanta, Ga, Centers for Disease Control and Prevention, 1996.
7. Waters RL, Adkins RH: Firearm versus motor vehicle related spinal cord injury: Preinjury factors, injury characteristics, and initial outcome comparisons among ethnically diverse groups. Arch Phys Med Rehabil 78:150–155, 1997.
8. Panjabi MM, White AA 3rd: Basic biomechanics of the spine. Neurosurgery 7:76–93, 1980.
9. Trafton PG: Spinal cord injuries. Surg Clin North Am 62:61–75, 1982.
10. Trafton PG, Boyd CA Jr: Computed tomography of thoracic and lumbar spine injuries. J Trauma 24:506–515, 1984.
11. Tator CH: Update on the pathophysiology and pathology of acute spinal cord injury. Brain Pathol 5:407–413, 1995.
12. Ditunno JF Jr, Graziani V, Tessler A: Neurological assessment in spinal cord injury. Adv Neurol 72:325–333, 1997.
13. Ditunno JF Jr, Young W, Donovan WH, et al: The international standards booklet for neurological and functional classification of spinal cord injury. Paraplegia 32:70–80, 1994.
14. Roberge RJ, Wears RC: Evaluation of neck discomfort, neck tenderness, and neurologic deficits as indicators for radiography in blunt trauma victims. J Emerg Med 10:539–544, 1992.
15. Scher AT: Spinal cord concussion in rugby players. Am J Sports Med 19:485–488, 1991.
16. Zwimpfer TJ, Bernstein M: Spinal cord concussion. J Neurosurg 72:894–900, 1990.
17. Mahoney BD: Spinal cord injuries. In Harwood-Nuss A (ed): The Clinical Practice of Emergency Medicine, 3rd ed. Philadelphia, Lippincott Williams & Wilkins, 2001, pp 495–501.
18. Levi AD, Tator CH, Bunge RP: Clinical syndromes associated with disproportionate weakness of the upper versus the lower extremities after cervical spinal injury. Neurosurgery 38:179–183, 1996.
19. Maroon JC, Abla AA, Wilberger JI, et al: Central cord syndrome. Clin Neurosurg 37:612–621, 1991.
20. Wilberger JE, Abla A, Maroon JC: Burning hands syndrome revisited. Neurosurgery 19:1038–1040, 1986.
21. Ferrera PC, Markowitz DB: Spinal cord injuries. In Ferrera PC, Colucciello SA, Marx JA, et al (eds): Trauma Management: An Emergency Medicine Approach. St. Louis, Mosby, 2001.

22. Hockberger RS, Kirshenbaum KJ, Doris PE: Spinal injuries. In Rosen P, Barkin R (eds): Emergency Medicine: Concepts and Clinical Practice, 4th ed. St. Louis, Mosby, 1998, pp 462–505.

23. Rathbone D, Johnson G, Letts M: Spinal cord concussion in pediatric athletes. J Pediatr Orthop 12:616–620, 1992.

24. Schneider RC: The syndrome of acute anterior spinal cord injury. J Neurosurg 12:95–122, 1955.

25. Dinning TA, Schaeffer HR: Discogenic compression of the cauda equina: A surgical emergency. Aust N Z J Surg 63:927–934, 1993.

26. Sayegh FE, Kapetanos GA, Symeonides PP, et al: Functional outcome after experimental cauda equina compression. J Bone Joint Surg Br 79:670–674, 1997.

27. Shapiro S: Cauda equina syndrome secondary to lumbar disc herniation. Neurosurgery 32:743–746, 1993.

28. American College of Surgeons: Advanced Trauma Life Support Program for Doctors, Student Course Manual, 6th ed. Chicago, American College of Surgeons, 1997, pp 26–30.

29. McGuire RA, Neville S, Green BA, et al: Spinal instability and the logrolling maneuver. J Trauma 27:525–531, 1987.

30. Vale FL, Burns J, Jackson AB, et al: Combined medical and surgical treatment after acute spinal cord injury: Results of a prospective pilot study to assess the merits of aggressive medical resuscitation and blood pressure management. J Neurosurg 87:239–246, 1997.

31. Jandreau SW, Gibbs MA: Vertebral injuries. In Ferrera PC, Colucciello SA, Marx JA, et al (eds): Trauma Management: An Emergency Medicine Approach. St. Louis, Mosby, 2001, pp 163–179.

32. Hoffman JR, Schriger DL, Mower W, et al: Low-risk criteria for cervical-spine radiography in blunt trauma: A prospective study. Ann Emerg Med 21:1454–1460, 1992.

33. Hoffman JR, Mower WR, Wolfson AB, et al: Validity of a set of clinical criteria to rule out injury to the cervical spine in patients with blunt trauma. National Emergency X-Radiography Utilization Group. N Engl J Med 343:94–99, 2000.

34. Samuels LE, Kerstein MD: 'Routine' radiographic evaluation of the thoracolumbar spine in blunt trauma patients: A reappraisal. J Trauma 34:85–89, 1993.

35. Terrigrino CA, Ross SE, Lipinski MF, et al: Selective indications for thoracic and lumbar radiography in blunt trauma. Ann Emerg Med 26:126–129, 1995.

36. Glass RBJ, Sivit CJ, Sturm PF, et al: Lumbar spine injury in a pediatric population: Difficulties with computed tomographic diagnosis. J Trauma 37:815–819, 1994.

37. Frankel HL, Rozycki GS, Ochsner MG, et al: Indications for obtaining surveillance thoracic and lumbar spine radiographs. J Trauma 37:673–678, 1994.

38. Kaye JJ, Nance EP Jr: Cervical spine trauma. Orthop Clin North Am 21:449–462, 1990.

39. Mahadevan S, Mower WR, Hoffman JR, et al: Interrater reliability of cervical spine injury criteria in patients with blunt trauma. Ann Emerg Med 31:197–201, 1998.

40. Roth EJ, Park T, Pang T, et al: Traumatic cervical Brown-Sequard and Brown-Sequard-plus syndromes: The spectrum of presentations and outcomes. Paraplegia 29:582–589, 1991.

41. Ross SE, Schwab W, David ET, et al: Clearing the cervical spine: Initial radiologic evaluation. J Trauma 27:1055–1060, 1987.

42. Fox JL, Wener L, Drennan DC, et al: Central spinal cord injury: Magnetic resonance imaging, confirmation and operative considerations. Neurosurgery 22:340–347, 1988.

42a. Lewis LM, Docherty M, Ruoff BE, et al: Flexion-extension views in the evaluation of cervical-spine injuries. Ann Emerg Med 20:117–121, 1991.

43. Kalfas I, Wilberger J, Goldberg A, et al: Magnetic resonance imaging in acute spinal cord trauma. Neurosurgery 23:295–299, 1988.

44. Bracken MB, Shepard MJ, Collins WF, et al: A randomized, controlled trial of methylprednisolone or naloxone in the treatment of acute spinal cord injury. N Engl J Med 322:1405–1411, 1990.

45. Bracken MB, Shepard MJ, Collins WF Jr, et al: Methylprednisolone or naloxone treatment after acute spinal cord injury: 1 year follow-up data (results of the Second National Acute Spinal Cord Injury Study). J Neurosurg 76:23–31, 1992.

46. Bracken MB, Shepard MJ, Holford TR, et al: Administration of methylprednisolone for 24 or 48 hours or tirilazad mesylate for 48 hours in the treatment of acute spinal

cord injury: Results of the Third National Acute Spinal Cord Injury Study. JAMA 277:1597–1604, 1997.
47. Yoshida GM, Garland D, Waters RL: Gunshot wounds to the spine. Orthop Clin North Am 26:109–116, 1995.
48. Manary MJ, Jaffe DM: Cervical spine injuries in children. Pediatr Ann 25:423–428, 1996.
49. Hadley MN, Zambramski JM, Browner CM, et al: Pediatric spinal trauma: Review of 122 cases of spinal cord and vertebral column injuries. J Neurosurg 68:18–24, 1988.
50. Lee C, Woodring JH, Goldstein SJ, et al: Evaluation of traumatic atlanto-occipital dislocations. Am J Neuroradiol 8:19–26, 1987.
51. Bohn D, Armstrong D, Becker L, et al: Cervical spine injuries in children. J Trauma 30:463–469, 1990.
52. McGrory BJ, Klassen RA, Chao EY, et al: Acute fractures and dislocations of the cervical spine in children and adolescents. J Bone Joint Surg Am 75:988–995, 1993.
53. Nitecki S, Moir CR: Predictive factors of the outcome of traumatic cervical spine fractures in children. J Pediatr Surg 29:1409–1411, 1994.
54. Kriss VM, Kriss TC: SCIWORA (spinal cord injury without radiographic abnormality) in infants and children. Clin Pediatr 35:119–124, 1996.
55. Grabb PA, Pang D: Magnetic resonance imaging in the evaluation of spinal cord injury without radiologic abnormality in children. Neurosurgery 35:406–414, 1994.
56. Atkinson PP, Atkinson JL: Spinal shock. Mayo Clinic Proc 71:384–389, 1996.
57. Rumana CS, Baskin DS: Brown-Sequard syndrome produced by cervical disc herniation: Case report and literature review. Surg Neurol 45:359–361, 1996.
58. Waters RL, Adkins RH, Yakura JS, et al: Motor and sensory recovery following incomplete tetraplegia. Arch Phys Med Rehabil 75:306–311, 1994.

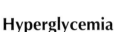
Chapter 20

Hyperglycemia and Hypoglycemia

Marjorie A. Bowman
John M. Howell

Hyperglycemia

Hyperglycemia is most commonly caused by diabetes mellitus. Occasionally, hyperglycemia is transient or results from a measurement error. There are many potential reasons for transient blood sugar elevations (Box 20–1), but diabetes should be considered as a diagnosis if recurrent hyperglycemia occurs in the setting of a potential cause of transient hyperglycemia. Less commonly, some patients develop secondary diabetes from Cushing's syndrome, acromegaly, hemochromatosis, or chronic pancreatitis.

Box 20–1. *Causes of Transient Hyperglycemia*

- Stress: Acute illnesses, pregnancy, trauma, seizures, acute pancreatitis
- Iatrogenic causes: Intravenous fluids, peritoneal dialysis, total parenteral nutrition
- Drugs: Steroids, estrogens, sympathomimetic agents (including epinephrine) nicotinic acid, phenytoin, thiazide diuretics, diazoxide, streptozotocin, pentamidine, alcohol, hypervitaminosis A

Severe hyperglycemia is associated with diabetic ketoacidosis (DKA) and diabetic hyperosmolar hyperglycemic syndrome (HHS).[1] These two conditions are similar except that the ketoacidosis of DKA causes more severe nausea; therefore, these patients seek care more quickly, with less dehydration. Metabolic acidosis causes deep (Kussmaul's) respirations, increases susceptibility to cardiac dysrhythmias, decreases myocardial contractility, and can lead to a decreased level of consciousness. DKA tends to occur in younger and type I diabetic patients; HHS tends to occur in the elderly and in type II diabetic patients. HHS often occurs in patients not previously diagnosed with diabetes. DKA and HHS may be part of the same disease spectrum. Consequently, features of both DKA and HHS can coexist in an individual patient.[1]

CLINICAL RECOGNITION ◄————

DKA presents with thirst, polyphagia, polyuria, nocturia, blurred vision, weight loss, hyperventilation, orthostatic hypotension, confusion, vomiting, abdominal pain (i.e., vague, diffuse discomfort), fruity odor on the breath, shock, and coma. These symptoms usually evolve relatively quickly. HHS tends to develop more subtly, sometimes over days to weeks. HHS leads to polyuria, polydipsia, increasingly abnormal mental status, confusion, and neurologic problems such as seizures, visual hallucinations, and focal neurologic findings. HHS can mimic stroke. Some patients have low-grade fever. Blurred vision is occasionally the presenting symptom of acute diabetic problems.

Common precipitants of DKA and HHS are emotional stress, noncompliance with a diabetic regimen, infection (often occult), gastrointestinal bleeding, acute myocardial infarction (AMI), and lack of adequate oral fluid intake. AMI may be silent (i.e., without chest pain) in elderly patients with DKA or HHS.

PHONE TRIAGE ◄————

Thirst and *frequency of urination* in a patient without known diabetes should precipitate an office visit, with timing based on chronicity (the longer the symptoms have been present without associated problems, the less urgent the visit). If thirst and urinary frequency are associated with *mental status changes or other neurologic symptoms*, the patient should be directed to be seen urgently, either at the office or in the emergency department, depending on local circumstances.

Any diabetic who is not feeling well or who has a fever should have his or her blood sugar checked. The patient can do this at home if the equipment is available there. Type I diabetic patients should be seen the same day, regardless of the home blood sugar measurement, if they have any of the following symptoms: *vomiting, abdominal pain, significant headache, fever, dysuria, significant malaise, dizziness or lightheadedness, chest pain, shortness of breath, confusion, or any other neurologic symptoms.* In patients with type II diabetes, usual protocols for determining the need for office visits can be followed for patients with home blood sugars lower than 300 mg/dL. For patients with type II diabetes who have blood sugars higher than 300 mg/dL, their usual blood glucoses should be discussed. At a minimum, the current blood sugar should be evaluated and the possible need for changes in management discussed, either over the telephone or at an office visit.

DKA is present when the glucose is greater than 250 mg/dL, the bicarbonate is less than 15 mEq/L, serum and urine ketones are positive, and there is a low pH (<7.3).[2, 3] Of course, some hyperglycemic states are intermediate between mild hyperglycemia and DKA.

In general, HHS is diagnosed in the face of both hyperglycemia and hyperosmolarity without significant ketosis. Coma may intervene when the serum osmlarity is greater than 350 mOsm/kg and the glucose is greater than 600 mg/dL. Other synonyms for HHS are hyperosmolar hyperglycemic nonketotic coma (HHNC), hyperosmolar hyperglycemic nonketotic state (HNNK), nonketotic hyperosmolar syndrome (NKHS), and nonketotic hypertonicity in diabetes. These terms are uncommonly used today. Serum osmolarity (normal 275–285 mOsm/L) is derived from the following formula:

$$2 (Na^+ + K^+) + glucose/18 + blood\ urea\ nitrogen\ (BUN)/2.8$$

 LABORATORY RECOGNITION ←

In most locations, the first determination of glucose is made from a fingerstick glucose test, which is now quite ubiquitously available. When the need for treatment is assessed, it must be remembered that there are many potential ways for a fingerstick glucose to be inaccurate. Fingerstick glucose measurements are about 15% lower than corresponding serum measurements.[4] Outdated test strips and inadequate control measures can lead to overreadings or underreadings. Falsely low readings are associated with too little blood placed on the test strip, high hematocrit (>55), and hypotension.[4] Falsely high readings are associated with low hematocrit (<25) and high uric acid.[4] In general, there is less accuracy at high (>350) or low (<50) glucose levels, although the general direction will be correct.[4]

Urine dipsticks are useful in the assessment of patients with hyperglycemia. However, urinary glucose can be falsely negative with ingestion of ascorbic acid. Ketonuria, a manifestation of diabetic ketoacidosis, also exists in starvation, pregnancy and lactaction, fever, hyperthyroidism, renal glycosuria, and glycogen storage disease, and with high-fat diets.[5]

If serum sodium is measured by the older flame photometric method, the sodium should be corrected up 1.6 mEq/L for each 100 mg/dL increase in glucose, or for each 1000 mg/dL increase in triglycerides. However, most laboratories measure serum sodium with ion-specific electrodes that do not require correction.

Dehydration, which occurs commonly with higher levels of hyperglycemia, is also associated with increases in albumin, bilirubin, calcium, total protein, lactate dehydrogenase, transaminase, and creatine phosphokinase.

Initial Management

Hyperglycemia without significant ketosis, dehydration, or hyperosmolarity can almost always be treated on an outpatient basis, even when the glucose seems significantly high (e.g., above 400 to 500 mg/dL). A high glucose value can be seen in chronically uncontrolled diabetic patients without acute symptoms or significant deterioration in electrolyte or fluid status. In these situations, the general goal should be to move toward improved overall control, rather than necessarily emphasizing the attainment of a normal glucose the same day. Daily doses of medications should be adjusted or new medications added, and these patients should be followed closely as outpatients through phone and office contacts.

If (1) the amount of acidosis is mild; (2) the hydration deficit can be corrected in the office; (3) the vital signs are normal; (4) there is good home support; and (5) there is no concurrent illness suggesting hospital admission, then either DKA or HHS can be treated on an outpatient basis.

Equipment and Medications

Equipment and medications for treating hyperglycemia are listed in Box 20–2.

Treatment of DKA, HHS, and Hyperglycemia with Significant Symptoms (Box 20–3)

Monitoring (Keep a Flow Sheet)
1. Check the patient's glucose level every 30 to 120 minutes. Fingerstick glucose can be used for some of these measurements if the patient is not hypotensive or does not have other factors that contribute to falsely aberrant fingerstick measurements. Correlate the initial fingerstick glucose with a serum determination.

Box 20–2. *Hyperglycemia and Hypoglycemia: Medications and Equipment*

- Glucagon
  - single-use vials can be stored at room temperature
  - Once reconstituted, use immediately
- Dextrose 50 ampules
- Human regular insulin
  - Store vials in the refrigerator. Insulin that has been frozen cannot be used. Comes in 1.5- and 10-mL vials, 100 units/mL
- U-100 syringes
- Fingerstick glucose reader
- Urine dipstick for ketones
- Electrocardiogram machine
- Intravenous fluids
- flow sheet

Box 20–3. *Treatment of Symptomatic Hyperglycemia*

Hyperosmolar Hyperglycemic Syndrome

- Hyperosmolar (usually >320 mOsm/kg)
- Hyperglycemia (usually >500 mg/dL)
- No significant ketosis
- No significant acidosis

Insulin. Can withhold until volume status improves. Can give 5–10 units bolus IV regular insulin, followed by 1–10 units per hour.

Fluids. Give normal saline or 0.45% saline with 1 ampule of sodium bicarbonate. Add glucose when glucose is <300 mg/dL. Give $1/2$ to 1 liter in the first hour, then $1/2$ liter per hour, until fluid deficit corrected, then 150 mL/hr.

Potassium. Withhold initially, then add 10 m Eq/hr in intravenous fluids. Increase to 15–20 mEq/hr if the potassium falls to 3.5 mEq/L. Be careful if renal failure exists.

Phosphate. Withhold initially, then alternate potassium chloride with potassium phosphate in the intravenous solution, then swittch to oral supplementation.

Calcium. May be needed. Give based on serum values.

Monitor. Electrocardiogram, blood glucose, electrolytes, BUN, creatinine, calcium, magnesium, phosphate, vital signs, mental state, urine output, anion gap.

Box continued on following page

Box 20–3. *Treatment of Symptomatic Hyperglycemia* Continued

Diabetic Ketoacidosis

- Blood sugar >250 mg/dL, pH <7.3
- Bicarbonate <15 mEq/L + serum and urine ketones

Insulin. May give 10–15 units (or 0.15 µ/kg) bolus regular insulin IV, followed by 10 unis (or 0.1 unit/kg) per hour. Taper insulin when glucose is dropping 50 mg/dL/hr.

Fluids. Give normal saline or 0.45% saline if Na^+ >155. Add glucose when glucose is <300 mg/dL. Give $1/2$ to 1 liter in the first hour, then $1/2$ liter per hour, until fluid deficit corrected, then 150–250 mL/hr.

Potassium. Add 10 m Eq/hr in intravenous fluids if adequate urine output and no tented T waves on the electrocardiogram. Increase to 15–20 mEq/hr if the potassium falls to 3.5 mEq/L. Be careful if there is renal failure.

Phosphate. Alternate potassium chloride with potassium phosphate in the intravenous solution to a total of 20 mEq of potassium phosphate, then switch to oral supplementation when feasible.

Monitor. Electrocardiogram, blood glucose, electrolytes, blood urea nitrogen (BUN), creatinine, calcium, magnesium, phosphate, vital signs, mental state, urine output, and anion gap.

---

2. Measure electrolytes every 2 to 6 hours.
3. Measure serum calcium, magnesium, and phosphate every 6 hours.
4. Document vital signs, mental status, and urine output every 30 to 60 minutes.
5. An electrocardiogram can be used as a screen for significant hyperkalemia and followed.
6. The anion gap should be followed in DKA, although it is less useful if there is concurrent lactic acidosis. Repeated serum ketones are not helpful.
7. Arterial blood gases should be done initially and repeated if the serum bicarbonate does not respond within a few hours.

Insulin

1. Insulin is more important in DKA than in HHS. Some HHS can be treated without insulin, and only with IV hydration. In fact, newly diagnosed diabetics with HHS may respond in a very brittle fashion to modest insulin dosages. Sometimes they also require large doses of insulin.
2. In DKA, initially give 10 to 15 units of regular insulin or 0.15 units/kg intravenously. Some physicians do not use a bolus for milder DKA,

especially in children (see the "Pediatrics" section). Insulin can be given intramuscularly, but it is best to avoid intramuscular administration in hypotensive patients in whom the absorption is particularly erratic. The maximum effect of an intravenous insulin bolus occurs at 10 to 30 minutes, and its duration is 1 to 2 hours. If a bolus is given, it is followed by 10 units/hr or 0.1 units/kg/hr in a drip. When a good response is obtained (e.g., the serum glucose drops by 50 mg/dL/hr), taper the drip to 1 to 2 units/hr. If there is an inadequate response, consider insufficient fluid repletion, insulin resistance, and inadequate insulin delivery.

3. In HHS, insulin can be withheld until the intravascular volume status is improved. Then, give a 5- to 10-unit bolus of regular insulin, followed by 1 to 10 units per hour, increasing or decreasing the dose to reach the goal of dropping the blood glucose by 50 mg/dL/hr. Remember that newly diagnosed diabetics with HHS may experience a precipitous drop in serum glucose with even modest insulin doses, and great care is required.

Fluids: DKA

1. In some patients, aggressive fluid resuscitation is required to normalize vital signs. Give normal saline unless the serum sodium is above 155 mEq/L, when 0.45% saline is appropriate. Add glucose to the intravenous fluids when the serum glucose is less than 300 mg/dL. Following fluid resuscitation, the intravenous rate should be $1/2$ to 1 liter over an hour, then $1/2$ liter per hour. After the fluid deficit is corrected clinically, the rate can be decreased to 150 to 250 mL/hr.

2. The use of bicarbonate is controversial. Intravenous bicarbonate is sometimes used for patients with severe hyperkalemia, a pH less than 6.9, cardiac arrhythmias, or instability. However, bicarbonate has not been shown to improve metabolic recovery and can be associated with metabolic alkalosis, hypokalemia, and cerebral edema. One ampule of sodium bicarbonate (i.e., 44 mEq) can be combined with 1 liter of 0.45% normal saline and infused as described under "Intravenous Fluids."

3. Hypokalemia develops with insulin therapy, and patients with DKA are usually total body deficient in potassium. In the face of hypokalemia, begin 10 mEq/hr in peripheral intravenous fluids when there is adequate urine output and no electrocardiographic evidence of hyperkalemia. Increase to 15 to 20 mEq/hr when the serum K^+ reaches 3.5 mEq/L.

4. Phosphate deficiences are associated with rhabdomyolysis and respiratory muscle weakness, but overzealous phosphate correction leads to hypocalcemia due to calcium-phosphate binding. Thus, it is reasonable to alternate potassium chloride and potassium phosphate

in the intravenous solutions until 20 mEq of potassium phosphate has been given; then switch to oral supplementation.

Fluids: HHS

1. Fluids are the mainstay of treatment. Resuscitate with normal saline until vital signs are normalized. Consider 0.45% normal saline after the patient is no longer dehydrated, or if the serum sodium is high. The rate can be up to 1 liter per hour. The total amount of fluid required may be large (e.g., 9 liters).
2. Just as for DKA, add 5% glucose when the serum glucose is below 300 mg/dL.
3. See the DKA recommendations for potassium repletion. Withhold phosphate initially.
4. Calcium is sometimes needed, and the amount should be based on serum values.

Complications

DKA is occasionally associated with cerebral edema, heralded by headache, altered mental status, and papilledema. The diagnosis is made by computed tomographic (CT) scan. If cerebral edema occurs, free water (i.e., deliver normal saline, not 0.45% saline) should be limited, the head of the bed elevated to at least 30 degrees, overhydration avoided, and consideration given to neurosurgical consultation for intracranial pressure (ICP) monitoring.

Arterial thrombosis occurs in both DKA and HHS and is associated with stroke, myocardial infarction, and limb ischemia. Subcutaneous heparin may help prevent arterial thrombosis, and treatment includes thrombectomy, intravenous anticoagulation, and thrombolysis.

Lactic acidosis can occur with either DKA or HHS and is more likely if there is concurrent sepsis, shock, or necrotizing fasciitis, or if the patient takes metformin. The anion gap and pH may not respond to insulin therapy alone. Consequently, aggressive fluid resuscitation and, occasionally, bicarbonate administration are needed.

Disposition and Transfer

Patients who need hospitalization should be transferred by ambulance (with advanced life support capabilities) with an intravenous line in place and appropriate fluids running. With DKA and significant hyperglycemia, consideration should be given to an insulin bolus followed by short-term monitoring (i.e., for hypoglycemia) in the office before transfer. Documentation of history, physical examination findings, medical history, office treatment procedures, and laboratory values should be sent with the patient. If possible, cardiac rhythm should be monitored during transfer.

Diabetic patients with significant hyperglycemia and either treated or mild dehydration may be discharged from the office if they understand the treatment plan, have support at home, and can return the next day for evaluation.

Pediatrics

Diabetic children are susceptible to DKA, and the treatment approach is similar to that for adults. The initial fluid bolus is in the range of 15 to 20 mL/kg. Children are usually dehydrated by 5% to 10% of body weight. In general, 5% to 7.5% dehydration can be replenished in the first 24 hours, with a more rapid intravenous rate in the first few hours. Dextrose should be added to the intravenous fluids as the serum glucose falls, but 10% dextrose is sometimes needed when the serum glucose falls below 200 mg/dL. For children, the standard insulin drip rate is 0.10 U/kg/hr. When the switch is made to subcutaneous administration, the first dose is 0.25 units/kg of regular insulin.

Intravenous potassium should be started at a rate of 10 to 20 mEq/hr as soon as the level is known not to be high and urine is produced. Intravenous bicarbonate should be considered for a pH less than 6.9 on arterial blood gas (ABG) measurement, cardiac dyshythmia or dysfunction, or severe hyperkalemia.[6]

Hypoglycemia

Hypoglycemia is usually caused by the medicines used to treat diabetes. Occasionally, patients get hypoglycemia from other medications, such as angiotensin-converting enzyme inhibitors.[7] Hypoglyemia can on occasion be caused by overexertion, surreptitious administration of diabetic agents, adrenocortical insufficiency, renal failure, and insulinomas. Hypoglycemia is associated with alcoholism through a convergence of mechanisms, and similarly, it can be seen in patients who are significantly ill. Some otherwise normal patients get postprandial hypoglycemia (usually several hours after eating), but this rarely requires urgent medical attention. Neonates, particularly those born to diabetic mothers, sometimes develop hypoglycemia shortly after birth.

CLINICAL RECOGNITION ◄

The symptoms of hypoglycemia[8] are anxiety, irritability, jitteriness, sweating, feeling of hunger or nausea, tiredness or fatigue, difficulty talking, weakness, high heart rate or palpitations, headache, blurred vision, and flushing or warmth. Later symptoms include confusion and coma. Occasionally, hypoglycemia occurs with other acute neurologic symptoms, such as seizures or weakness in an arm and leg, a cerebrovascular accident–like complex, but almost any neurologic symptom is possible. Patients who have had previous episodes of hypoglycemia, such as diabetic patients, often recognize the symptoms and initiate treatment, although some diabetic patients have unawareness of hypoglycemia with fewer symptoms occurring. If untreated, hypoglycemia can lead to permanent neurologic impairment or death. Patients may not remember a hypoglycemic event. Patients who are under the influence of drugs or alcohol, who take β-blocking agents, or who are lying down at rest may also have fewer symptoms.

 ## PHONE TRIAGE ◄

Any patient with diabetes who has the symptoms described previously may have hypoglycemia. Blood sugar should be checked, if this can be done quickly and the patient is not seriously ill. Treatment should be provided urgently if the patient has neurologic symptoms or seems acutely ill.

 ## LABORATORY RECOGNITION ◄

Fingerstick glucose measurements are often not accurate at low readings. Whereas a low reading generally suggests that hypoglycemia is present, it may not be accurate as an exact reading. The reasons for false-positive and false-negative fingerstick glucose measurements are discussed in the "Hyperglycemia" section. Serum glucose measurements are much more accurate.

Box 20–4. *Treatment of Hypoglycemia*	
Responsive, cooperative patient	Oral glucose tablet or solution **OR** Glucagon 1 mg IM, may repeat in 20 minutes, plus glucose May use juice if others not available
Unresponsive or uncooperative patient	Intravenous 10%, 20%, or 50% dextrose **OR** Glucagon 1 mg IV or IM plus glucose

Treatment

Acute changes in blood sugar tend to be less well tolerated than chronically low blood sugar, as can occur in adrenocortical insufficiency.

In general, acute hypoglycemia should be treated urgently, preferably after blood has been drawn for a serum glucose assessment. Oral glucose should be provided for patients who are able to cooperate; otherwise, they should be treated parenterally (Box 20–4). A dose of 15 to 20 g of oral glucose should be given, preferably in the form of solution or tablets, which diabetics can carry with them. Glucose gel[9] and orange juice may be less effective.[9, 10] Diabetic patients can also keep glucagon on hand and give it to themselves or have others give it to them intramuscularly for emergencies. Glucagon use should be accompanied by the administration of glucose. For unresponsive patients without nearby glucagon or intravenous glucose, some honey or syrup can be placed along the patient's gumline.

Intravenous dextrose (i.e., 1 ampule or 20 to 50 mL of $D_{50}W$) is preferred to 1 mg of intravenous glucagon.[11] Some recommend using 10% to 25% dextrose solutions to prevent the local damage that can occur from extravasation of 50% glucose, especially in children. Dextrose 10% or 25% is made by diluting D_{50} with sterile water. Glucagon can be given intramuscularly and repeated in 20 minutes if needed; it is often used in non-office situations or during transport if intravenous access has not been obtained. Some form of glucose should be given soon after glucagon administration. Some patients lose their responsiveness to glucagon.

Intravenous dextrose is routinely given to comatose patients for whom the diagnosis is unknown. Neonatal hypoglycemia should be treated in the hospital.

After acute dextrose or glucagon therapy is provided, blood glucose should be repeated and is usually corrected. With long-acting hypoglycemic agents, insulinomas, or neonatal hypoglycemia, patients may need intravenous glucose for prolonged periods.

Equipment and Medications

Equipment and medications for treating hypoglycemia are listed in Box 20–2.

Pediatrics

The general treatment for pediatric patients is similar to that for adults. Most children are given intravenous D_{25} to prevent both tissue inflammation and the rebound hypoglycemia that might follow D_{50} administration. The dextrose dose for children is 0.5 to 1.0 g/kg, or 2 to 4 mL/kg of D_{25}. D_{10} should be given to neonates in the dose of 5 to 10 mL/kg/dose. The glucagon dose for children is 20 µg/kg.

References

1. Ennis ED, Stahl EJ, Kreisberg RA: The hyperosmolar hyperglycemic syndrome. Diabetes Rev 2:115–126, 1994.
2. Lebovitz HE: Diabetic ketoacidosis. The Lancet 345:767–772, 1995.
3. Bell DSH, Alele J: Diabetic ketoacidosis. Postgrad Med 101:193–204, 1997.
4. Bennett BD: Blood glucose determination: Point of care testing. South Med J 90:678–680, 1997.
5. Wallach J: Interpretation of Diagnostic Tests: A Synopsis of Laboratory Medicine, 5th ed. Boston, Little, Brown, 1992.
6. Raney LH: Disorders of glucose metabolism. In Howell JM, (ed): Emergency Medicine. Philadelphia, WB Saunders, 1997.
7. Morris AD, Boyle DI, McMahon AD, et al, and the DARTS/MEMO Collaboration: ACE inhibitor use is associated with hospitalization for severe hypoglycemia in patients with diabetes. Diabetes Care 20:1363–1367, 1997.
8. Hepburn DA, Deary IJ, Fier BM, et al: Symptoms of acute insulin-induced hypoglycemia in humans with and without IDDM. Factor-analysis approach. Diabetes Care 14:949–957, 1991.
9. Slama G, Traynard PY, Desplanque N, et al: The search for an optimized treatment of hypoglycemia: Carbohydrates in tablets, solution or gel for the correction of insulin reactions. Arch Intern Med 150:589–593, 1990.
10. Brodows RG, Williams C, Amatruda JM: Treatment of insulin reactions in diabetics. JAMA 252:3378–3381, 1984.
11. Collier A, Steedman DJ, Patrick AW, et al: Comparison of intravenous glucagon and dextrose in treatment of severe hypoglycemia in an accident and emergency department. Diabetes Care 6:712–715, 1987.

Chapter 21

Electrolyte Disturbances

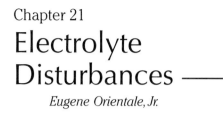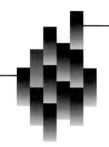

Eugene Orientale, Jr.

Hyponatremia

 ### CLINICAL RECOGNITION

The signs and symptoms of hyponatremia correlate with the underlying disorder and the rapidity and extent of the fall in serum sodium concentration.[1] Mild hyponatremia (sodium > 125 mmol/L) is usually asymptomatic.[2] Musculoskeletal symptoms of mild to moderate hyponatremia include weakness, easy fatigability, or cramps. Central nervous system symptoms from brain swelling tend to occur with more profound acute hyponatremia and include apathy, nausea and vomiting, headache, seizure, coma, and respiratory arrest.[1] The symptoms of chronic hyponatremia are generally milder and more heterogeneous, and include lethargy, confusion, malaise, and, more rarely, seizures.[2]

 ### PHONE TRIAGE

Electrolyte disturbances cannot be diagnosed over the phone but can be suspected. Patients with a history of hyponatremia are more likely to have this condition recur. Answers to questions regarding fluid status (e.g., swelling, dry mouth, lack of urination, or orthostatic hypotension [dizziness with standing]) may suggest hyponatremia. Generally, milder symptoms suggest an office appointment, and serious symptoms, such as coma or seizures, suggest the need for evaluation in an emergency room associated with a hospital.

Box 21-1. *Differential Diagnoses of True Hyponatremia*
Hypovolemic: Excessive diuretics, vomiting, diarrhea, sweating, mineralocorticoid deficiency (Addison's disease), salt-losing nephritis, burns
Euvolemic: Syndrome of inappropriate antidiuretic hormone secretion (SIADH), hypothyroidism, polydipsia (psychogenic), pain/emotion, postsurgical drugs (e.g., exogenous antidiuretic hormone)
Hypervolemic: Congestive heart failure, cirrhosis, nephrotic syndrome, acute renal failure, chronic renal failure, hypoalbuminemia

Epidemiology and Pathophysiology

Hyponatremia is a common electrolyte disturbance. The differential diagnoses of hyponatremia are provided in Box 21-1. Although hyponatremia implies that serum sodium concentration is less than normal, patients with hyponatremia may be hypovolemic, euvolemic, or even hypervolemic. Similarly, the total body sodium content may be decreased. Sodium, as the body's dominant cation, has the greatest impact on plasma osmolality, or concentration of solutes, which ultimately defines the concentration of fluid in intracellular and extracellular compartments.

$$\text{Osmolality (mOsm/kg)} =$$

$$2 \, (\text{sodium, mEq/L} + \text{potassium, mEq/L}) + (\text{BUN, mg/dL} / 2.8)$$

$$+ \, (\text{glucose, mg/dL} / 18)$$

Initial Management

Measurement or calculation of serum osmolality helps in the differentiation of true hypotonic hyponatremia from that situation in which another osmotically active solute, such as glucose or cholesterol, is present in excess. With true hypotonic hyponatremia, the serum osmolality is low (<270 to 290 mOsm/kg).

Treatment considers the underlying cause, degree of hyponatremia, acuity of the electrolyte disturbance, and degree of symptoms. Asymptomatic hyponatremia generally does not require aggressive treatment, whereas symptomatic hyponatremia might require immediate and carefully measured intervention. Rapid infusion of saline can precipitate cerebral swelling and its sequelae; thus, in most cases, sodium should not be corrected by more than 1 mEq/L/hr, and then only when the hyponatremia is symptomatic. Once symptoms are relieved, sodium correction may be reduced further to no more than 12 mEq/L/day.

The patient's volume status should be determined and corrected if indicated. Orthostatic hypotension, reduced skin turgor, decreased central venous pressure, tachycardia, and dry mucous membranes are all consistent with a hypovolemic state. Conversely, congestive heart failure, edema, ascites, stigmata of renal failure, hypoalbuminemia, and cirrhosis are typically more consistent with a state of fluid overload.

The initial work-up of hyponatremia requires ready access to laboratory studies not usually available quickly in the office. First, other osmotically active solutes (such as glucose) are eliminated as causes of hyponatremia. Then, urine osmolality is examined; if urine osmolality is low, dilutional hyponatremia exists caused by excessive water intake (psychogenic polydipsia) or advanced renal failure with inability to concentrate urine. If urine osmolality exceeds serum osmolality, urine sodium level is checked; if urine sodium is low (<20 mEq/L) or high, attention is given to the patient's volume status. Therapeutic interventions are aimed at correcting the underlying cause of the electrolyte disturbance.

Euvolemic Hyponatremia. This condition may arise in the syndrome of inappropriate antidiuretic hormone excretion (SIADH), glucocorticoid deficiency, severe hypothyroidism, and thiazide diuretic use. SIADH is characterized by inappropriately concentrated urine (urine osmolality > 100 mOsm/kg) in the setting of hypotonic hyponatremia. Diagnostic criteria for SIADH include hypotonic hyponatremia; urine osmolality greater than 200 mOsm/kg, usually with elevated urine sodium (>20 mEq/L); euvolemic state with no evidence of volume contraction or expansion; and normal thyroid, adrenal, cardiac, hepatic, and renal function.[3]

Short-term treatment of SIADH is initiated for those patients with severe symptomatic hyponatremia, typically with sodium in the range of 115 to 120 mEq/L. In such cases, a forced diuresis with intravenous furosemide followed by replacement of renal sodium and potassium losses is indicated. Although electrolyte losses may be addressed with administration of isotonic or hypertonic saline, true correction of serum sodium cannot be achieved until the underlying cause is addressed. Initially, a sodium level of 125 to 130 mEq/L is desirable.

Hypovolemic Hyponatremia. Treatment is directed at restoring intravascular volume. Intervention should begin in the urgent care or office setting, but management may need to be continued in the inpatient setting. Focus is directed at restoring hemodynamic stability rather than correcting serum sodium per se through appropriate saline infusion (usually isotonic saline) that restores hemodynamic stability. Some clinicians may opt for hypertonic saline (3%) when very rapid correction of sodium is required. In such cases, hourly monitoring of serum electrolytes in the intensive care setting may be indicated.

Hypervolemic Hyponatremia. Urine sodium levels greater than 20 mEq/L are more consistent with renal disease, whereas urine sodium levels lower than 20 mEq/L are seen with congestive heart failure, nephrotic syndrome, or liver insufficiency. Treatment is aimed at restoring the sodium deficit relative to the water overload by careful water and salt restriction. This is usually accomplished by administration of diuretics such as furosemide. Attention should be directed at mitigating or eliminating the underlying cause of the hypervolemic state.

Equipment and Medications

Equipment and medications are listed in Table 21–1.

Table 21–1. Equipment/Medication for Hyponatremia, Hypernatremia, or Hypercalcemia

Supplies	Cost	Storage	Shelf Life
$1/4$ Normal saline, 500 mL	$0.75/bag	Room temperature, cool & dry area	2 yr
$1/2$ Normal saline, 500 mL	$0.75/bag	Room temperature, cool & dry area	2 yr
D5 $1/2$ Normal saline, 500 mL	$0.60/bag	Room temperature, cool & dry arrea	2 yr
Normal saline, 500 mL	$0.51/bag	Room temperature, cool & dry area	2 yr
D_5W, 500 mL	$0.53/bag	Room temperature, cool & dry area	2 yr
Lactated Ringer's, 500 mL	$0.64/bag	Room temperature, cool & dry area	2 yr
IV tubing (Basic infusion set)	$1.08	Room temperature, cool & dry area	Indefinite, if sealed
IV angiocatheters (16–24 gauge)	50 per box, $35.35/box	Room temperature, cool & dry area	Indefinite, if sealed
14G	50 per box, $35.35/box		
20G	50 per box, $81.79/box		
22G	50 per box, $81.79/box		
24G	50 per box, $81.79/box		
Furosemide (Lasix)	20 mg $0.03/pill 40 mg $0.03/pill 20-mg vial	Controlled room temperature Oral tablets/solution stored in light-resistant containers	Parenteral (tubex) cartridges)— potent for 3 mo Oral solutions are discarded 60 days after opening Tablets expire 1–2 yr from date of issue

Note: Costs obtained from Purchasing Department, St. Francis Hospital, Hartford, Conn, 2002.

ELECTROLYTE DISTURBANCES

Disposition and Transfer

Management of acute or severe hyponatremia is generally performed in the inpatient setting. Interventions for hyponatremia that occurs with hypovolemia or hypervolemia should be initiated in the office. However, prompt transfer from the office or urgent care setting should be initiated shortly thereafter.

Pediatrics

The algorithm for treating hyponatremia in children is similar to that used in adults. Establishing the underlying cause of hyponatremia is even more important given the smaller total body fluid compartments and the increased sensitivity to fluid shifts seen in children.

Euvolemic Hyponatremia. These patients, similar to their adult counterparts, require water restriction. Those children who present in this manner with edema also require sodium restriction and possibly forced diuresis with furosemide.[1]

Hypovolemic Hyponatremia. Table 21–2 illustrates helpful clinical criteria for estimating the degree of dehydration in children; an accurate estimate of percent dehydration is needed to calculate fluid requirements in the hyponatremic/hypovolemic child. Volume expansion is begun with fluids that raise the sodium by no more than 10 mEq/L/day.

Table 21–2. Estimation of Dehydration on Children

Extent of dehydration	Mild	Moderate	Severe
Weight loss—infants	5%	10%	15%
Weight loss—children	3%–4%	6%–8%	10%
Pulse	Normal	Slightly increased	Greatly increased
Blood pressure	Normal	Normal to orthostatic, >10 mm Hg change	Orthostatic to shock
Behavior	Normal	Irritable, more thirsty	Hyperirritable to lethargic
Thirst	Slight	Moderate	Intense
Mucous membranes	Normal	Dry	Parched
Tears	Present	Decreased	Absent, sunken eyes
Anterior fontanelle	Normal	Normal to sunken	Sunken
External jugular vein	Visible when supine	Not visible except with supraclavicular pressure	Not visible even with supraclavicular pressure
Skin (less useful in children >2 yr)	Capillary refill >2 sec	Slowed capillary refill, 2–4 sec (decreased turgor)	Greatly delayed capillary refill (>4 sec) and tenting; skin cool, acrocyanotic, or mottled
Urine specific gravity (SG)	>1.020	>1.020; oliguria	Oliguria or anuria

With permission from Jospe N. Fluids and electrolytes—Clinical aspects. *Pediatr Rev* 17:397, 1996.

ELECTROLYTE DISTURBANCES

Hypervolemic Hyponatremia. Sodium and water restriction is attempted first; diuresis is considered second, except in the setting of cardiopulmonary or renal failure. In the latter, dialysis may be a consideration for those with oliguria or anuria.

Hypernatremia

 ## CLINICAL RECOGNITION ◄───────────────

The patient with hypernatremia may vary in appearance from asymptomatic to confused or obtunded. Signs of volume depletion may be present in the symptomatic elderly patient or the neonate with severe diarrheal illness. Nervous system manifestations of hypernatremia include restlessness, spasticity, muscle twitching, tremor, lethargy, confusion, seizures, and coma. Many of these symptoms are more likely to occur in those experiencing a rapid rise in serum sodium concentration.

For the asymptomatic office patient who is found to have hypernatremia, repeat electrolyte testing can eliminate the possibility of a falsely positive test. For the bedridden nursing home patient, immediate repeat testing is probably unnecessary, given the high prevalence in this setting.

Determination of the underlying cause of this disturbance is based on an appropriate medical history, physical examination, and determination of volume status, urine volume, and urine osmolality. Because the majority of patients with this condition are hyperosmolar, reduced urine output and high urine osmolality are typical.

 ## PHONE TRIAGE ◄───────────────

Patients with a history of hypernatremia are more likely to have a recurrence of this condition. Patients who report excessive thirst may have polydipsia caused by poorly controlled diabetes mellitus or, more rarely, diabetes insipidus. Nursing home patients with reduced free water intake are prone to hypernatremia.

Box 21–2. *Causes of Hypernatremia*
Pure water loss: Increased insensible loss, impaired thirst mechanism, impaired access to free water (e.g., coma, intubation, altered mental status)
Excess sodium intake: Iatrogenic causes (excess saline or sodium bicarbonate), excess ingestion (seawater, drowning), adrenal disorder (Cushing's syndrome or primary hyperaldosteronism)
Loss of water exceeding loss of sodium: Gastrointestinal (vomiting, diarrhea, intestinal fistula), central diabetes insipidus, nephrogenic diabetes insipidus

Epidemiology and Pathophysiology

Hypernatremia is a relatively common clinical electrolyte disturbance with a broad differential diagnosis (Box 21–2). Hypernatremia more commonly occurs in the inpatient than the outpatient setting. It is a hyperosmolar state occurring by pure water loss, excess sodium intake, or loss of water in excess of sodium loss. Whereas hyponatremia results from problems in water handling, hypernatremia typically arises from problems of inadequate water intake. Included in the differential diagnosis is diabetes insipidus (DI), a condition of impaired production of ("central" DI) or responsiveness to ("nephrogenic" DI) antidiuretic hormone (ADH).

Hypernatremia is associated with mortality rates of 42% to 60% in geriatric patients,[4] although these figures may be more representative of underlying disease than of sodium imbalance. Patients who are admitted with hypernatremia are often elderly nursing home patients with an underlying infection such as pneumonia or a urinary tract infection.

Initial Management

Office treatment of newly diagnosed hypernatremia is mostly limited to recognition of the disorder; definitive evaluation and treatment commonly occur in the inpatient setting. It is tempting but incorrect to advise fluid resuscitation for all patients with hypernatremia. Effective treatment is dependent on determination of the underlying cause and whether or not the patient is volume depleted. Free water can be replaced enterally (either by mouth or nasogastric tube), or intravenously with D_5W or hypotonic saline. For those hypernatremic patients who present with volume depletion and hemodynamic compromise, fluid resuscitation first with normal saline can be safely advised. Fluid resuscitation with isotonic saline continues until the patient stabilizes; then, consideration of administering D_5W or hypotonic saline is made. The free water deficit may be estimated from the following formulas[5]:

Current total-body water (TBW) (liters) = 0.6 × current body weight (kg)

$$\text{Desired TBW} = \frac{\text{Serum Na (mEq/L)} \times \text{current TBW}}{\text{Normal serum Na (mEq/L)}}$$

Body water deficit = Desired TBW - current TBW

The rate of administration and choice of hypotonic fluids should be decided judiciously to avoid overly rapid correction of serum sodium. This usually equates to one half of the deficit being given over the first 24 hours, with the remaining deficit given over the following 1 to 2 days. Care should be taken not to correct sodium at a rate faster than 1 mEq/L/hr.

Equipment and Medications

Equipment and medications are listed in Table 21–1.

Disposition and Transfer

Definitive evaluation and care of hypernatremic patients is commonly an inpatient task. Therefore, arranging transfer should be done expeditiously. In the patient with mental confusion or hemodynamic instability, such transfer is made emergently. Before transfer is provided, fluid administration should be started.

Pediatrics

The hypernatremic pediatric patient is also usually dehydrated. Free water is usually lost in excess to that of sodium, even though sodium stores are also reduced. The leading differential diagnosis in children would include diarrheal illness, followed by diabetes insipidus (both central and nephrogenic). Premature infants are more prone to develop hypernatremia owing to their inability to regulate water consumption, intake of high solute–containing formula, and hyperpnea (leading to increased insensible fluid losses).

Management of hypernatremia in a pediatric patient does not significantly differ from that in an adult patient. Free-water loss relative to sodium is replaced with normal saline or Ringer's lactate to restore an effective plasma volume.[1] Thereafter, a hypotonic solution (relative to "physiologic" solution for the pediatric age in question) is used for fluid replacement. Sodium concentrations of 150 to 160 mEq/L may be corrected over 24 hours provided this electrolyte disturbance arose acutely. Rapid rehydration in the setting of chronic hypernatremia may result in devastating cerebral edema caused by the protective development of idiogenic osmoles in the brain. For sodium levels above 160 mEq/L, "the rehydration should be spread out over the number of days necessary to lower the Na^+ concentration to 150 mEq/L by 10 mEq/day (e.g., 2 days for a Na^+ concentration of 170 mEq/L)."[1]

Hypercalcemia

 ## CLINICAL RECOGNITION ◄————————————

Hypercalcemia is a condition in which total calcium exceeds the normal reference range, which is both laboratory and assay dependent, but is usually within 8.9 to 10.1 mg/dL.[6] The biologically active component of calcium is the ionized fraction, which has a reference range of 4.75 to 5.3 mg/dL[6]; however, in practice, the quality control of ionized calcium measurements is less reliable,[7] so most laboratories report the former. Total calcium must be corrected for serum albumin because a large fraction (40%) of calcium is bound to plasma proteins. Total calcium should be inversely adjusted by 0.8 mg/dL for every 1.0 mg/dL that the albumin deviates from the normal of 4.0 mg/dL. Thus, a patient with an albumin of 3.0 and a total calcium of 10.1 (upper limit of normal) actually has a corrected total serum calcium of 10.9 mg/dL and is, by definition, hypercalcemic.

Presenting symptoms are nonspecific and dependent on the underlying cause, the severity of hypercalcemia, and the rate of rise of calcium. Symptoms may include nausea, anorexia, constipation, polyuria, abdominal pain, and bone pain. Severe volume depletion and mental obtundation are more characteristic of hypercalcemic crisis. Cardiologic manifestations of severe hypercalcemia include bradyarrhythmias, bundle branch block, complete heart block, and cardiac arrest.

A thorough history and physical examination are needed to establish the cause. Questions regarding history of cancers, medications, infectious exposures, vitamin intake, family history of hypercalcemia, and corresponding symptoms should be asked. The following diagnostic tests should be considered:

- Parathyroid hormone (PTH) level
- Age- and sex-appropriate search for malignant disease (e.g., chest radiography, mammography, complete blood count and smear, colorectal evaluation, prostate examination/prostate-specific antigen [PSA], Pap smear)[8]
- Multiple myeloma evaluation: Serum and urine electrophoresis
- Vitamin A and D levels
- Corticotropin (Cortrosyn) stimulation test
- Serum calcitriol (1,25-dihydroxyvitamin D) and 25-hydroxyvitamin D levels
- Urine vanillylmandelic acid (VMA) and metanephrine levels

PHONE TRIAGE

Hypercalcemia should be considered in patients with a history of malignancy. Nonspecific gastrointestinal symptoms (e.g., nausea, anorexia, vomiting, abdominal pain), dehydration, polyuria, or bone pain should alert phone personnel to the possibility of hypercalcemia.

Epidemiology and Pathophysiology

Hypercalcemia is found in approximately 1.5% of healthy patients[9] and 0.5% of hospitalized patients.[10] Hypercalcemia may result from increased bone resorption, increased intestinal absorption, or reduced excretion. Excessive PTH secretion secondary to hyperparathyroidism is the most common cause of hypercalcemia, resulting from increased bone resorption. Uncommonly, vitamin D intoxication, sarcoidosis, and milk-alkali syndrome cause hypercalcemia through increased intestinal absorption. Reduced excretion of calcium is the least common cause of hypercalcemia; usually, the ensuing dehydration of severe hypercalcemia causes reduced renal excretion because of increased sodium (and calcium) reabsorption that preserves intravascular volume.

The differential diagnosis for this disorder is presented in Box 21–3.[11] More than 90% of cases of hypercalcemia are caused by either primary hyperparathyroidism or malignancy,[12] particularly in patients with advanced solid tumors of the head and neck, lung, breast, stomach, kidney, uterus, cervix, and, more rarely, colon. Hematologic malignancies such as lymphoma, multiple myeloma, and leukemia may also manifest with hypercalcemia.

> ### Box 21–3. *Causes of Hypercalcemia*
>
> Primary hyperparathyroidism
> Malignant disease
> Medications: Thiazide diuretics, lithium, estrogens, antiestrogens, vitamin D toxicity, vitamin A toxicity, theophylline toxicity
> Granilomatous diseases: Sarcoidosis, tuberculosis, histoplasmosis, coccidioidomycosis, leprosy, berylliosis, silicotic granuloma
> Nonparathyroid endocrine disorders: Hyperthyroidism, adrenal insufficiency, pheochromocytoma
> Familial hypocalciuric hypercalcemia
> Immobilization
>
> Reprinted with permission from Kaye TB: Hypercalcemia—How to pinpoint the cause and customize treatment, *Postgrad Med* 97:154, 1995.

Initial Management

Although it is usually reasonable when treating the asymptomatic patient to "electively" establish the cause first, the patient with significant symptoms or severe hypercalcemia (calcium level > 14 mg/dL)[11] requires urgent treatment.

These patients are typically volume depleted, and initial measures are directed at volume expansion with normal saline, which can begin in the office setting. Volume expansion is begun at the rate of 2 to 4 L/day for the first 24 hours.[7] Patients are carefully observed for fluid overload; if this occurs, consideration should be given to forced diuresis with a potent loop diuretic, such as furosemide (Lasix), which leads to both sodium and calcium diuresis. Because loop diuretics cause renal loss of sodium in excess of calcium, a forced diuresis may incur renally mediated sodium conservation and thus limit calcium diuresis. Therefore, "standing orders for furosemide therapy should not be part of the initial therapy for hypercalcemic crisis."[7] Initial therapy with fluid resuscitation does not succeed in patients with renal impairment for reasons other than volume contraction; patients with severe preexisting renal disease may require dialysis with a low-calcium dialysate to correct their hypercalcemia.

Only one pharmacologic agent—calcitonin—has any place in the urgent or acute care setting. When given exogenously, calcitonin-salmon (Calcimar, Miacalcin) exerts its calciuretic effect within a few hours and its anti-osteoclastic effect shortly thereafter.[13] Presumably because of lack of office availability of the drug, administration of calcitonin in the setting of severe hypercalcemia usually takes place in the inpatient setting. Further therapy aimed at limiting bone resorption can be initiated, almost invariably in the inpatient setting. These therapies include bisphosphonates, glucocorticoids, gallium nitrate, or, more rarely, plicamycin. These measures to reduce calcium have a slower onset of action than does diuresis, but they have a more sustained duration of action; thus, such measures should be begun as soon as is feasible. A summary of the agents for hypercalcemia is found in Table 21–3. Starting doses for these agents are found in Table 21–4.[7] With the exception of furosemide and normal saline, these agents are not cost effective for maintenance in the primary care office setting.

Hypercalcemia associated with hyperparathyroidism commonly takes an indolent course, permitting planned rather than emergent surgery. Even without symptoms, the long-term effects of untreated hypercalcemia include abnormalities such as renal calculi, osteoporosis, peptic ulcer disease, hypertension, and neuropsychiatric disease.

Table 21–3. Treatment of Hypercalcemia—Summary

Treatment	Brand Name	Onset of Action	Duration of Action	% Normalized	Advantages	Disadvantages
Saline		Hours	During infusion	0–10	Rehydration	Cardiac decompression, intensive monitoring, electrolyte disturbance, hypokalemia, hypomagnesemia
Saline + loop diuretic (furosemide)	Lasix	Hours	During treatment	0–10	Enhanced renal calcium exretion	Cardiac decompensation, intensive monitoring, electrolyte disturbance, hypokalemia, hypomagnesemia
Calcitonin	Calcimar Miacalcin	Hours	2–3 days	10–20	Nontoxic, rapid onset of action in life-threatening hypercalcemia	Lowers calcium by only 2–3 mg/dL; tachyphylaxis not prevented glucocorticoids
Plicamycin	Mithracin	24–48 hr	5–7 days	40–60	20-yr experience	Renal insufficiency, liver abnormalities, platelet defects with repeated administration
Etidronate	Didronel	24–48 hr	7–10 days	20–40		Hyperphosphatemia, 3-day infusion
Gallium nitrate	Ganite	48–72 hr	10–14 days	70–80	Potency	Length of intravenous administration, renal impairment precludes its use
Pamidronate	Aredia	24–48 hr	10–14 days	70–100	Potency, relatively nontoxic	Fever in 20%, hypophosphatemia, hypomagnesemia

Adapted from Nussbaum SR: Pathophysiology and management of severe hypercalcemia. Endocrinol Metab Clin North Am 22:351, 1993; with permission.

Table 21–4. Pharmacologic Treatment of Hypercalcemia—Dosages

Treatment	Brand Name	Recommended Starting Dose
Saline		200–250 mL/hr, 2.5 to 4 L/day
Saline + loop diuretic furosemide)	Lasix	As above: Lasix 10–80 mg IV q6–12h, as needed (maximum single dose 6 mg/kg)
Calcitonin	Calcimar Miacalcin	4 IU/kg body weight every 12 hr SC/IM
Plicamycin	Mithracin	25 mcg/kg body weight/day IV for 3–4 days
Etidronate	Didronel	7.5 mg/kg body weight/day for 3 days
Gallium nitrate	Ganite	200 mg/m^2 (body surface area)/day for 5 days
Pamidronate	Aredia	60–90 mg IV over 24 hr

In the setting of malignancy-associated hypercalcemia, the disease is usually not occult.[14] More commonly, symptoms of the malignancy bring the patient to the doctor and, as a result, hypercalcemia is found incidentally. Thus, definitive treatment of malignancy-associated hypercalcemia should be directed at treatment of the underlying cause. Even if treatment is aggressive, the interval between diagnosis of hypercalcemia and death is often less than 6 months.[14] It should be noted that aggressive treatment of hypercalcemic crisis in all patients with underlying advanced malignancy may not be warranted; some argue that this deprives the patient of a "compassionate" death.[4]

Equipment and Medications

Equipment and medications are listed in Table 21–1.

Disposition and Transfer

Mild or asymptomatic hypercalcemia is an outpatient disease. Diagnostic evaluation may take place electively. Clear cases of acute hypercalcemia with metabolic encephalopathy or cardiac arrhythmias constitute a medical emergency, requiring immediate transfer to an inpatient setting. Administration of saline infusion or combination saline infusion/forced diuresis may be begun in the office or urgent care setting while transfer of the patient is being arranged.

Pediatrics

Hypercalcemia is a rare occurrence in pediatric patients, except for cases of malignancy-associated hypercalcemia. The furosemide (Lasix) dose, given parenterally, for infants and children is 1 mg/kg/dose every 12 hours intravenously or intramuscularly as needed.

Hyperkalemia

CLINICAL RECOGNITION ◄————————————

Hyperkalemia is typically defined as potassium above 5.5 mEq/L. Clinical manifestations of hyperkalemia are rare, unless it is severe. Symptoms comprise muscle weakness, including dyspnea due to respiratory muscle weakness, tingling, paresthesias, and, rarely, flaccid paralysis. The effect of hyperkalemia on the heart is generally insignificant at below 6 mEq/L.[15] However, severe hyperkalemia can induce lethal cardiac arrhythmias, including atrioventricular dissociation, ventricular tachycardia, and ventricular fibrillation. Concomitant hypocalcemia, hyponatremia, and acidemia enhance cardiac toxicity. Electrocardiographic (ECG) findings include peaked T waves, prolonged PR interval, second-degree atrioventricular (AV) block, loss of P-wave amplitude (or complete loss), and intraventricular conduction delay. The formation of "sine waves"—a widened QRS blended with a widened T wave—is ominous and portends poorly for impending cardiac function.[15]

PHONE TRIAGE ◄————————————

Symptoms of hyperkalemia are unlikely unless the hyperkalemia is severe. Patients with a history of renal disease or chronic renal failure are prone to hyperkalemia. Because of the myriad of drugs that affect potassium (e.g., nonsteroidal anti-inflammatory drugs [NSAIDs], angiotensin-converting enzyme [ACE] inhibitors, and diuretics), a drug history of the patient is of some value; any patient with renal disease who has taken one of the aforementioned medications is a possible candidate for further office evaluation.

Epidemiology and Pathophysiology

Hyperkalemia is not as common as hypokalemia. Renal failure accounts for more than 75% of cases of hyperkalemia; in fact, if one eliminates hyperkalemia due to acute and chronic renal failure, the incidence of this electrolyte abnormality is very low.[16] Elderly patients are somewhat more predisposed to hyperkalemia owing to certain high-risk medications, innate disturbances in potassium handling, and comorbid disease.

Potassium is the principal intracellular cation; it plays a paramount role in maintaining the electrical potential of those cells that undergo spontaneous depolarization. Although extracellular potassium accounts for a mere 1% to 2% of body stores, its extracellular concentration is critical to electrically excitable tissues such as those found in the cardiac and skeletal muscles. Hyperkalemia causes an increase in the resting potential of the cell, moving the resting potential closer to the threshold potential for depolarization; as a result, cells are more electrically excitable and thus are more likely to depolarize.

The causes of hyperkalemia can be discretely divided into four major categories (Box 21–4): Pseudohyperkalemia, increased intake, transcellular shift from intracellular fluid (ICF) to extracellular fluid (ECF), and decreased renal excretion.[16]

Pseudohyperkalemia. This condition results from the release of potassium by cells within the blood specimen, particularly in the setting of thrombocytosis, hemolysis, or leukocytosis. It is a function of laboratory error and does not signify a disease condition. Pseudohyperkalemia is suggested by the absence of other electrolyte abnormalities, such as elevated renal indices (blood urea nitrogen [BUN], creatinine) or decreased bicarbonate; in such cases, a promptly repeated potassium assay typically yields a normal result.

Increased Intake. This is a rather unusual occurrence, resulting from either iatrogenic causes or, more rarely, dietary causes. Iatrogenic causes

---

Box 21–4. *Causes of Hyperkalemia*

Pseudohyperkalemia (Release of Potassium by Cells in a Test Tube). Thrombocytosis, leukocytosis, hemolysis, abnormal leaky red blood cell (RBC) membrane

Increased Intake. Oral (including salt substitutes), intravenous, exchange transfusion, use of aged packed RBCs

Transcellular Outward Movement of Potassium. Metabolic and acute respiratory acidosis, insulin deficiency and hyperglycemia in uncontrolled diabetes mellitus, increased tissue catabolism (trauma, chemotherapy, hemolysis, and rhabdomyolysis), exercise, medication-related symptoms (digoxin, β blockers, succinylcholine, and arginine), familial hyperkalemic periodic paralysis

Decreased Renal Excretion of Potassium. Acute oliguric renal failure, acute glomerulonephritis or acute tubular necrosis, oliguric end-stage renal failure, hypovolemia, hypoaldosteronsim, medications (potassium-sparing diuretics and angiotensin-converting enzyme [ACE] inibitors), distal renal tubular acidosis (type IV renal defect in potassium excretion—familial or obstructive)

include excessive intravenous potassium or oral supplements, as well as hemolysis from aged transfused blood, both of which are more common with rapid intravenous infusions or in neonates. High potassium loads may also come in the form of potassium-containing salt substitutes or antibiotics such as potassium penicillin G. Generally, this category represents a rare cause of hyperkalemia due to rapid excretion of excess potassium by intact kidneys.

Transcellular Shift from Intracellular to Extracellular Fluid. Factors that affect cellular potassium balance include acid-base balance, insulin, mineralocorticoids, and sympathetic (adrenergic) activity. Acidosis results in efflux of potassium from cells into the extracellular fluid, causing hyperkalemia; alkalosis causes the opposite, resulting in hypokalemia. Metabolic disorders have a more profound effect on potassium shift than do respiratory disorders.[17] Insulin activates influx of potassium into the ICF; accordingly, insulin (administered with glucose) is a treatment option for acute hyperkalemia. Mineralocorticoids such as aldosterone have the opposite effect on potassium, and they reduce serum potassium. Aldosterone augments potassium excretion in the urine, feces, saliva, and sweat. Sympathetic activity also affects potassium; β-adrenergic activity tends to reduce extracellular potassium, whereas α-adrenergic activity increases potassium levels in the serum. Extreme hyperkalemia impedes sodium transport across the cell membrane, thus preventing depolarization; this explains the clinical manifestations of flaccidity and paralysis associated with marked hyperkalemia.

Decreased Renal Excretion. Decreased renal excretion is the most common cause of true hyperkalemia. Renal failure, both acute and chronic, represents the most frequent cause in this category. Drug adverse effects are also extremely common; mechanisms of action and examples of such drugs include the following:

- Decreased aldosterone secretion: Heparin, ACE inhibitors
- Decreased tubular potassium excretion: Potassium-sparing diuretics, lithium, trimethoprim
- Both decreased aldosterone and tubular potassium excretion: NSAIDs, cyclosporine[18]

Initial Management

In patients with no other electrolyte abnormality, a repeat potassium assay should be done to exclude pseudohyperkalemia. Because an immediate electrolyte assay may not be available in the office setting, an ECG may be performed in selected patients. However, the ECG is an insensitive means of detecting hyperkalemia[19]; one study found abnormal ECG results in 64% of patients with potassium levels above 5.5 mEq/L. In severe hyperkalemia, the specificity of abnormal ECG findings is more impressive; all patients with potassium levels above 6.7 mEq/L had one or more ECG abnormalities.[20]

For patients with significant hyperkalemia (>6.0 mEq/L), the condition is a potentially life-threatening emergency. To stabilize such patients, continuous cardiac monitoring is instituted, along with measures to either increase elimination of potassium or shift ECF stores to the intracellular space. Emergency therapy for hyperkalemia is summarized in Table 21–5. One author recommends the administration of calcium to all patients with

Table 21–5. Emergency Therapy of Hyperkalemia

Therapy	Indication	Mechanism	Dose	Onset	Duration	Note
Ca gluconate (10%)	Severe hyperkalemia with ECG changes	Antagonism of cardiac conduction abnormalities	10 mL (1 amp) IV over 5 minutes	1–3 min	30–50 min	Usually only with K > 7; dose may be repeated after 1–2 minutes
Ca chloride (10%)	Severe hyperkalemia with ECG changes	Antagonism of cardiac conduction abnormalities	10 mL (1 amp) IV over 5 minutes	1–3 min	30–50 min	As above; more rapidly absorbed vs gluconate
Insulin & glucose	Moderate hyperkalemia	Redistributes K into cells	50 g glucose, 10 U Reg Insulin (both given IV), or 50 mL D₅W	30 min	4–6 hr	Glucose unnecessary if blood sugar is elevated; may repeat insulin every 15 min with glucose infusion, if needed
Cation-exchange resin (Kayexalate)	Moderate hyperkalemia	Excretion/ exchange for Na ions	Oral: 15–50 g with a 70% sorbitol soln (50–100 mL) Rectal: 30–50 g in aqueous medium 1.25 g/5 cc; 60-, 120-, 200-, 500-cc suspensions available	1–2 hr	4–6 hr	Can lead to CHF. Enema is retained for 30–60 min
Loop diuretic	Moderate hyperkalemia	Renal excretion	Lasix 10–80 mg IV	With diuresis	With diuresis	May work even in severe renal disease
Bicarbonate	Moderate hyperkalemia	Antagonizes metabolic acidosis, redistributes K into cells	1 amp (50 mEq) IV	Rapid	Variable	Not routinely recommended, controversial
Albuterol		Redistributes K into cells	10 mg[12] in saline by nebulizer	30 min	2 hr	Contraindicated in coronary disease patients
Dialysis	Hyperkalemia with renal failure	Excretion, improves acidosis		Rapid	Variable	

amp, ampule; CHF, congestive heart failure; ECG, electrocardiogram; IV, intravenous.

ELECTROLYTE DISTURBANCES

ECG abnormalities; calcium antagonizes the membrane effect of hyperkalemia and reverses the ECG changes within minutes, for up to 1 hour.[19]

For mild to moderate hyperkalemia (serum K^+ 5.5 < 7 mEq/L), therapeutic measures include exchange resins, insulin and glucose, intravenous diuretics, β agonists such as albuterol, and, rarely, sodium bicarbonate. The mechanism of action, dosage, onset of action, and duration of effect for each of these measures are summarized in Table 21–5. Close monitoring of adverse effects of cation-exchange resins and serum electrolytes is required if treatment is provided outside the inpatient setting. Although it is safe when administered in the general population, resin/sorbitol treatment in elderly patients with end-stage renal disease has resulted in intestinal necrosis and perforation[21]; therefore, it should be administered with caution in such patients. Because of its effect on sodium retention, care must be observed in those patients receiving exchange resins who are prone to fluid overload or hypernatremia.

The effects of calcium, insulin, β agonists, and bicarbonate are all temporary; these interventions are typically followed by cation-exchange

Table 21–6. Medications for Hyperkalemia

Therapy	Cost	Storage	Shelf-Life
Calcium gluconate (10%)	10-mL single-use vial = $0.34–0.36	Room temperature	Stable indefinitely when maintained at room temperature
Calcium chloride (10%)	10-mL single-use vial =$0.33	Room temperature	Stable indefinitely when maintained at room temperature
Insulin, Regular	10-mL vial, 100 units/mL $9.00	Refrigerate unused containers (controversial); room temperature for vial in use	Vial in use at room temperature stable 24 to 30 mo
Cation-exchange resin (Kayexalate)	15 g/60 mL unit dose bottle = $2.30	Room temperature	Stable indefinitely, freshly prepared suspension should be used within 24 hr
Furosemide (Lasix)	20 mg $0.03/pill 40 mg $0.03/pill 20 mg/2 mL vial $0.22/vial	Room temperature, oral tablets/ solution stored in light-resistant containers	Parenteral (tubex cartridges)—potent for 3 mo Oral solutions are discarded 60 days after opening Tablets expire 1–2 yr from date of issue
Sodium bicarbonate 8.4%	50-mL single-use vial = $0.45	Airtight container, avoid extremes in temperature	Stable indefinitely
Albuterol	Solution for inhalation— 2.5 mg/3 mL unit dose = $0.14	Room temperature	Stable indefinitely

Note: Costs obtained from Purchasing Department, St. Francis Hospital, Hartford, Conn, 2002.

resins, diuretics, or, in the setting of severe renal disease, dialysis.[19] Calcium administration and dialysis are generally reserved for severe hyperkalemia or conditions refractory to other measures. Definitive care is directed at establishing, mitigating, and, if possible, eliminating the cause of this electrolyte disturbance.

Equipment and Medications

Equipment and medications are listed in Table 21–6.

Disposition and Transfer

Because of its potential to produce lethal cardiac arrhythmias without warning, significant hyperkalemia (K^+ > 6.0 mEq/L) warrants transfer to the inpatient setting. Mild hyperkalemia (K^+ 5.5–6.0 mEq/L) may be addressed in the outpatient setting, depending on the acuity of the disorder and its underlying cause. It is conceivable that patients in institutionalized settings, such as nursing homes or rehabilitation hospitals, might be treated for moderate hyperkalemia without inpatient transfer; again, caution must be taken to observe adverse effects of therapy and to closely monitor serum potassium.

Pediatrics

Pseudohyperkalemia is most common in children owing to frequently hemolyzed specimens. Neonates are more prone to iatrogenic hyperkalemia if given rapid intravenous infusion of potassium with IV fluids. Congenital disorders, such as 21-hydroxylase deficiency, and other inborn errors of metabolism must be considered during the neonatal period.

The same treatment options exist for treatment in children and in adults. Dosage variations are significant; these are summarized in Table 21–7.

Table 21–7. Pediatric Dosage Considerations: Hyperkalemia

Therapy	Pediatric Dosage
Calcium gluconate	0.5 mL/kg Ca gluconate 10% solution IV over 5–10 min, while monitoring for bradycardia and hypotension
Insulin & glucose	Administer IV over 2 hr: 0.5 g/kg of glucose, with 0.3 units regular insulin per gram of glucose
Bicarbonate	1–2 mEq/kg IV over 5–10 min
Cation-exchange resin retention (Kayexalate)	1–2 g/kg/day orally in 20% sorbitol solution; enema in similar dosage
	Note: 1 g Kayexalate per kg body weight should lower serum potassium by 1 mEq/L

References

1. Josepe M, Forbes G: Fluids and electrolytes—Clinical aspects. Pediatr Rev 17:395–403, 1996.
2. Fried LF, Palevsky PM: Hyponatremia and hypernatremia. Med Clin North Am 81:585–609, 1997.
3. O'Shea MH: Fluid and electrolyte management. In Woodely M, Whelan A (eds): Manual of Medical Therapeutics, 27th ed. St. Louis, Little, Brown 1992, p 48.
4. Palevsky PM, Bhagrath R, Greenburg A: Hypernatremia in hospitalized patients. Ann Intern Med 124:197–203, 1996.
5. Berl T, Schrier RW: Disorders of water metabolism. In Schrier RW (ed): Renal and Electrolyte Disorders, 4th ed. Boston, Little, Brown, 1992.
6. Freidman GD, Goldberg M, Bassis ML, et al: Biochemical screening tests: Effect of panel size on medical care. Arch Intern Med 129:91, 1972.
7. Edelson GW, Kleerekoper M: Hypercalcemic crisis. Med Clin North Am 79:79–92, 1995.
8. Bilezikian JP: Management of hypercalcemia. J Clin Endocrinol Metab 77:1445–1449, 1993.
9. Palmer M, Jakobsson S, Akerstrom G, et al: Prevalence of hypercalcemia in a health survey: A 14 year follow up study of serum calcium values. Eur J Clin Invest 18:39–46, 1988.
10. Fisken RA, Heath A, Bold AM: Hypercalcemia: A hospital survey. Q J Med 196:405–418, 1984.
11. Kaye TB: Hypercalcemia—How to pinpoint the cause and customize the treatment. Postgrad Med 97:155, 1995.
12. Bilezikian JP: Etiologies and therapy of hypercalcemia. Endocrinol Metab Clin North Am 18:389–414, 1989.
13. Deftos LJ: Hypercalcemia—Mechanisms, differential diagnosis, and remedies. Postgrad Med 100:119–126, 1996.
14. Potts JT: Hyperparathyroidism and other hypercalcemic disorders. Adv Med 41:165–212, 1996.
15. Williams ME: Hyperkalemia. Crit Care Clin 7:155–174, 1991.
16. Mandal AK: Hypokalemia and hyperkalemia. Med Clin North Am 81:611–639, 1997.
17. Androgue HJ, Madias NE: Changes in potassium concentration during acute changes in acid-base disturbances. Am J Med 71:456–467, 1981.
18. Clark BA, Brown RS: Potassium homestasis and hyperkalemic syndromes. Endocrinol Metab Clin North Am 24:573–591, 1995.
19. Greenburg A: Hyperkalemia: Treatment options. Semin Nephrol 18:46–57, 1998.
20. Dreifus LS, Pick A: A clinical correlative study of the electrocardiogram in electrolyte imbalance. Circulation 14:815–825, 1956.
21. Perazella M, Mahnen Smith RL: Hyperkalemia in the elderly: Drugs exacerbate impaired potassium homeostasis. J Gen Intern Med 12:646–656, 1997.

Chapter 22
Anaphylaxis
Steven Larson

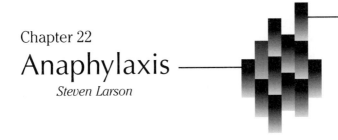

Anaphylaxis is a rapidly progressing, life-threatening medical emergency that requires prompt clinical recognition and treatment. The term *anaphylaxis* is used to describe the rapid, generalized, and often unanticipated series of immunoglobulin E (IgE)-mediated events that occur following exposure to foreign substances in previously sensitized individuals. The term *anaphylactoid reaction* is used to describe a clinically indistinguishable syndrome not mediated by IgE antibody or before exposure to inciting antigens.[1] Clinically, manifestations of anaphylaxis and anaphylactoid reactions range from minor rashes and pruritus to upper airway obstruction and shock.

Exposure to a foreign substance can elicit anaphylaxis or an anaphylactoid reaction in three ways: (1) Exposure to a foreign protein with resultant IgE antibody response; (2) complement cascade activation via immune complexes; and (3) direct release of mediators independent of IgE or complement.[1]

The necessary components of the classical IgE-mediated anaphylactic response are as follows: (1) a sensitizing antigen; (2) an IgE-class antibody response, resulting in systemic sensitization of mast cells (and basophils); (3) reintroduction of the sensitizing antigen; (4) mast cell degranulation with generation and/or release of mediators of inflammation; and (5) production of a disease response by the mast cell–derived mediators manifested by anaphylaxis.[2]

Complement-mediated anaphylaxis is seen following administration of whole blood or its products. In this scenario, immune complexes activate the complement cascade, which in turn produces C3a, C4a, and C5a. These complement factors are capable of causing mast cell (and basophil) degranulation, mediator generation and release, and consequent systemic reactions.

Nonimmunologic or anaphylactoid reactions are produced by agents capable of direct mast cell activation, including medications such as opiates and narcotics, radiocontrast dye, dextrans, neuromuscular blocking agents, and other low-molecular-weight chemicals.

IgE-mediated anaphylaxis has been implicated in reactions to drugs, chemicals, insect envenomations, foods, preservatives, and environmental

315

agents. Of patients receiving penicillin therapy in the United States, 1% to 2% experience a course complicated by systemic allergic reactions.[2] Allergic reactions are generally manifested by urticaria alone; however, an estimated 1 to 5 per 10,000 patients treated with penicillin develop a severe anaphylactic reaction. One of this number dies.[3] Other beta-lactam antibiotics may cross-react with penicillin; approximately 8% of penicillin-sensitive subjects react to cephalosporins.[3] Hymanoptera venoms contain protein antigens capable of IgE antibody responses. After bee stings, 0.5% to 4% of the population experiences a systemic reaction; at least 40 patients die annually.[2] Foods (e.g., peanuts, nuts, shellfish) appear to be the most common cause of anaphylaxis, accounting for more than 30% of cases overall.[4] Over the past 10 years, IgE-mediated allergy to natural rubber latex (NRL) has come to be recognized as a serious potential health problem among health care providers; about 10% of health care workers are sensitized to NRL.[5]

Non–IgE-mediated anaphylactoid responses can occur in response to a variety of agents. Anaphylactoid reaction to contrast dye occurs in 1% to 2% of patients, with 1 to 10 fatalities per 100,000 patients. It is estimated that 40 to 50 deaths occur annually secondary to dye exposures.[4]

 ## Clinical Recognition ←

ANAPHYLAXIS

Anaphylaxis is manifested clinically by a variety of cutaneous, respiratory, cardiovascular, and gastrointestinal symptoms. Clinical manifestations are dependent on the specifics of antigen exposure (i.e., quantity and route), the degree of hypersensitivity, and the target end-organ response to mediator release. Most reactions occur within 30 minutes, but they may take only seconds to minutes, depending on the route of exposure. Symptoms may persist 2 to 4 hours following exposure, rarely extending beyond 24 hours. In approximately 3% of patients, a biphasic course with recurrent symptoms of anaphylaxis is noted within 24 hours.[4]

Symptoms such as pruritus of the palms and soles, perioral tingling, sneezing, rhinorrhea, a feeling of impending doom, and generalized warmth are characteristic early warning symptoms of anaphylaxis. More than 90% of patients develop urticaria and/or angioedema, typically of the face or lips.[4] Frequently, patients complain of mild respiratory symptoms that are described as a dry cough, chest tightness, wheezing, or dyspnea. Laryngeal or supraglottic edema, manifested by throat tightness, hoarseness, or the sensation of a "lump in the throat," is the primary cause of death in anaphylaxis. Refractory hypotension, associated with tachycardia and arrhythmia, may herald complete cardiovascular collapse. Gastrointestinal symptoms of nausea, vomiting, cramping, and diarrhea reflect angioedema of the bowel mucosa.

Phone Triage ◄────────────

As was noted earlier, anaphylaxis typically occurs with vague premonitory symptoms. Individuals involved in phone triage must be trained to recognize the variable, mild symptoms of a potential hypersensitivity reaction. Early therapeutic intervention clearly improves clinical outcome. All patients must be asked whether they have a known history of allergies, or previous hypersensitivity reaction. If there is concern for exposure, therapy should not be delayed; patients should be instructed to use their epinephrine (Epi Pen) if available, as well as to take 50 mg of diphenhydramine orally, if that is available. They should call 911 and be transported to the nearest emergency facility for further management

Laboratory Recognition ◄────────────

Anaphylaxis is a clinical diagnosis. In the short-term care setting, there is no indication for laboratory testing.

Initial Management

Most fatalities associated with anaphylaxis are secondary to upper airway obstruction caused by angioedema, respiratory failure from bronchospasm, or cardiovascular collapse. Successful treatment and management of anaphylaxis are dependent on prompt recognition and early initiation of therapy. The goal of patient management is to reduce or reverse the pathophysiologic process.

Epinephrine, with both α- and β-adrenergic action, is the first-line drug of choice in the treatment of anaphylaxis. Its α-agonist action increases peripheral resistance while reversing peripheral vasodilatation, vascular leak, and resultant systemic hypotension. Its β-adrenergic effects result in increased production of cyclic adenosine monophosphate (cAMP) and subsequent bronchodilatation while blocking further release of chemical mediators. It also serves as both a positive inotropic and a chronotropic agent with respect to cardiac activity.

Patients who present with signs of possible anaphylaxis should be given epinephrine immediately. The recommended dose of epinephrine for the adult population is 0.3 mL 1:1000 dilution administered subcutaneously. For the pediatric population, 0.01 mL/kg 1:1000 is administered. The sub-

ANAPHYLAXIS

cutaneous dose may be repeated at 20-minute intervals.[6] While awaiting clinical response to the epinephrine, IV access should be established and if possible, the patient should be placed on a cardiac monitor.

If there is no response to subcutaneous epinephrine, as manifested by refractory hypotension or impending airway collapse, resuscitation with normal saline solution is begun, and intravenous infusion of epinephrine is the next treatment option. The recommended dose is 1 mL 1:10,000 dilution of epinephrine diluted in 10 mL of normal saline solution, given over 5 minutes as an intravenous push. This may be repeated as clinically indicated. Patients with impending airway compromise from supraglottic or laryngeal edema may benefit from aerosolized racemic epinephrine, which assists in decreasing the amount of airway swelling.[4]

Several key adjunct therapies are available for the management of anaphylaxis; these include antihistamines and corticosteroids. Although antihistamines do not diminish histamine release from mast cells, they play a key role in blocking the action of circulating histamines at target tissue cell receptors. Many of the signs and symptoms of anaphylaxis such as flushing, hypotension, bronchospasm, pruritus, and tachycardia are associated with histamine release and can be diminished through antagonists to histamine receptors.[2] An H_1 blocker such as diphenhydramine 25 to 50 mg should be given to all patients with anaphylaxis. An H_2 blocker such as cimetidine is particularly useful if hypotension is a prominent feature. Corticosteroids are recommended for all patients with anaphylaxis and are felt to diminish the risk for a biphasic course in anaphylaxis, although their actual real benefit has been controversial. They are particularly useful for patients with underlying asthma and coincidental bronchospasm resulting from anaphylaxis.

Patients concurrently using β-adrenergic agents may present with a more severe, prolonged, and refractory anaphylactic reaction. The traditional first-line therapeutic agent—epinephrine, an α and β agonist—is less effective in the setting of β-receptor blockade. Owing to its positive inotropic and chronotropic effects, glucagon 1 to 2 mg given intravenously over 5 minutes may be of great benefit.[4]

Disposition and Transfer

Close monitoring of the patient with anaphylaxis is warranted, with particularly close attention to the principal tenets of basic life support: Airway, Breathing, and Circulation (ABC). Early Advanced Cardiac Life Support (ACLS) intervention may be necessary in the face of significant laryngeal edema or hypotension. Patients manifesting airway or hemodynamic instability must be transferred to the nearest emergency department for close observation and further management. Patients with life-threatening symptoms on initial presentation should be admitted and observed for 24 hours.

Patients managed in the outpatient office setting, who demonstrate only minor symptoms that resolve with initial therapy, may be observed over a 2- to 4-hour period. If symptoms resolve without progression or recurrence, the patient may be treated in the office and sent home on steroids and H_1/H_2 blockers for a 3-day course. Given the risk of a biphasic reaction over the next 24 hours, patients must understand their disease and be instructed to return if symptoms recur or worsen.

Patients with established sensitivity reactions must be cautioned to avoid known causative agents. At all times, they should carry an emergency treatment kit that includes epinephrine and diphenhydramine. Family members or caregivers should be instructed in its use. A medical alert bracelet is also recommended.

Complications

The most imposing threat of anaphylaxis is respiratory compromise from airway edema. Rapid loss of airway patency due to edema complicates attempts at airway management through direct laryngoscopy. Clinicians must respect the pathophysiology and be prepared to obtain a surgical airway via crichothyroidotomy. Hypotension presents another significant source of morbidity; early intravenous access and volume resuscitation, along with early use of epinephrine, remains the best treatment for patients in this setting.

Pediatrics

In general, management of anaphylaxis in pediatric patients requires adherence to the same principles as in the adult population. Early use of epinephrine 0.01 mL/kg 1:1000 administered subcutaneously, as well as intravenous fluid, is the principal therapy in pediatric anaphylaxis. As in the adult population, H_1 blockers (diphenhydramine) and steroids play an equally important role in the management of pediatric anaphylaxis. Supplemental oxygen and albuterol nebulizer therapy is useful for bronchospasm.

References

1. Bochner BS, Lichtenstein LM: Anaphylaxis. N Engl J Med 324:1785, 1991.
2. Atkinson TP, Kaliner MA: Anaphylaxis. Med Clin North Am 76:841, 1992.
3. Lin RY: A perspective on penicillin allergy. Arch Intern Med 152:930, 1992.
4. Zull D: Anaphylaxis. In Harwood-Nuss A (ed): The Clinical Practice of Emergency Medicine, 3rd ed. Philadelphia, Lippincott Williams & Wilkins, 2001, pp 1053–1057.
5. Brehler R: Natural rubber latex allergy: A problem of interdisciplinary concern in medicine. Arch Intern Med 161:1057, 2001.
6. Freeman TM: Anaphylaxis: Diagnosis and treatment. Prim Care 25:809, 1998.

ANAPHYLAXIS

Chapter 23

Acute
Poisonings

Francis DeRoos

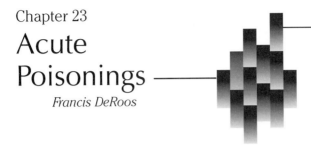

Poisoning, either unintentional or deliberate, is a significant problem in the United States. The American Association of Poison Control Centers (AAPCC) collects and publishes data on over 2 million exposures reported to poison control centers annually.[1] These exposures involve thousands of different compounds from pharmaceutical drugs to insecticides to illicit drugs to botanicals. Although clinical manifestations of acute poisoning from this vast array of compounds are diverse, patients can be assessed initially in a similar manner. The primary focus of this chapter is the management of acutely poisoned patients; however, many of the concepts presented here can be used to assess patients poisoned by chronic exposures as well.

 CLINICAL RECOGNITION

History (Identification of the Toxin)

As with other medical conditions, such as an acute myocardial infarction and major trauma, the first few hours of managing an acute overdose are the most critical. Patients who have been poisoned with highly toxic compounds may be verbal and "asymptomatic" initially, only to be moribund 1 hour later. Because of this, many management decisions must be based primarily on the exposure history and the patient's presenting signs and symptoms. In fact, in most cases, these clinical parameters are all the information that is needed for the clinician to narrow the differential diagnosis to a small list of potential toxins and to design an effective treatment strategy.

The most critical part of the assessment is an accurate history that focuses on the specific agents involved. Other key historical points that should be documented include the quantity ingested, whether the drug formulation was regular or sustained release, and what symptoms have developed. The timing of the ingestion is helpful because it allows application of known pharmacokinetic and toxicokinetic principles to predict onset and/or peak of toxicity. Time of ingestion is also important when one is deliberating whether to induce emesis with syrup of ipecac or to perform orogastric lavage. Finally, the patient's underlying medical condition is one of the most important prognostic indicators in cases of poisoning. A healthy adult tolerates physiologic stress far better than one who has multiple medical problems. Additional clues in the history may help in the identification of emotional stressors or occult depression that may place the patient at risk for suicide.

Documenting this history may initially appear straightforward; however, one must remember that it may not always be reliable. Suicidal patients are notoriously unreliable historians.[2] Caretakers often rush a toddler to health care after a household product exposure and forget to read the label or grab the bottle. Some product names are very similar, and this can be quite confusing. The similarities among clozapine, Clonipin, and clonidine are an excellent example. Sometimes exposures are misidentified because the pills are not stored in the original prescription bottle, or they are simply stored loosely in a bag or other plastic container. Because illicit, herbal, and botanical products have not been regulated in any way, people have been poisoned by unknown adulterants and contaminants.[3, 4]

Despite these potential pitfalls, there are some effective resources and strategies that can aid in identification of exposures. Perhaps the most overlooked strategy is direct observation of the pill containers or the tablets themselves. Sending family members back to the home or calling for another family member to bring the product in ensures accurate identification. In addition, if the patient has a history of hypertension, his or her chances of ingesting an antihypertensive are great. This method of using the patient's or the family's medical history may be extremely enlightening to the physician as he or she develops a list of possible exposures.

Sometimes the method of obtaining the history can affect the success of poisoning identification. For example, patients who are profoundly suicidal often do not give specifics when asked, "What did you take?" However, if the physical examination reveals a dramatic physical finding that narrows the differential diagnosis and a few historical clues focus on one or a few toxins, many patients will tell you the specific pills taken, when they realize, by your focused questioning, that you have "figured it out." Other clues that you may identify during a patient encounter that place poisoning on your differential list are signs of depression, including alterations in sleep or eating patterns, difficulties in interpersonal situations, poor eye contact, and significant stressors.

The regional poison center is an invaluable resource, not only for assistance in the clinical management of poisoned patients but also for the identification of products. All regional poison centers can be contacted through one national toll-free phone number: 1-800-222-1222. Poison centers have access to multiple databases, including Poisondex, which contains the trade names of thousands of products, their active/toxic ingredients, manufacturer contacts, and recommendations for treatment. In addition, if only a tablet formulation is available, this program may be able to identify the product simply from its shape and color and any imprints added to the tablet.

Physical Examination

Sometimes, history may be unavailable or unrevealing and the physical examination must direct initial therapy. A toxin-specific physical examination (Box 23–1) can provide valuable clues about the agent ingested and can guide management. This focused physical examination includes vital signs, neurologic status that emphasizes the mental status, pupillary and oculomotor functions, and diaphoresis and skin color. Obviously, if a patient has respiratory depression or hypotension, he or she should be resuscitated to maintain the airway with positioning, oxygen supplementation, and IV access, while 911 notification is made for assistance and monitored transport to the nearest hospital.

Box 23–1. *Toxicology-Focused Physical Examination*

Vital signs (the most valuable part)
Neurologic examination (mental status, reflexes, muscle tone)
Eyes (movement, pupils)
Skin and mucosa (color, moisture, and markings)
Bowel sounds

Fortunately, this is an uncommon occurrence; however, vital sign changes can help with differential diagnosis and direct therapy. For example, if a patient has bradycardia with a heart rate of 50 beats per minute, only a handful of toxins can induce this, including β blockers, calcium channel blockers, cardiac glycosides, clonidine, phenylpropanolamine, organophosphates, and sedative-hypnotics.[5] The possible toxins may be clarified further by looking for other findings associated with poisoning from these agents. For example, clonidine and sedative-hypnotics also induce somnolence and stupor; organophosphates cause nausea, vomiting, diarrhea, fasciculations, and weakness; and phenylpropanolamine induces a reflex bradycardia secondary to peripheral vasoconstriction and profound hypertension.[5] Table 23–1 lists agents associated with various vital sign abnormalities. This list is not meant to be exhaustive but rather is a quick reference tool for identification of the most common and significant toxins involved.

ACUTE
POISONINGS

Table 23–1. Toxins Associated with Vital Sign Abnormalities

Temperature

Hyperthermia (increased temp)	Hypothermia (decreased temp)
Cocaine/amphetamines/PCP	Ethanol, benzodiazepines, barbiturates
Theophylline/caffeine	Hypoglycemic agents
Antihistamines	Opioids
Salicylates (aspirin)	Clonidine
Phenothiazines	
Serotonin syndrome	

Heart Rate

Tachycardia (increased HR)	Bradycardia (decreased HR)
Cocaine/amphetamines	β blockers
Theophylline/caffeine	Calcium channel blockers
Ethanol/benzodiazepine withdrawal	Digoxin
Tricyclic antidepressants	Clonidine
Antihistamines	Antidysrhythmics, including lidocaine
Iron	Cholinergics, including organophosphates
	Phenylpropanolamine (w/d from U.S. market)

Blood Pressure

Hypertension (increased BP)	Hypotension (decreased BP)
Cocaine/amphetamines	β blockers
Theophylline/caffeine	Calcium channel blockers
Phenylpropanolamine (w/d from U.S. market)	Clonidine
	Tricyclic antidepressants
Ergotamines	Ethanol, benzodiazepines, barbiturates
Lead	Nitrates/nitroprusside
MAO inhibitor interactions	Iron
	Sildenafil (Viagra) drug interaction
	MAO inhibitor overdose

Respiratory Rate

Tachypnea (increased RR)	Bradypnea (decreased RR)
Salicylates (aspirin)	Opioids
Cocaine/amphetamines	Ethanol/benzodiazepines/barbiturates
Theophylline/caffeine	Clonidine
Ethylene glycol/methanol	Botulism
Methemoglobin inducers	
Hydrocarbons (aspiration)	
Cyanide/hydrogen sulfide/carbon monoxide	

BP, blood pressure; HR, heart rate; MAO, monoamine oxidase; PCP, phencyclidine; RR, respiratory rate.

After the initial poisoning-directed physical examination, vital sign abnormalities and a constellation of signs and symptoms may refine the differential diagnosis. These symptom complexes have been called *toxidromes*. Five major toxidromes describe cholinergic, anticholinergic, opioid, sedative-hypnotic, and sympathomimetic findings (Table 23–2).

Table 23–2. Classic Toxidromes—Clinical Manifestations and Agents Commonly Involved

Toxidromes	Clinical Manifestations	Agents Commonly Involved
Opioid	Hypopnea/bradypnea Lethargy, obtundation Mioisis (pinpoint pupils)	Opioids Clonidine/guanabenz Phenothiazines Hypoglycemic agents
Sympathomimetic	Hyperthermia, tachycardia, hypertension Agitation, delirium, seizures Mydriasis (dilated pupils) Increased bowel sounds Diaphoresis (sweating)	Cocaine/amphetamines Theophylline/caffeine Salicylates MAO inhibitors (adrenergic interaction)
Anticholinergic	"Hot as Hades, mad as a hatter, blind as a bat, dry as a bone, and red as a beet" Hyperthermia, tachycardia, hypertension, agitation, delirium, seizures Mydriasis Decreased bowel sounds Dry, flushed skin	Diphenhydramine, hydroxyzine Tricyclic antidepressants Traditional antipsychotics Benzetropine Scopolamine, atropine Plants: Jimson weed (*Datura* genus), deadly nightshade (*Atropa belladonna*), henbane (*Hyoscyamus niger*)
Cholinergic	Bradycardia (muscarinic), tachycardia (nicotinic), hypertension (nicotinic) Miosis Bronchorrhea SLUDGE—*s*alivation, *l*acrimation, *u*rination, *G*I upset, *e*mesis	Organophosphates/carbamates Physostigmine Pilocarpine Betel nut (*Areca catechu*) Mushrooms: *Clitocybe dealbata*, *C. illudens, Inocybe lacera*
Sedative-hypnotic	Hypothermia, bradypnea/hypopnea Rarely hypotension Lethargy, stupor, obtundation	Ethanol Benzodiazepines Barbiturates Others: Ethchlorvynol, meprobamate, chloral hydrate, glutethimide

GI, gastrointestinal; MAO, monoamine oxidase.

PHONE TRIAGE ◄

Perhaps the most challenging aspect of clinical toxicology is assessment of situations and patients over the phone (Box 23–2). Two types of emergency phone calls are made to a physician's office. The first involves an accidental exposure of a toddler to a relatively small quantity of a household product or prescription medication, and the second involves a despondent adult who has, within several hours, either contemplated or actually ingested a large quantity of one or several substances in a suicide attempt. Each of these situations should be handled differently.

Box 23–2. *Key Components of Phone Triage*

Assess for overall mental state (anxious, lethargic, despondent?)
Specifics about what agent involved—exact wording and spelling,
    quantity ingested
When did it happen?
Any symptoms currently?
Contact the regional poison control center: 800-222-1222

In the accidental exposure situation, it is important to reassure the care provider so that an accurate assessment of the situation can be made. Careful assessment of the exposure quantity and product can prevent misinformation and possibly serious triaging errors. The physician should have the person get the product involved and elicit the complete product name and manufacturer. Seemingly unimportant advertising descriptors such as "super," "professional," or "extra strength" may be useful for determining actual concentrations or doses of the compounds involved. Then, the caller should be asked about the exact timing and circumstances of the exposure, including any symptoms that the child may have. A child who was found with an open cleaning product and appears well may not even have ingested the product; however, a toddler who is actively vomiting pills after being found with an open prescription is much more of a concern. Any child who demonstrates significant symptoms and more than one or two episodes of emesis or crying, and now appears well, should probably be evaluated by a physician. The caller should be instructed that any chemicals spilled on the patient's skin must be washed off immediately and before a physician is seen. The care provider should always be instructed to bring in the actual substance containers with the patient. Because of the vast numbers of drugs and chemicals found in homes today, the decision to manage a patient at home or to refer him or her into the office or the emergency department is a difficult one, and it can be made in consultation with the regional poison center.

In the setting of an intentional adult ingestion, patient history may be unreliable because of shame or guilt, and patients may be reluctant to inform you that they have ingested something. Clues to possible intentional ingestion include an altered level of concentration or slurred speech, unexpected tears, or a fairly withdrawn or terse conversation. Patients with a history of depression, substance abuse, and stressful financial difficulties or relationships are at high risk for intentional overdose. If any of these things is detected and there is concern about possible overdose, the clinician should ask patients directly whether they have tried to harm themselves. This relieves the patients of this burden and demonstrates compassion on the part of the physician. One must remember that the patient has taken a very difficult step and has reached out by calling the office and seeking assistance. Immediately after an intentional ingestion has been detected, the emergency medical system (911) should be contacted to transport the patient to the nearest hospital. Most poisoned patients who are going to die do so in the first few hours after the ingestion, so time to supportive care is critical.

Equipment and Medications

In the majority of poisoned patients, timely and vigilant supportive care is all that is required. Basic airway management equipment (including suction, nasal and oral airways, and a bag-valve mask), IV catheters and crystalloid solution, and a few intravenous medications (including glucose and naloxone) should be available (Box 23–3). Although antidotes are available for some poisonings, such as digoxin-specific FAB fragments (cardiac glycosides) and fomepizole (toxic alcohols), many are expensive and all are rarely used, making it illogical for these to be stocked in an office practice facility.

Box 23–3. *Office Equipment Required for the Treatment of Poisoning*

Airway equipment, including nasal trumpets, oral airways, bag-valve mask with appropriate variety of sizes
IV catheters and crystalloids (normal saline or lactated Ringer's)
Medications—syrup of ipecac, oxygen, glucose, naloxone

Initial Management

In the treatment of patients who present after an acute substantial poisoning, the first priority should be adequate resuscitation and transfer to the hospital for a higher level of care. The two major causes of morbidity in poisoning are airway or ventilatory compromise and cardiovascular compromise. Patients who are becoming progressively lethargic or who are developing signs of shock, such as cool, clammy skin, diaphoresis, tachycardia, or frank hypotension, should be stabilized with supplemental oxygen, possibly an airway-assist device, and a large-bore IV catheter with a wide open (1- to 2-L bolus in first 15 to 30 min of care) crystalloid infusion while arrangements are made for transfer to the hospital. In addition, all patients with altered mental status or new neurologic findings or complaints should have a rapid glucose determination.[6]

A focused history and physical examination, as discussed earlier, should help narrow the differential diagnosis and aid in determination of possible specific treatments. Information obtained should be communicated to the emergency department staff so they can prepare to continue the evaluation or resuscitation with appropriate laboratory assays and mobilization of unique antidotes or specialized therapies, such as hemodialysis, immediately. One must remember to send any and all tablets or containers to the hospital with the patient.

After initial assessment of the patient's airway, breathing, and circulation (ABCs) and initial resuscitation, the care of the poisoned patient turns to gastrointestinal (GI) decontamination. The goal of GI decontamination is to remove the harmful compound before it causes systemic toxicity. GI decontamination can be accomplished by induction of emesis with syrup of ipecac, by orogastric lavage after placement of a large-bore orogastric tube, by prevention of further absorption with oral activated charcoal (which adsorbs many toxins), or by whole bowel irrigation, which is used to flush slowly absorbed compounds through the GI tract before systemic absorption occurs.[7]

Syrup of ipecac contains cephaeline and emetine, both of which act on the gastric mucosa and the medullary chemoreceptor trigger zone to induce emesis. It is highly effective, inducing more than 90% of patients to vomit; in human experimental models, if syrup of ipecac is given within 1 hour of ingestion, an average of 30% of the ingested toxin is removed.[8] Its effects last for at least 2 hours, limiting the ability of the clinician to administer activated charcoal or oral antidotes such as *N*-acetylcysteine.[9, 10] Use of syrup of ipecac should be considered in the treatment of patients who have not already vomited and who present within 1 hour of a potentially life-threatening ingestion. Numerous contraindications exist, limiting its role in overdose management primarily to home use for pediatric ingestions. Contraindications to ipecac include:

- Age younger than 6 months
- Caustic or hydrocarbon ingestion
- Presentation hours after ingestion, and most importantly
- Compounds with the potential to induce altered mental status, including lethargy, seizures, and/or hypotension.[7] This is because it takes an average of 20 to 30 minutes for emesis to be induced, and during this time, the drug can be absorbed and patients may develop signs such as lethargy and most have difficulty in protecting their airway during the induced vomiting[11]

In general, the difficulties and risks associated with the use of orogastric lavage and oral activated charcoal in the outpatient setting far outweigh any potential benefit, and their use should not be attempted.

Disposition and Transfer

In patients who do not require immediate resuscitation, the keys to appropriate triage lie in the focused history and physical examination. Patients with signs or symptoms of poisoning such as confusion, tachycardia, abdominal pain, or persistent vomiting should be either referred directly to the hospital, if at home, or prepared for ambulance transport to the hospital, if in the office.

In an acute, intentional ingestion, regardless of the agents involved or the symptoms they may cause, immediate transfer to the hospital is also recommended. It must be remembered that depressed and suicidal patients are well known to provide inaccurate histories.[2] A seemingly harmless handful of ampicillin may evolve within the next hour into a polypharmacy poisoning that cannot be appropriately managed in the office setting. Even patients with seemingly benign and relatively remote (12- to 24-hour) ingestions should probably be screened for occult acetaminophen poisoning. This is because acetaminophen is readily available and its toxicity is not manifest for up to 24 to 36 hours after ingestion when significant hepatic necrosis has occurred.[12]

Children, on the other hand, can often be managed at home or after a brief office visit, depending on the compounds involved, the timing of the exposure, and whether any symptoms have developed. This is because the history tends to be more accurate, the quantities ingested tend to be smaller, and the exposures involve only one substance. This is where the regional poison center can assist in assessment of the risk after individual exposures.

Because they do not manifest severe toxicity after their overdoses, many patients, both adults and children, can be discharged to home with close physician follow-up from the emergency department after several hours of observation; alternatively, they can be transferred to a psychiatric inpatient facility. Exceptions to the "4- to 6-hour observation rule" are drugs or compounds with a known delayed onset of toxicity. These compounds may not manifest significant toxicity for 8 to even 12 hours after ingestion; the only prudent disposition is gastrointestinal decontamination and hospital admission (Box 23–4).

Pediatrics

Pediatric patients account for the vast majority of exposures reported to poison centers nationwide. This is because at between 1 and 2 years of

---

Box 23–4. *Late-Presenting Drugs*

Acetaminophen
Sustained-release preparations—Lithium, β blockers, calcium channel blockers
Oral hypoglycemic agents (sulfonylureas)
Monoamine oxidase inhibitors
Compounds taken concomitantly with anticholinergic agents
Some heavy metals, including elemental lead and mercury

Box 23–5. *Deadly in a Dose*—Listing of Drugs That Can Kill a Toddler in 1 or 2 Doses*

Benzocaine (maximum strength Orajel)
β blockers
Calcium channel blockers
Camphor
Chloroquine
Clonidine
Cyclic antidepressants
Methadone
Methylsalicylate (oil of wintergreen)
Phenothiazines
Sulfonylureas
Theophylline

*Dose refers to a single pill or roughly a 5-mL swallow.
Adapted from Osterhoudt KC: The toxic toddler: Drugs that can kill in small doses. Contemp Pediatr 17:73–88, 2000.

age, toddlers develop adequate pincer grasp, a strong desire to explore new objects with their mouths, and mobility that enables them to roam the home and surroundings. Fortunately, less than 5% of severe or fatal poisonings occur in children younger than 6 years of age. This is because most pediatric exposures involve only one or two tablets or a small swallow of chemicals at a time. However, with a few highly toxic compounds, including oral hypoglycemic agents (sulfonylureas), calcium channel blockers, and methadone, this limited amount can be fatal.[13, 14] In addition, small mouthfuls of topical agents containing benzocaine, camphor, and methylsalicylate, as well as other essential oils, can also kill a toddler. Box 23–5 provides a list of compounds; physicians should be aware of these as being possibly life threatening to a toddler, even if only 1 or 2 tablets or a mouthful is ingested.

Following any accidental exposure in a child, there is an excellent opportunity for parent education and anticipatory guidance. These "teaching moments" rarely present themselves and should be taken advantage of whenever possible. Schedule a follow-up visit shortly after the episode, and sit down with the family and discuss poison proofing the home. It is important that the clinician not appear judgmental during this visit because most parents harbor guilt surrounding this event. A discussion about simple interventions, such as moving cleaning supplies into elevated cabinets, putting a lock on the medicine cabinet, and being careful not to leave daily doses of medications on the nightstand, can go a long way to minimize future exposures. Many regional poison centers have materials for families and physicians with tips about poison proofing the home; these may be beneficial for the reader as well.

ACUTE
POISONINGS

References

1. Litovitz TL, Klein-Schwartz W, White S, et al: The 1999 annual report of the American Association of the Poison Control Toxic Exposure Surveillance System. Am J Emerg Med 18:517–574, 2000.
2. Wright N: An assessment of the unreliability of the history given by self-poisoned patients. J Toxicol Clin Toxicol 16:381–384, 1980.
3. Schauben JL: Adulterants and substitutes. Emerg Med Clin North Am 8:595–611, 1990.
4. Waien SA, Hayes D Jr, Leonardo JM: Severe coagulopathy as a consequence of smoking crack cocaine laced with rodenticide. N Engl J Med 345:700–701, 2001.
5. Nelson L, Hoffman RS: Effective strategies for drug-induced bradycardia and heart block. J Crit Illness 9:916–930, 1994.
6. Hoffman RS, Goldfrank LR: The poisoned patient with altered consciousness: Controversies in the use of a "coma cocktail." JAMA 274:562–569, 1995.
7. Perrone J, Hoffman RS, Goldfrank LR: Special considerations in gastrointestinal decontamination. Emerg Med Clin North Am 12:285–299, 1994.
8. Tenebein M, Cohen S, Sitar DS: Efficacy of ipecac-induced emesis, orogastric lavage, and activated charcoal for acute drug overdose. Ann Emerg Med 16:838–841, 1987.
9. Curtis RA, Bartone J, Giacona N: Efficacy of ipecac and activated charcoal/cathartic: Prevention of salicylate absorption in a simulated overdose. Arch Intern Med 144:48–52, 1984.
10. Kornberg AE, Dolgin J: Pediatric ingestions: Charcoal alone versus ipecac and charcoal. Ann Emerg Med 20:648–651, 1991.
11. Roberston WO: Syrup of ipecac—A slow or fast emetic. Am J Dis Child 103:136–139, 1962.
12. Sporer KA, Khayam-Bashi H: Acetaminophen and salicylate serum levels in patients with suicidal ingestion or altered mental status. Am J Emerg Med 14:443–447, 1996.
13. Koren G: Medications which can kill a toddler with one tablet or teaspoonful. Clin Toxicol 31:407–411, 1993.
14. Osterhoudt KC: The toxic toddler: Drugs that can kill in small doses. Contemp Pediatr 17:73–88, 2000.

Chapter 24

Chemical
Terrorism

Marilyn V. Howarth
Iris M. Reyes

Threats of chemical terrorism and chemical use are very familiar to those in the military. Unfortunately, recent events and threats of terrorism have heightened the awareness of the general public. Although rare thus far, chemical terrorism has the potential for catastrophic consequences. It is essential that physicians in the community have an understanding of the nature and scope of the chemicals that could be used for terrorist acts. Physicians in the community frequently serve as an early warning system to public health professionals nationwide. Early recognition by community-based physicians is invaluable to early management of events of chemical terrorism. This discussion focuses on the chemicals most likely to be used in terrorist acts, possible modes of delivery of these chemicals, the strategies for early identification of chemical-related injury and illness, and preventive measures taken by individuals, physicians' offices, and hospital emergency departments to minimize exposure and cross contamination of other patients and staff.

Numerous countries around the world have stockpiles of chemical and biological weapons. It has been confirmed that Saddam Hussein in Iraq has a large stockpile of chemical weapons and was poised to use them.[1] Fortunately, the Persian Gulf War was brief and these weapons were not employed. The breakup of the Soviet Union and a variety of effects on political alignments thereafter have increased the threat of biological and chemical proliferation and possible use. The availability (due to changing political power) and security of these stockpiles have increased the threat that even small terrorist groups might gain access to previously well-secured stockpiles. The Iraqis used chemical weapons containing cyanide, mustard, and nerve agents against Kurdish Iraqi citizens in the region of Iraq that borders Turkey and Iran. U.S. military physicians examined these casualties and confirmed the reports by identifying lesions consistent with the use of nitrogen mustard.

By gaining an understanding of the exposure mechanisms of chemical and biological agents, those preparing for potential terrorist events may gain insight. With rare exceptions, biological agents are not dermally active but require ingestion or inhalation for infection. Most chemical agents are dermally active. Infectious agents that are spread from person to person can cause mass illness. Chemical agents can affect only those exposed to them. With the exception of caretakers and bystanders who approach and physically contact contaminated individuals, there is little opportunity for secondary exposure. Most chemical agents are volatile and disperse through the air for inhalation exposure as well. The dispersion of infectious agents for inhalation exposure is dependent on the generation of a respirable aerosol (1- to 10-μm-diameter particles), which requires a high level of sophistication.[2] Generating respirable particles in a sufficient quantity requires a high-energy generating system. Once generated, the respirable particles require appropriate weather or environmental conditions to enable the aerosol cloud to remain in the breathing zone of the targeted individuals. Given the complexities of distribution, infection of large numbers of people with microbial agents is more difficult to attain than exposure of large numbers of people to toxic chemicals.

Many of the chemical agents that are considered likely for use in chemical terrorist attacks were used for chemical warfare as early as World War I. Chlorine and phosgene were among the first to be used. Cyanide was introduced later in the war. The greatest number of casualties was caused by the vesicant mustard, which was introduced late in the war. Only during World War II did German scientists develop the first nerve agents. The nerve agents are considered up to 100 times more potent than the chemical agents previously used in World War I. Two classes of military chemical agents are differentiated by their persistence in the environment. Persistent agents (i.e., vesicant mustard and nerve agent VX) have low volatility and evaporate slowly. Nonpersistent agents are those that are quite volatile and are expected to persist in the environment for only a few hours. These agents include phosgene, cyanide, and the G series of nerve agents.

More likely than the seizure and use of stockpiled chemical warfare agents in acts of terrorism is the use of stockpiled chemicals that exist for legitimate purposes. Thousands of tons of cyanide and phosgene are manufactured annually for legitimate purposes. These chemicals are shipped back and forth across the United States and are vulnerable to attack and hijacking. The use of an unsophisticated explosive device placed at a strategically important location would put thousands of civilians in jeopardy of chemical exposure.

The threat of unintentional release of chemical agents from military stockpiles has prompted a preparedness initiative called the Chemical Stockpile Emergency Preparedness Program. This program has been implemented in communities around the stockpiles. The Environmental Protection Agency has developed the Risk Management Program, designed to evaluate the risks of chemical release by American industry. Originally, the data contained in the Risk Management Program were to have been freely available on the worldwide web. Successful legal challenges, however, have restricted access to this information to emergency response personnel, researchers, and government officials.[3]

The protection and treatment of first responders and other health care workers depend on the rapid identification of chemical agents involved in terrorist or unintentional releases. When a chemical is identified, one must remember that multiple chemical agents may be involved. First responders have not routinely carried chemical detection equipment. Even Hazardous Materials (HazMat) units may not have equipment capable of detecting the chemical warfare agents used in terrorist incidents.[4]

Agents with Potential Use for Chemical Terrorism

Nerve Agents

Nerve agents were developed for military use during the Second World War. Other similar agents are used for legitimate purposes in medicine and as insecticides, but their potency is much lower than that of the pure agents used by the military. Five organophosphorus compounds are generally regarded as nerve agents. They are tabun, which the North Atlantic Treaty Organization designates as GA, sarin (GB), soman (GD), GF, and VX. These agents were produced mostly during research efforts designed to identify new insecticides (Table 24–1).

In recent memory, the most infamous of terrorist attacks using chemical agents occurred in June of 1994 when members of a Japanese cult released sarin in Japan. There were 7 deaths, 300 casualties, and many more hospitalizations. In March of 1995, the same cult released

Table 24–1. Chemical and Physical Properties of Nerve Agents

Property	Tabun (GA)	Sarin (GB)	Soman (GD)	VX
Vapor pressure (compared with air)	5.6	4.86	6.3	9.2
Appearance	Colorless/brown liquid	Colorless liquid	Colorless liquid	Colorless/straw-colored liquid
Odor	Fruity	Odorless	Fruity: Oil of camphor	Odorless
Persistency in soil (half-life)	1–1.5 days	2–24 hours	Relatively persistent	2–6 days
LD-50* (liquid on skin of 70-kg man)	1 g	1.7 g	350 mg	10 mg
LCt-50[†] (vapor inhalation)	400 mg/min/m³	100 mg/min/m³	50 mg/min/m³	10 mg/min/m³

*Dose necessary to cause death in 50% of population with skin exposure.
[†]Vapor or aerosol dose necessary to cause death in 50% of exposed population.
Adapted from Sidell F: Nerve agents. In Zatchuk R (ed): Textbook of Military Medicine. Washington, DC, U.S. Department of the Army, the Surgeon General, and the Borden Institute, 1997, p 141.

sarin in the Tokyo subways. More than 5500 people sought medical care, and there were 12 deaths.[5] The vast majority of the 5500 people seeking medical care (4000) had no effects from the agent but were scared and worried about exposure. Many lessons were learned from these events that have shaped the current recommendations for hospital and prehospital triage, decontamination, and care.[6]

Nerve agents can be absorbed through the skin at a rate directly related to temperature. Even after thorough decontamination, the nerve agent that remains on the skin can lead to increased absorption and exposure. The most important route of exposure for nerve agents is inhalation, which results in more rapid evolution of symptoms than does dermal contact.

Nerve agents act by inhibiting acetylcholinesterase (AChE). Acetylcholinesterase catalyzes the hydrolysis of esters, in particular esters of choline. The variable toxicity of nerve agents may be due to their variability in inhibition of biological enzymes. The cholinergic synapses include the neurons to the skeletal muscle, the preganglionic autonomic nerves, and the postganglionic parasympathetic nerves. Exogenous acetylcholine stimulates muscles and other structures innervated by cholinergic synapses (i.e., the glands of the mouth, the respiratory and gastrointestinal systems, the musculature of the pulmonary and gastrointestinal systems, the organs innervated by the efferents of the cranial nerves).[7]

Cholinesterase inhibition can occur within minutes. An immediate test would be helpful for confirming an exposure; diagnosis must be made before the laboratory confirmation is received if appropriate treatment is to be instituted. There is no correlation between the red blood cell (RBC) cholinesterase level and the nerve gas vapor exposure that causes only irritative symptoms. When systemic symptoms such as vomiting occur, however, the RBC cholinesterase is often inhibited by as much as 25%. The number is variable; however, systemic effects predict the depression of RBC cholinesterase activity.

Local irritation of the eyes, nose, and airways can be caused by low levels of nerve gas vapor. As the dose of nerve agents increases, the triad of eye, nose, and lung involvement is usually seen. There may be a subjective sense of dim vision and tightness in the chest, which may occur in the absence of physical findings. At higher exposures, there may be marked diaphoresis, miosis, and copious secretions from the nose, mouth, lungs, and gastrointestinal tract. In severe exposures, the initial effects may not be reported before the patient loses consciousness. In very high concentrations, loss of consciousness may occur within a minute after exposure. Convulsions and limb spasms are generally apparent soon after the patient loses consciousness.

Dermal effects of liquid nerve agents are concentration dependent. There may be a delay of several minutes to several hours followed by localized sweating and possibly vesiculation at the site of skin contact.

Very high level dermal exposures can result in gastrointestinal symptoms of nausea, vomiting, and diarrhea, as well as generalized sweating and fatigue. Symptoms may occur despite appropriate decontamination. Not readily appreciated are the subacute effects, which can include depression, social withdrawal, antisocial thoughts, and restless sleep with nightmares for days after the exposure. Exposures to sarin have resulted in electroencephalographic (EEG) changes such as slowing of activity with bursts of high voltage in the temporal lobes lasting for longer than a week after exposure. Long-term effects on the central nervous system (CNS) have been reported in humans after poisoning with nerve agents or organophosphate insecticides. The pathologic findings in the brain are similar to those seen in hypoxia or with the type of lesions seen after status epilepticus.

The principles of treatment of nerve gas poisoning include terminating the exposure, maintaining the airway, establishing and maintaining breathing, administering an antidote if one is available, and correcting cardiovascular abnormalities. Medical care providers and rescuers must protect themselves from contamination. Terminating the exposure does not simply mean leaving an exposed area. It refers to the very specific practice of decontamination, which is performed for the purpose of preventing further absorption and spread of the agent to others. In the event of an inhalation exposure alone, the exposure can be terminated using appropriate personal protective equipment (i.e., respirators). Because atropine is a cholinergic blocking therapy, it blocks the effects of the accumulated acetylcholine in the synapse. When its effect is worn off, however, the acetylcholine remains in the synapse and continues to be active. A more effective strategy is the combination of atropine with pralidoxime (2-PAM) and diazepam. The effective dose of atropine is a matter of judgment. In a conscious person with mild to moderate effects who is not in severe distress, 2 mg of atropine should be given intramuscularly at 5- to 10-minute intervals until dyspnea and secretions are minimized. Usually, 2 to 4 mg is sufficient. In unconscious patients, however, the atropine dose may exceed 10 times this amount. Convulsions caused by nerve gas can be treated with traditional anticonvulsants of the benzodiazepine family.

Vesicants

A vesicant is a chemical that produces vesicles or blisters. First used as a chemical weapon in World War I, sulfur mustard is the most well-known chemical warfare agent in this category. Unlike sulfur mustards, nitrogen mustards are useful for chemotherapy of neoplasms such as mycosis fungoides, among others. The arsenical, lewisite, is also a vesicant.

Sulfur Mustard

A precursor of sulfur mustard, thioglycol, is widely commercially available.[8] In general, mustards act as alkylating agents that form a highly reactive sulfonium or ammonium electrophilic center. The reactive electrophile modifies the normal functioning of a variety of cellular and subcellular constituents, including peptides, ribonucleic acid (RNA), deoxyribonucleic acid (DNA), and membrane components.

The skin, the eyes, and the airways are the most commonly affected organs. One of the key clinical differences among vesicants is their onset of clinical effects. Those in the mustard group have an onset of clinical effects (i.e., fluid-filled blisters and pain) that occurs up to hours following initial exposure. Other vesicants, such as lewisite and phosgene, cause immediate pain. One of the unique properties of mustard vapor is that it has a density 5.4 times greater than air, causing it to hug the ground, sink into trenches, and remain active in the air for some time. One to one and one-half teaspoons of liquid is enough to cover 25% of the body surface area. This degree of dermal exposure constitutes the potential for a lethal dose. Therefore, erythema with or without blisters covering 25% or more of the body is a matter of great concern.[9]

Reactions to sulfur mustard vary, depending on temperature, humidity, site on the body, and amount of moisture on the skin. Warm, moist areas are much more sensitive than others. The effects from liquid mustard appear more rapidly than do the effects from mustard vapor. Vesication begins about 2 to 18 hours after exposure and may not be complete for several days. The typical bulla is thin and superficial and appears yellowish or translucent. There is a surrounding erythema. It may be up to 5 cm in diameter. A central zone of coagulation necrosis with blister formation at the periphery may occur with extremely high doses.

The eyes are more sensitive than the skin to the effects of mustard. Erythema, blepharospasm, and conjunctivitis are all common. Corneal opacity can occur when the cornea undergoes revascularization after injury. Scarring between the iris and the lens may occur, restricting pupillary movement and predisposing to glaucoma. Direct introduction of liquid mustard to the eye can result in immediate corneal disruption and loss of vision, including panophthalmitis. Miosis can occur because of the cholinergic activity of mustard.[10]

Mustard has little effect on the lung beyond the airways. The upper airways, including the trachea, bronchi, and smaller bronchioles, are most often affected. Atelectasis occurs owing to bronchial secretions. Effects on the gastrointestinal tract can occur within the first few hours after exposure. Early nausea and vomiting can be caused by the cholinergic activity of mustard. In addition, mustard has a very unpleasant odor, which may itself lead to nausea and vomiting. Those who have died from mustard exposure died generally of massive pulmonary damage, not because of primary parenchymal damage, but rather by complications of infection and sepsis.

The diagnosis of mustard exposure is clinical. There is no specific laboratory test or antidote. Mustard destroys the precursor cellular elements of the bone marrow. Leukopenia may begin at day 3 through day 5 and reaches its nadir at 6 to 9 days. The long-term effects of mustard exposure include changes of pigmentation of the skin, sometimes with scarring. Chronic bronchitis is more common among those with mustard exposure. A causal relationship has been discerned between exposure to mustard and various cancers and chronic diseases of the respiratory system and the skin. Certain chronic eye conditions and psychological disorders, as well as sexual dysfunctions, have also been linked causally to mustard and lewisite effects.

Lewisite

Lewisite is an arsenical vesicant that damages the skin, eyes, and airways. Its clinical effects appear within seconds of exposure. The antidote for lewisite is British anti-lewisite (or BAL). The biochemical mechanism of injury includes inhibition of enzymes such as pyruvic oxidase and alcohol dehydrogenase. Despite its clear effects on these enzymes, the exact mechanism of injury has not been identified. Lewisite, liquid or vapor, produces pain and irritation immediately after contact with the skin. The pain caused by lewisite is much less severe than that caused by mustard, and it decreases once the blisters are present. Erythema precedes the blisters, occurring within 15 to 30 minutes after exposure to liquid. Blisters may emerge within several hours. Similar progression with a longer time course is expected after vapor exposure. Lewisite vapor is extremely irritating to mucous membranes. Fortunately, inhalation exposure to lewisite leads instinctively to attempts to immediately extricate oneself from exposure. Lewisite can cause pulmonary edema in addition to airway effects. "Lewisite shock" is an important cardiovascular effect of lewisite overexposure, characterized by protein leakage from capillaries with resultant hypotension. There is no specific laboratory test for lewisite. Urinary arsenic excretion might be helpful as a confirmatory test. Clinically ill patients require diagnosis and management well before laboratory confirmation. The antidote, BAL, decreases the severity of skin and eye lesions if applied topically soon after exposure. Intramuscular BAL reduces the severity of the systemic effects. Very few data are available regarding the long-term effects of lewisite because it has rarely been used.

Pulmonary Toxicants

Phosgene and Chlorine

Phosgene and chlorine have legitimate commercial uses. Neither phosgene nor chlorine produces vesicles; rather, each presents with urticaria and erythema on skin exposure. Pure phosgene is a colorless liquid. Its military formulation may be a yellowish-brown liquid. The biochemical mechanism of injury for both phosgene and chlorine involves their reaction with water on mucous membranes to form hydrochloric acid. The skin, eyes, and lungs are affected immediately, and severe tissue damage can ensue. Phosgene affects an additional mechanism of injury involving amino, hydroxyl, and sulfhydroxyl groups in tissues.

The clinical effects of pulmonary toxicants vary with the concentration and duration of exposure. Acute effects of chlorine vapor exposure may include mucous membrane irritation with hypersalivation, laryngeal edema, and bronchospasm. The ocular lesions include conjunctivitis and keratitis. Pulmonary edema can result after several hours, following inhalation or skin exposure, even with appropriate decontamination. There is no antidote for phosgene or chlorine. Supportive therapy with oxygen, bronchodilators, and steroids may be helpful.[10] Necrotic lesions of the skin should be débrided, cleansed, and disinfected; other lesions should be cared for in a way similar to lesions caused by corrosives.

Cyanide

Cyanide is present and is used in a variety of products in industry, mostly in the form of sodium, potassium, or calcium salt. The volatile liquid, cyanic acid, may be an important form in chemical terrorism. The use of cyanide, more than other chemical agents, has a high likelihood of leading to rapid mortality. The vapor inhalation dose necessary to cause death in 50% of the exposed population (LCt=50) is 2500 to 5000 mg/min/m^3 for the vapor, and the liquid skin exposure dose necessary to cause death in 50% of the exposed population (LD=50) for liquid on the skin is 100 mg/kg.[11]

Cyanide is known to bind and activate several enzymes. Its lethal effect is due to its interference with aerobic cell metabolism caused by binding to cytochrome oxidase. The systemic effects of cyanide exposure can be seen in most organ systems. Prominent early signs and symptoms of cyanide poisoning include transient hyperpnea, headaches, dyspnea, and findings of general CNS excitement, including anxiety, changes in personality, agitation, and seizures. Flushing, weakness, and vertigo can also occur. Coma and dilated, unresponsive pupils are late-appearing signs of CNS depression. An odor of bitter almonds has been associated with cyanide poisoning; however, many in the population cannot detect it. The skin may become cherry red in appearance owing to the increased oxygenation of venous blood, but this is not an essential feature.[12]

Increased epinephrine and histamine release results in profoundly decreased blood pressure, decreased visual focus with mydriasis, and increased frequency and depth of inspiration. Emesis, defecation, urination, and salivation can often occur. Decreased awareness and consciousness can be followed by convulsions. Cardiac arrhythmias and depression of the sinoatrial (SA) node are also important.

Laboratory findings reveal progressive lactic acidosis. Cyanide has a rapid onset of action. Lethal doses achieve their effects in minutes. Cyanide-exposed patients who are conscious require supportive therapy alone. Available antidotes are themselves toxic. The antidotes that may be useful if given before cardiac arrest include amyl nitrite and sodium nitrite with or without sodium thiosulfate. The use of these agents causes significant vasodilation, necessitating careful blood pressure monitoring.

Hospital Preparedness

Recent tragic events have forced our nation to deal with terrorism. Heightened awareness of our vulnerabilities has led to the development of emergency systems specifically designed to address terrorism. In the past, the focus has been on preparedness of the military and out-of-hospital emergency and fire services.[13]

Hospitals and health care workers are likely to be among the first responders to terrorist acts. The development of a plan to handle such an incident should be institution-specific, coordinated with governmental and local emergency medical services and community-based agencies. A bioterroristic event is likely to be covert, with no previous notification of the release of a pathogen. It is likely that the first clues will be sick and dead victims.

Unlike bioterrorism, chemical terrorism is not likely to be covert. Although chemical exposures can have worsening and even permanent effects, the expression of symptoms is fairly prompt. Hospitals and other medical providers might experience an onslaught of patients at the same time or in a very short period. Preparedness plans must account for this rapid onslaught of patients.[14]

For 30 years, the Joint Commission on Accreditation of Healthcare Organizations (JCAHO) has required hospitals to meet established disaster plan standards.[15] These disaster plans are designed to establish standard operating procedures for mobilizing resources for specific incidents that could jeopardize the community, disrupt services, or cause an influx of large numbers of patients into the hospital. A well-designed and well-implemented plan can promote an effective response with minimal confusion and disruption of hospital services.

Two recent studies examined hospital preparedness for biological and chemical weapons.[16, 17] Wetter and colleagues[16] found in his survey of 224 hospitals that fewer than 20% had plans in place to handle a biological or chemical terrorist incident. Approximately half had an outdoor decontamination unit with isolated shower, ventilation, and water containment systems. Only 12% had 1 or more self-contained breathing apparatuses or respirators. Six percent had the minimum required physical resources for a hypothetical sarin incident. Approximately half reported having sufficient ciprofloxacin or doxycycline for 50 anthrax victims.

Treat and colleagues[17] interviewed personnel at 30 hospitals to assess their level of preparedness, including mass decontamination capabilities, training of the staff, and facility security capabilities. She found that no respondents believed that their sites were fully prepared to handle a biological incident. Seventy-three percent believed that they were ill prepared to handle a chemical incident and the same percent could not handle a nuclear event. Although 87% reported that their emergency rooms could handle 10 to 50 casualties at once, only one had stockpiled any medications for treatment of terrorist incidents.

The findings that a significant number of hospitals are unprepared to treat victims in the event of a terrorist act are disturbing. Although the studies have revealed that busier urban hospitals are better prepared, very few met the criteria for handling a theoretical sarin or anthrax exposure involving 50 victims. During the Tokyo sarin incident, one 520-bed hospital received 640 victims who had bypassed any prehospital responders and had undergone no decontamination procedures.[18]

Effective preparedness depends on the prompt availability of resources at the local level. Federal response teams will not be the first responders to incidents of terrorism. Hospitals play a vital role in the early and ongoing response to terrorist incidents. They have not received the level of funding for preparedness commensurate with this important role. The secretary of Health and Human Services has recently proposed $125 million to help U.S. hospitals and local public health agencies become prepared. To date, the Domestic Preparedness Program has provided only limited funding for state and local responders. Hospitals have not been included in the response plans, nor have they received funding to move forward on their own. A tremendous gap exists between government efforts and the true level of individual preparedness at the local level.

Preparedness according to guidelines recently proposed by the JCAHO should include:

- Training health care workers to become familiar with pathogens that may be used, their symptoms, and routes of transmission.
- Creating a single integrated system of response to address a range of possible diseases and disasters.
- Analyzing the preparedness of all regional medical facilities.
- Establishing a surveillance system to promptly detect incidents of bioterroristic activity.

Since the attacks of September 11 on the World Trade Center and the Pentagon and the subsequent release of anthrax-contaminated letters, health care providers have revisited their disaster plans. Disaster plans have been revised to include the recommendations of the Centers for Disease Control and Prevention.[19]

Medical Office Preparedness

It is not reasonable to expect individual physicians' offices to stockpile medications and equipment to prepare for large numbers of patients exposed to chemical or biological agents. Preparation designed for early recognition, containment, contamination reduction, and transport is reasonable, however.[20, 21]

Physicians whose offices are located in close proximity to industry may see patients involved in chemical exposure incidents. Generally, companies working with hazardous chemicals will have established a referral pattern to medical providers who care for work-related injury and illness. Even physicians not usually involved in the care of work-related injury, however, may see exposed patients in the event of off-site contamination of community residents. The prepared clinician should become knowledgeable about area industry and should consider the potential presentations of patients who may have exposure.[22, 23] Chemical exposure can cause a variety of symptoms and signs, and it should be considered in all patients presenting to the physician's office with unexplained symptoms of nausea, dizziness, itching or burning eyes or skin, or cyanosis.[24] Similarly, patients' reports of clouds of vapor, odors, dead animals or fish, or fire should also raise the suspicion of chemical exposure.

The physician's office staff must be trained to act quickly if a patient presents who is visibly contaminated with a chemical agent. They must immediately sequester the affected individual to minimize the possibility of exposure to others in the office. When decontamination is necessary, transport of the patient to a hospital is required. Only facilities with decontamination plans in place should attempt to decontaminate patients. A safe area for keeping the patient while he or she is undergoing decontamination, a method for washing contaminants off the patient, a means of containing the rinsate, and adequate protection for personnel treating the patient are required before decontamination can be initiated.[25, 26] Recognizing that decontamination is not feasible for most physicians' offices, contaminated patients able to change clothing on their own should do so. All contaminated clothing and objects should be bagged by the patient or a medical professional with the use of appropriate personnel protective equipment. Changing clothes may be helpful for reducing contamination if not eliminating it. The use of sinks to wash eyes and mucous membranes may be helpful. Initial assessment should include gathering as much information as possible about the exposure. While containment is occurring, transportation to a hospital with appropriate decontamination and treatment facilities should be arranged.

Conclusions

To date, acts of chemical terrorism have been rare. However, prudent primary care clinicians should be vigilant for patterns of illness that may be sentinel events of chemical terrorism. Assembling resources that may be useful in the event of a chemical attack is important for all community-based providers. The extent and sophistication of preparation vary widely according to the role of the clinical site and the proximity of other resources.[27] Planning for the management of chemically contaminated patients in an office setting is important. Staff should learn about the risks posed by contaminated patients and how to contain and minimize them.

Explosives remain the most likely method of terrorist attack. Placement of explosives near community sources of hazardous chemicals may have catastrophic consequences. For physicians, becoming knowledgeable about the agents of chemical warfare may be important. The catastrophic release of industrial chemicals such as phosgene, chlorine, and ammonia remains more likely, however. The well-prepared clinician will research community hazardous chemical stores through local Emergency Medical Services, the Environmental Protection Agency, and the Agency for Toxic Substances and Disease Registry.[3, 23]

References

1. Dunn P: Chemical Aspects of the Gulf War 1984–1987. Investigations by the United Nations. Ascotvale, Australia, Materials Research Laboratories, 1987.
2. Centers for Disease Control and Prevention: Biological and chemical terrorism: Strategic plan for preparedness and response. Recommendations of the CDC Strategic Planning Workgroup. MMWR Morb Mortal Wkly Rep 49:1–14, 2000.
3. Environmental Protection Agency: Risk management program. Available at http://www.epa.gov/swercepp/acc-pre.html
4. Detection and management of chemical agents. In Chemical and Biological Terrorism: Research and Development to Improve Civilian Medical Response. Washington, DC, National Academy Press, 1999, pp 43–64.
5. Nozaki H, Aikawa N, Shinozawa Y, et al: Sarin gas poisoning in the Tokyo subway. Lancet 345:980–981, 1995.
6. Nozaki H, Hori S, Shinozawa Y, et al: Secondary exposure of medical staff to sarin vapor in the emergency room. Intensive Care Med 21:1032–1035, 1995.
7. Sidell F: Nerve agents. In Zatchuk R (ed): Textbook of Military Medicine. Washington, DC, U.S. Department of the Army, the Surgeon General, and the Borden Institute, 1997, pp 129–180.
8. Detection and management of chemical agents. In Chemical and Biological Terrorism: Research and Development to Improve Civilian Medical Response. Washington, DC, National Academy Press, 1999, p 122.
9. Sidell F, Urbanetti J, Smith W, Hurst C: Vesicants. In Zatchuk R (ed): Textbook of Military Medicine. Washington, DC, U.S. Department of the Army, the Surgeon General, and the Borden Institute, 1997, pp 197–228.
10. Borak J, Diller WF: Phosgene exposure: Mechanisms of injury and treatment strategies. J Occup Environ Med 43:110–119, 2000.
11. Baskin SI, Brewer TG: In Zatchuk R (ed): Textbook of Military Medicine. Washington, DC, U.S. Department of the Army, the Surgeon General, and the Borden Institute, 1997, pp 271–286.
12. Detection and management of chemical agents. In Chemical and Biological Terrorism: Research and Development to Improve Civilian Medical Response. Washington, DC, National Academy Press, 1999, pp 125–126.
13. Richards CF, Burstein JL, Waeckerle JF, Hutson HR: Emergency physicians and biological terrorism. Ann Emerg Med 34:183–190, 1999.

14. Macintyre AG, Christopher GW, Eitzen E, et al: Weapons of mass destruction events with contaminated casualties: Effective planning for health care facilities. JAMA 283:242–249, 2000.
15. Joint Commission on the Accreditation of Healthcare Organizations. Available at http://www.jcaho.org
16. Wetter DC, Daniell WE, Treser CD: Hospital preparedness for victims of chemical or biological terrorism. Am J Public Health 91:710–716, 2001.
17. Treat KN, Williams JM, Furbee PM, et al: Hospital preparedness for weapons of mass destruction incidents: An initial assessment. Ann Emerg Med 38:562–565, 2001.
18. Okumura T, Suzuki K, Fukuda A, et al: The Tokyo subway sarin attack: Disaster management, part 2: Hospital response. Acad Emerg Med 5:618–624, 1998.
19. Centers for Disease Control and Prevention. Available at 1-800-311-3435; http://www.cdc.gov
20. Agency for Toxic Substances and Disease Registry: Managing Hazardous Materials Incidents. Emergency Medical Services: A Planning Guide for the Management of Contaminated Patients. Washington, DC: U.S. Department of Health and Human Services, 2000.
21. Hospitals and Community Emergency Response: What You Need to Know. Washington, DC, United States Department of Labor—OSHA, 1997.
22. Hall H, Dhara V, Price-Green P, Kaye W: Surveillance for emergency events involving hazardous substances—United States, 1990–1992. MMWR Morb Mortal Wkly Rep 43:1–6, 1994.
23. Agency for Toxic Substances and Disease Registry. Available at http://www.atsdr.cdc.gov
24. Agency for Toxic Substances and Disease Registry: Managing Hazardous Materials Incidents. Medical Management Guidelines for Acute Chemical Exposures. Washington, DC, U.S. Department of Health and Human Services, 2000.
25. Agency for Toxic Substances and Disease Registry: Managing Hazardous Materials Incidents. Hospital Emergency Departments: A Planning Guide for the Management of Contaminated Patients. Washington, DC, U.S. Department of Health and Human Services, 2000.
26. Hurst C: Decontamination. In Zatchuk R (ed): Textbook of Military Medicine. Washington, DC, U.S. Department of the Army, the Surgeon General, and the Borden Institute, 1997, pp 351–359.
27. Chemical Terrorism Pocket Guide. Available at http://www.oqp.med.va.gov/cpg/cpg.htm

Chapter 25
Environmental Emergencies

Amy J. Behrman

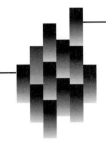

Environmental hazards can cause or exacerbate a wide variety of injuries and illnesses in all age groups. Physician recognition of environmental causation is critical to appropriate medical management of many conditions. Without a careful exposure history, the causative diagnosis may be missed, the treatment may be wrong, and the hazardous exposure may continue. Key components of the environmental history are summarized in Box 25–1; more detailed discussions can be found in many easily accessible sources.[1-3]

Box 25–1. *Key Components of the Occupational/Environmental Exposure History*

Current/recent symptoms
Time course (onset, duration, pattern, relation to activities)
Location of onset and events preceding onset
Prior history of similar symptoms
Similar symptoms in others (family, coworkers, contacts)
Home environment/location/hazards (includes heat and water
  sources)
Work environment/location/hazards (includes school)
Recreational environment/location/hazards (includes travel)
Recent changes in activities/exposures
Use of personal protective equipment
Current/medical history
Social/lifestyle (includes smoking, alcohol, illicit drugs)
Medications (includes alternative and nonprescription)
Allergies (includes animal and plant sensitivities)

It may be useful for the clinician to think of potential environmental hazards as physical, chemical, and biological (Table 25–1). The epidemiology of exposures seen in ambulatory practice reflects local conditions,

Table 25–1. Examples of Common Environmental Hazards

Physical	Chemical	Biological
Heat	Pesticides	Animal/plant allergens
Cold	Fertilizers	Water contaminants
High altitude	Heavy metals	Food-borne pathogens
Water (drowning risk)	Asbestos	Respiratory pathogens
Ionizing radiation	Household cleaners	Blood-borne pathogens
Electricity	Acids/alkalis	Molds
Height	Carbon monoxide	Envenomations
Noise	Hydrocarbons	Zoonoses
Ergonomic stresses	Solvents	Laboratory agents

as well as the demographics and habits of the patient population. A comprehensive discussion of environmental emergencies is beyond the scope of this text. This chapter focuses on a few common exposures that may present in office settings.

Cold-Related Injury

Epidemiology and Pathophysiology

Primary hypothermia is defined as a core temperature less than 35°C due to cold exposure. Hypothermia due to extreme cold may occur during recreational activities such as hiking, climbing, and swimming; during occupational activities such as construction work or military training; or accidentally, if children or adults are unable to obtain adequate shelter. Hypothermia may also result from prolonged exposure to only moderate cold. Risk factors include old or young age, altered mental status, and underlying medical conditions that impair thermoregulation, such as endocrine insufficiencies, malnutrition, stroke, substance abuse, and extensive skin disease. Most cases in this country occur in urban areas and affect the elderly, the intoxicated, and the homeless.[4] Body heat may be lost by conduction (as during cold water immersion), convection (as during windy, cold conditions), radiation (with inadequate insulating clothing), and evaporation.

Mild hypothermia is defined as core temperature between 32° and 35°C.[5] Patients in this range exhibit physiologic adjustments for conservation of body heat, such as peripheral vasoconstriction and shivering. Heart rate, cardiac output, and blood pressure may rise in this "excitation" phase. Below 32°C, hypothermia is called *severe*. Metabolic excitation gives way to depression of cardiac and central nervous system (CNS) function with bradycardia, hypotension, depressed mental status, and dysrhythmias. Fatality is common in patients with severe hypothermia.

Localized cold injuries may occur with or without hypothermia. Cold injuries with freezing of tissue (frostbite) results in some degree of permanent injury, in contrast to nonfreezing injuries, which are due to chronic cold exposure (chilblains, trench foot) that may resolve fully. The epidemiology of frostbite mirrors that of hypothermia. Extremities and facial areas are most vulnerable. The pathophysiology of frostbite begins with cycles of cold-induced vasospasm. When the core temperature is threatened, peripheral blood flow may be completely cut off, allowing ice formation in extracellular and (eventually) intracellular spaces. Secondary intracellular fluid depletion disrupts enzymes and cell membranes. When rewarming allows renewed blood flow, damaged endothelium triggers prostaglandin and thromboxane release with resultant thrombosis and necrosis.[6] Frank gangrene may result. Refreezing increases permanent tissue loss. Frostbite classifications mirror burn terminology: First-degree injury is restricted to the epidermis, second-degree injury to the full skin thickness, and third-degree injury to subcutaneous tissues; fourth-degree injury extends to muscle, tendon, and bone.

 ## CLINICAL RECOGNITION

Mildly hypothermic patients may present with an exposure history, shivering, lethargy, or confusion. Severely hypothermic patients present with cold skin and depressed mental status. Bradycardia and hypotension may occur. Presentation may mimic other conditions such as stroke or intoxication. Medical illness (e.g., sepsis, pneumonia, endocrine dysfunction) and trauma often complicate hypothermia. The electrocardiogram (ECG) may reveal a variety of dysrhythmias. Cold-induced myocardial irritability may lead to fatal ventricular dysrhythmias, spontaneously or after minimal stimulation. The diagnosis is confirmed by documentation of a low core temperature. Unfortunately, many office thermometers are inaccurate below 34°C.[5] Primary care physicians who are likely to see hypothermia in the office setting should obtain a thermometer that is capable of monitoring low core temperatures.

Frostbite victims may present with complaints of numbness or pain in affected regions. With first-degree frostbite, the skin may appear red, hard, waxy, and cold. Second-degree frostbite causes edema and blister formation. (The blister fluid is high in inflammatory mediators.) Third-degree frostbite causes bluish skin, hemorrhagic blister formation, and localized necrosis. Fourth-degree frostbite involves little edema; the skin may be cyanotic, black, or frankly necrotic. Areas of irreversible versus reversible tissue injury cannot be reliably identified on initial presentation.

Nonfreezing injuries present with pain, pruritus, and paresthesias. Initially, chilblains and trench foot cause pale, cool, hypesthetic skin. Later erythema, edema, bullae, and nodules (in chilblains) develop. Permanent tissue loss is rare.

PHONE TRIAGE ◄

> Patients with mild hypothermia or frostbite may call the office complaining of pain or numbness. If the history is consistent with severe or prolonged exposure to cold, if there are visible skin lesions, or if the patient appears confused, he or she should be seen immediately. If the patient has more severe hypothermia, the phone call is likely to be made by a family member or caregiver. A history of mental status change, unresponsiveness, or deteriorating status should trigger a call in most settings for Emergency Medical Services (EMS) transfer to the nearest emergency department.

Initial Management

Hypothermia. The primary concern in the treatment of severely hypothermic patients is to avoid malignant dysrhythmias. **Patients with very low core temperatures should be handled gently to avoid jarring of the irritable myocardium.** All unnecessary procedures involving the thorax should be avoided. If the patient is truly pulseless, cardiopulmonary resuscitation (CPR) should be initiated. Intravenous access should be established peripherally. Advanced Cardiac Life Support (ACLS) should be initiated for ventricular dysrhythmias. Bretylium (5 mg/kg) is probably the most effective drug used to prevent and treat ventricular tachycardia (VT)/ventricular fibrillation (VF) in this setting.[7] If bretylium remains unavailable, current ACLS guidelines for VT/VF should be followed. Although the hypothermic heart is resistant to defibrillation, hypothermia may protect the CNS and other organs from ischemic damage, so full neurologic recovery is possible even after prolonged arrest. Therefore, ACLS should be maintained until a pulse or normothermia is achieved. (Hence the tag, "You're not dead until you're warm and dead.")

In all cases of potential hypothermia, ongoing heat loss should be stopped: Wet clothing should be removed and replaced with warm, insulating clothing and/or blankets. Heat lamps and/or hot water bottles should be used, if available. Active internal re-warming with heated oxygen and intravenous saline is appropriate in all but the mildest of cases, and it has the advantage of preferentially warming the heart and other organs while avoiding potential "core temperature afterdrop."[5] (Dextrose-free saline can be warmed with a blood warmer, an office heater, or even a microwave.) Known or suspected alcoholics should receive intravenous thiamine. Hypoglycemic patients should receive D_{50}.

Frostbite. Optimal initial treatment of frostbite can minimize tissue loss and long-term disability. The first consideration is to treat potentially fatal associated conditions, including hypothermia. The second priority is to avoid refreezing of the injured parts, which worsens permanent tissue loss. The third priority is to begin rapid rewarming. Patients may erroneously believe that slow warming or snow rubbing will be helpful. In fact, prompt immersion in warm water is the most effective way to warm frostbitten limbs. The water should be clean to minimize infection risk, and it should not be warmer than 42°C so that thermal injury can be avoided. Warm compresses may be used on facial injuries. Re-warming pain can be intense and should be treated. Nonsteroidal anti-inflammatory drugs (NSAIDs) should be included in the regimen if possible because of their potential impact on inflammatory mediators of cell injury. It is reasonable for the clinician to drain fluid-filled blisters to remove collections of inflammatory mediators. Topical aloe vera and/or topical antibiotics should be applied to skin lesions to minimize inflammatory injury and prevent superinfection. Systemic antibiotic prophylaxis is more controversial. Frostbite constitutes a tetanus-prone wound, and tetanus immunization should be urgently brought up to date. Nonfreezing injuries do not require acute care and are managed supportively, with an emphasis on avoiding further cold exposure. Equipment and medications needed for initial management of hypothermia and frostbite are listed in Table 25–2.

Table 25–2. Office Equipment and Medications

Cold Exposure	Heat Exposure	Carbon Monoxide Exposure
Thermometer capable of reading low temperatures	Thermometer capable of reading high temperatures	Oxygen
Blankets, blanket warmers	Intravenous saline or lactated Ringer's solution	Non-rebreather masks
Heat lamps	Intravenous tubing	Electrocardiogram (ECG) machine/monitor
Intravenous tubing	Sponges or spray bottles for wetting patient	
Intravenous saline	Fans for evaporative cooling	
Warming device for saline	Ice packs	
Thiamine ampules		
D_{50} ampules		
ECG machine/monitor		
Defibrillator		
Bretylium		
Tetanus toxoid (store in refrigerator)		
Hot water tub/sink		
Dry sterile dressings		
Aloe vera ointment		
Bacitracin ointment		
Nonsteroidal anti-inflammatory drugs (NSAIDs)		
Narcotic pain medications		

Disposition and Transfer

Patients with mild hypothermia, who have no complicating medical conditions and become asymptomatic with office re-warming, can be discharged if they have a warm environment available. Severe hypothermia is a medical emergency. Patients with core temperatures below 32°C on presentation (or for whom the true core temperature cannot be determined), patients with serious underlying illnesses, patients with abnormal ECGs, and patients who remain symptomatic must be transferred to an emergency department for definitive care, including invasive re-warming procedures. As has been noted, stimulation of the irritable myocardium should be avoided during transfer, and cardiac monitors should be used. Active internal re-warming should continue during transfer. Copies of ECGs, relevant medical history, and exposure history should accompany the patient.

Patients with frostbite should also be transferred for further wound management, but ACLS capability is not required. Injured areas should be covered with dry sterile dressings during transfer. Refreezing must be avoided during the process. Pain medications should be maintained during the transfer process. Nonfreezing injuries may be discharged.

Pediatrics

Small children are susceptible to hypothermia because of their increased surface area-to-volume ratio and their relative inability to adjust to their environment. Severe hypothermia can develop insidiously in infants who are exposed to cold environments with inadequate insulation. Cold water immersions are a particular risk in toddlers who may fall into lakes or swimming pools. Hypothermia and frostbite may occur during winter sports. Treatment does not differ from that given to adults. Deep frostbite may result in permanent growth plate injuries.

Complications and Sequelae

The chief complications of hypothermia are death and morbidity from coexistent illnesses and injuries. As has been noted, the neurologic sequelae of coma and cardiac arrest may be less than expected because of the protective effects of extreme cold on the brain and other organs. The potential sequelae of frostbite include necrosis, gangrene, other bacterial infections, amputation, chronic cold sensitivity, chronic pain, hyperhidrosis, arthritis, and increased vulnerability to further cold injury. Great emphasis should be placed on educating patients to prevent further cold injuries.

Heat-Related Illness

Epidemiology and Pathophysiology

Heat emergencies are most common in warm climates, but they may occur in any situation wherein the body produces and/or absorbs more heat than it can dissipate. Heat-related morbidity and mortality are most common among the elderly[8] and those with underlying medical conditions or drugs that inhibit physiologic cooling mechanisms (e.g., obesity, cardiovascular disease, extensive skin disease, sympathomimetic use, anticholinergics, antihistamines, tricyclic antidepressants, lithium, salicylates, phenothiazines, and dehydration) or behavioral accommodation to heat (e.g., psychosis, intoxication, disability, forced labor). Small children are also at some increased risk, and heatstroke is the second leading cause of death among young athletes.[9] Certain occupational groups such as steelworkers, firefighters, and military recruits are at increased risk owing to exertion in hot environments. Acclimatization lowers the risk of heat-related illness by improving the body's ability to dissipate heat by sweating and increased peripheral blood flow. Inadequate ventilation, high humidity, and lack of wind contribute to the risk of heatstroke.

Heat-related illnesses include heat edema, heat cramps, heat syncope, heat exhaustion, and heatstroke. Only heatstroke constitutes a medical emergency; the others may be treated by the patient's moving to a cool environment, resting, and drinking cool fluids. Heatstroke is defined as a core temperature greater than 40.5°C with CNS dysfunction.[9] Other causes of elevated temperature and altered mental status (e.g., infection, drug reaction, alcohol withdrawal) must be excluded because their treatment differs markedly. Heatstroke mortality ranges from 10% to 70% in different populations. The pathophysiology of heatstroke involves complete decompensation of normal heat-regulatory mechanisms. Multiple organs are involved, but the CNS is particularly sensitive to heat injury; therefore, most presenting symptoms involve central neurologic dysfunction. The prognosis depends on the peak temperature, the duration of exposure, and underlying medical conditions.

CLINICAL RECOGNITION ◄————————————

Patients present with fever and a variety of CNS symptoms, which may include confusion, irritability, bizarre behavior, hallucination, seizures, ataxia, or coma. Sweating may be increased, decreased, or absent. Patients may complain of nausea and vomiting. They are likely to be tachycardic with orthostatic hypotension and other signs of dehydration. They may be able to give a history of exertion and/or exposure. The primary care physician is likely to be familiar with medical and social conditions predisposing to heatstroke and its complications. Laboratory studies are useful for monitoring organ damage, but they are nonspecific with regard to diagnosis. Head computed tomography (CT) and lumbar puncture may be necessary to rule out trauma or CNS infection in patients with altered mental status.

PHONE TRIAGE ←

Patients who manifest or complain of CNS dysfunction in a setting consistent with major heat exposure and/or exertion should be emergently evaluated. Depending on the practice setting and access to acute care facilities, reception staff should be instructed to send patients to the ED or bring them immediately to the office. EMS transport should be called for any patient at risk who does not have a reliable source of transportation.

Initial Management

The key to initial treatment is interruption of heat exposure and reduction of the patient's core temperature to 40°C. The patient should be placed in a cool room. Warm, constricting, and occlusive clothing should be removed. Airway protection and ventilatory support should be provided, if needed. Intravenous access should be obtained, and fluid resuscitation should begin with normal saline or lactated Ringer's solution. Flow rates can be initiated at 250 mL/hr, but the rate may need to be adjusted higher if the patient is markedly dehydrated, or lower if underlying cardiovascular disease is present. Fluids should be adjusted as electrolyte abnormalities are documented and carefully monitored to avoid overload.

Simple cooling techniques should be initiated in the office if the patient presents there. Evaporative cooling consists of wetting the patient with tepid water and blowing fans over his or her body. It is effective and well tolerated. (Depending on the ambient humidity, the patient will need re-wetting at intervals.) Ice packs can be placed on pulse points such as the groin and neck, but these may be poorly tolerated by patients. Cool water immersion and ice packing are effective but cumbersome and poorly tolerated. Immersion may be feasible in the office for small children. Invasive cooling techniques such as peritoneal lavage and gastric lavage are inappropriate for the outpatient setting. Cardiac monitoring should be maintained during cooling for patients with known or suspected heart disease. Core temperature should be monitored throughout the cooling process, and efforts should cease when the temperature reaches 40°C. Equipment and medications useful in the initial management of heatstroke are listed in Table 25–2.

Disposition and Transfer

Transfer to an acute care facility is indicated for all patients with a clinical diagnosis of heatstroke. Transfer is not necessary for most patients with a history of heat exposure who do not have a high temperature and CNS findings. (Exceptions should be made for medially fragile patients and those who lack access to a safe, cool environment at home.) Transfer is urgent in heatstroke because end-organ complications, including congestive heart failure, rhabdomyolysis, acute tubular necrosis, coagulopathies, and liver dysfunction, may occur early or late. In addition, fluid management may be problematic in infants and in elderly and fragile patients. Active cooling measures should continue during transport. Copies of laboratory test results, relevant medical history, and exposure history should accompany the patient.

Pediatrics

Infants may have immature regulatory mechanisms, as well as an inability to obtain fluids, remove clothing, and move out of hot environments. The physician should elicit a clear history of the exposure circumstances to rule out abuse/neglect and to counsel the parent on prevention of heat illness. Children left in cars on hot days are at enormous risk.

Carbon Monoxide

Epidemiology and Pathophysiology

Carbon monoxide (CO) is a highly toxic, colorless, odorless gas produced by the incomplete combustion of carbon-containing material.[10] It causes the largest number of toxic deaths in most industrialized countries. Common environmental sources include furnace and heater fumes, vehicle exhaust, house fires, foundries, paper mills, and solvent fumes containing methylene chloride (which is metabolized to CO by the liver after inhalational exposure).[11] Accidental exposure rates are highest in northern states, during winter months, and in industrialized areas.

CO binds avidly to intracellular proteins, including hemoglobin, myoglobin, and the cytochromes.[12] It displaces oxygen from hemoglobin and alters the oxyhemoglobin dissociation curve, thereby dually impairing tissue oxygen delivery in exposed persons. CO binding to cytochromes disrupts oxidative phosphorylation. CO binding to cardiac myoglobin depresses stroke volume and cardiac output. Thus, the most obvious effect of CO exposure is tissue anoxia, although additional mechanisms may contribute to illness. Cardiac and CNS functions are most severely disrupted. Most CO deaths probably result from cardiac arrest. Mortality is highest among the elderly and those with underlying cardiac and pulmonary disease.[13]

CLINICAL RECOGNITION ◄

Presenting symptoms are nonspecific and can be extremely subtle, even in life-threatening exposures. Patients typically complain of a flulike syndrome, fatigue, nausea, headache, dyspnea, or worsening angina. Chest pain and dyspnea may become more frequent and exertional. Patients may be confused, drowsy, lethargic, or comatose. They may collapse suddenly after brief or chronic exposure. Physical examination is also nonspecific. Patients may have tachycardia or hypotension. "Cherry red" skin and flame-shaped retinal hemorrhages are classic findings but are rarely found. Neurologic findings are more common and may include memory deficits, confusion, stupor, apraxia, weakness, dizziness, and subtle neuropsychiatric abnormalities.

Recognition of CO exposure is crucial to treatment and to the prevention of fatalities in the patient and others. Clues to CO poisoning are found in the environmental history. Patients may have exacerbation of symptoms only in the vicinity of a faulty or poorly vented engine exhaust. Patients may be sicker on weekends or may awaken with morning headache and nausea if the source is at home. They may have an occupational history suggestive of exposure sources. They may have been in a house fire. Family members or coworkers may have similar symptoms. Historically, CO toxicity has been associated with poorly ventilated, confined spaces, but recent reports indicate that high concentrations (as from outboard motors) may be toxic even outdoors.[14] The primary care physician must be alert for patterns indicative of environmental exposures so that this and other toxicants can be identified.

The most useful laboratory test is carboxyhemoglobin (HbCO). Elevated HbCO can confirm a diagnosis of CO toxicity, although results may not be available in the office setting and must be interpreted carefully within the clinical context. For example, smokers can have chronically elevated HbCO levels of 5% to 10% without other CO exposure; persons with dangerous CO exposures may have normalized their HbCO after waiting several hours to be tested. Furthermore, levels of HbCO do not correlate well with short-term outcomes or long-term sequelae.[15] Treatment decisions are made on the basis of cardiac and neurologic symptoms after the toxic exposure is established by history and HbCO level (see later).

PHONE TRIAGE ←

Clinical recognition of environmental CO toxicity is difficult, and phone triage is even more difficult. Office staff responsible for triage should understand the local epidemiology and timing of CO exposures (e.g., industrial exposures might occur year-round, home-heating exposures during cold weather, recreational exposures during good weather, and automobile exposures sporadically). They should realize that flulike syndromes and nonspecific GI symptoms may be due to toxicity. They can arrange urgent evaluation for anyone with new or worsening chest pain, dyspnea, or CNS symptoms. Patients can and should be educated to recognize and avoid exposure risks for CO during routine visits.

Initial Management

Patients with suspected CO intoxication should be observed and monitored. Cardiac monitoring is essential for patients with underlying coronary artery disease who may decompensate with ischemic stress. Supportive care includes treatment of anginal symptoms, airway protection if needed, and avoidance of exertion. When the diagnosis of significant CO exposure is established, treatment with 100% O_2 is indicated; this is ideally given by non-rebreather mask. If HbCO levels to confirm the diagnosis will not be available before ED transfer, it may be advisable to start oxygen therapy presumptively. Patients should be followed with serial neurologic checks and cardiac monitoring. Standardized tests of neurologic function may be useful in documenting the acute course and sequelae of CO toxicity.[16] Equipment and medications for the initial management of CO toxicity are listed in Table 25–2.

Disposition and Transfer

Most patients with known or strongly suspected CO poisoning will need transfer for definitive diagnosis and care. In mild exposures without neurologic or cardiovascular compromise, 100% O_2 for at least 4 hours is sufficient therapy. It is critical for the clinician to ensure that the environment where the CO exposure took place has been remediated before the patient returns and that other exposed individuals have access to care. Patients who develop neurologic or cardiovascular instability and all patients with a history of unconsciousness related to CO exposure are candidates for hyperbaric oxygen therapy (HBO) at the nearest hyperbaric chamber. HBO chambers can be located by calling the Divers Alert Network (DAN) at 919-684-2948. Patients should be transferred on 100% O_2 and cardiac monitors. Copies of ECGs, relevant medical history, and exposure history should accompany the patient.

Complications and Sequelae

As has been noted, the most serious sequelae are adverse cardiac events (e.g., infarcts, arrhythmias) and neurologic injuries (e.g., cerebral edema, seizures, cognitive dysfunction, memory loss). Noncardiogenic pulmonary edema may also occur. Delayed neurologic sequelae may develop in up to 10% of patients. Children, pregnant women and their fetuses, the elderly, and those with underlying illnesses are most vulnerable.[15] HBO may decrease the incidence of delayed neurologic sequelae.[17] HBO may be complicated by barotrauma to the airways and ears. Pneumothorax is a contraindication to HBO.

Pediatrics

Young children and fetuses may be particularly vulnerable to CO toxicity. Fetal hemoglobin has a higher affinity for CO than does adult hemoglobin. Treatment decisions do not differ from those for adults.

Conclusion

Primary care and emergency medicine physicians should become familiar with the evaluation and treatment of environmental/occupational exposures typical of their local climate, fauna, industries, and recreational activities. They should know how to access local and national public health resources to gain information and to report environmental exposures and problems (see Box 25–2 for a partial listing). Many allergic and infectious emergencies can also be considered environmental (reference chapters on asthma, anaphylaxis, and infectious emergencies). Physicians treating patients with environmental diseases should consider how to treat them, how to triage them, how to refer them for tertiary care, how to prevent discharge back to an unsafe environment, and how to prevent exposures within their communities.

> ## Box 25–2. *Public Health Resources for Investigating and Reporting Environmental and Occupational Emergencies*
>
> Centers for Disease Control and Prevention
> 1-800-311-3435
> http://www.cdc.gov/netinfo.htm
>
> American College of Occupational and Environmental Medicine
> 847-818-1800
> http://www.acoem.org/
>
> Association of Occupational and Environmental Clinics
> 202-347-4976
> http://www.aoec.org
>
> The Environmental Health Information Service
> 919-541-3841
> http://ehis.niehs.nih.gov/
>
> CA Dept of Health Services' Hazard Evaluation System and
>   Information Service
> http://www.dhs.ca.gov/ohb/HESIS/hesfact.htm
>
> Agency for Toxic Substances and Disease Registry
> 1-888-422-8737
> http://www.atsdr.cdc.gov/atsdrhome.html
>
> Occupational and Environmental Medicine Resources
> http://occenvmed.net/

References

1. Pope AM, Ball DP (eds): Environmental Medicine. Washington, DC, National Academy Press (Institute of Medicine), 1995.
2. Goldman RH, Peters JM: The occupational and environmental history. JAMA 246:2831–2836, 1981.
3. Sanborn M, Abelson A: Environmental Health in Family Medicine (a curriculum). Available at http://www.ijc.org/boards/hptf/modules/content
4. Danzl DF, Pozos RS: Accidental hypothermia. N Engl J Med 331:1756–1760, 1994.
5. Besser HA: Hypothermia. In Tintinalli JE, Kelen GD, Stapczynski JS (eds): Emergency Medicine: A Comprehensive Study Guide, 5th ed. New York, McGraw-Hill, 2000, pp 1231–1235.
6. McCauley RL, Smith DJ, Robson MC: Frostbite and other cold-induced injuries. In Auerbach PS (ed): Wilderness Medicine, 3rd ed. St Louis, Mosby, 1995, pp 129–145.
7. Murphy K, Nowak RM, Tomlanovich MD: Use of bretylium tosylate as prophylaxis and treatment in hypothermic ventricular fibrillation in the canine model. Ann Emerg Med 15:1160–1165, 1986.
8. Centers for Disease Control and Prevention: Heat-related mortality: United States, 1997. MMWR 47:473, 1998.
9. Walker JS, Barnes SB: Heat Emergencies. In Tintinalli JE, Kelen GD, Stapczynski JS

(eds): Emergency Medicine: A Comprehensive Study Guide, 5th ed. New York, McGraw-Hill, 2000, pp 1235–1242.

10. Gochfeld M: Fire and pyrolysis products. In Broods S (ed): Environmental Medicine. St Louis, Mosby Year Book Medical Publishers, 1995.

11. Rioux JP, Myers RAM: Methylene chloride poisoning: A paradigmatic view. J Emerg Med 6:227–238, 1988.

12. Van Meter KW: Carbon monoxide poisoning. In Tintinalli JB, Kelen GD, Stapczynski JS (eds): Emergency Medicine: A Comprehensive Study Guide, 5th ed. New York, McGraw-Hill, 2000, pp 1302–1306.

13. Centers for Disease Control and Prevention: Unintentional carbon monoxide poisonings in residential settings. MMWR 44:765–767, 1995.

14. Centers for Disease Control and Prevention: Houseboat-associated carbon monoxide poisonings on Lake Powell–Arizona and Utah, 2000. MMWR 49:1105–1108, 2000.

15. Thom SR, Keim L: Carbon monoxide poisoning: A review. Clin Toxicol 27:141–156, 1989.

16. Seger D, Welch L: Carbon monoxide controversies: Neuropsychologic testing, mechanism of toxicity, and hyperbaric oxygen. Ann Emerg Med 24:242–248, 1994.

17. Thom SR, Taber RL, Mendiguren II, et al: Delayed neuropsychologic sequelae after carbon monoxide poisoning: Prevention by treatment with hyperbaric oxygen. Ann Emerg Med 25:474–480, 1995.

Chapter 26

Transport and Transfer of Emergency Patients

Raymond H. Lucas
Eugene Orientale, Jr.

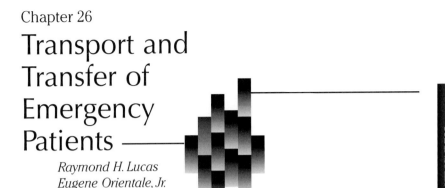

For the office or out-of-hospital emergency, transferring the patient safely to a hospital emergency department (ED) or other appropriate setting becomes of paramount importance soon after initial lifesaving interventions have been undertaken. The physician should be familiar with available transport options, the capability and scope of practice provided by ambulance personnel, and ways to access patient transportation systems. In addition, for the patient who is already hospitalized but needs transfer to a different hospital for a special procedure or a higher level of care, specific federal regulations exist to which he or she must adhere.

Additionally, it is not uncommon for patients, once they have been admitted to the hospital, to require transfer to another facility. Thus, the second part of this chapter discusses how to arrange a medically safe transfer that meets federal guidelines.

Emergency Medical Services (EMS) and Ambulance Transport Systems

"Is an Ambulance Necessary?"

Whether or not an ambulance is necessary is the first question that the clinician must answer when transferring a patient. Many patients in the office or clinic who need hospital admission may safely drive themselves or be driven by a family member. For example, an otherwise healthy patient who has stable vital signs and cellulitis and who has not responded to outpatient antibiotic therapy may not need an ambulance or arranged transport to a hospital ED. Other, sicker patients could deteriorate, however, if they drive themselves. The following guidelines will help the clinician to determine when ambulance transport is necessary:

361

1. Patients in shock or with unstable vital signs
   Example: Patients who are hypotensive
2. Patients with an altered mental status
   Example: Patients who are comatose, acutely psychotic, or delirious
3. Patients with acute respiratory emergencies that require oxygen or
   that create the possibility that the patient will need assisted ventilation
   Example: Asthmatic patients with labored respirations, anyone with
   low oxygen saturation, patients with stridor
4. Patients with unstable or potentially unstable cardiac arrhythmias
   Example: Someone with ventricular tachycardia, paroxysmal
   supraventricular tachycardia (PSVT), and concurrent chest pain; rapid
   atrial fibrillation; and pulmonary edema
5. Patients with a diagnosis that includes a short window of time for
   therapeutic intervention
   Example: Acute myocardial infarction, acute stroke, a pulseless
   extremity, toxin ingestion
6. Patients with physical impairments, acute or chronic, that make
   traveling otherwise impossible or difficult
   Example: Patients with certain back or hip injuries, hemiparesis,
   amputees, etc.
7. Patients who require immediate intervention that the office cannot
   provide but that is available from the Emergency Medical Services
   (EMS) system
   Example: Patients who require defibrillation, antiarrhythmic therapy,
   IV glucose, β-agonist therapy, immobilization of the spine, or a
   fractured extremity
8. Patients in active labor with imminent delivery
   Example: A multiparous woman 8 cm dilated with contractions
9. Any patient with the likelihood that one of the previously listed
   conditions could exist in the immediate future
   Example: Suspected acute myocardial infarction (MI)

In addition to patient clinical factors, other variables affect the decision
of whether to call 911 or another ambulance. These include time of day,
distance to the hospital, weather and traffic conditions, and typical response
time of the local EMS system. For example, it may take 5 to 20 minutes for
an ambulance to respond to a scene and another 10 minutes to get to the
hospital. However, if the office is only two blocks from the hospital, the
patient may get there faster if driven by family or staff with the physician
in attendance. On the other hand, a patient who presents to a rural office
setting with an acute MI may be best served by a helicopter landing in the
parking lot that transports patients directly to a cardiac referral center.

To make the best decisions for the patient, the physician should have
an understanding of the response time and the capabilities of the local
EMS system and private ambulance companies, as well as other factors

that can affect time of transport. When in doubt, a phone call to the emergency physician at the intended receiving hospital can provide valuable advice on the most appropriate form of transport.

"Should I Call 911 or a Private Ambulance Company?"

Once the decision to call an ambulance is made, the urgency of the situation dictates whom to call. Anyone with an acute life-threatening situation likely deserves a call to the EMS system for that community, usually by calling 911. When calling 911, an emergency medical dispatcher screens the call and determines the level of ambulance—Advanced Life Support (ALS) or Basic Life Support (BLS)—that will respond. Additionally, a first responder, usually a firefighter or sometimes a police officer, may be the initial person to respond before the ambulance. Most suburban and urban EMS systems strive for a 4-minute response time for BLS ambulances and an 8-minute response time for ALS ambulances. These response intervals are based on early EMS system research, which suggested that cardiopulmonary resuscitation (CPR) within 4 minutes and defibrillation within 8 minutes improved the patient's odds of surviving out-of-hospital cardiac arrest.[1, 2] Response times vary widely, however, from community to community and at different times of the day.

One should be aware that when emergency medical technicians (EMTs) or paramedics respond, they have their own medical protocols that they follow; these have been developed by their medical director. Also, many municipal EMS systems have a policy of transporting only to the closest hospital, which may not be the intended destination for your patient.

Private ambulance companies may be better suited for some patients, especially if the situation is not truly emergent. Private companies may take longer to respond to the scene but may be more flexible. They usually transport patients to any destination and may add additional personnel, such as a nurse or respiratory therapist, if needed for certain patients. Some commercial or hospital-based transport services may specialize in pediatric, perinatal, or neonatal transportation. Commercial ambulance companies may require a guarantee of payment up front; the 911 system will bill later or sometimes not at all.

"What Do BLS, ALS, EMT, and Paramedic Really Mean?"

Ambulances are equipped and staffed to various levels of patient care. Although it may be "safe" to always request the highest level of care available, it is also more costly and sometimes not necessary. In most locations, ambulances are staffed and equipped according to the prehospital provider curriculum levels approved by the U.S. Department of Transportation (DOT). Some variability exists from state to state in the exact scope of practice for prehospital providers.

First Responders

First responders do not staff transport ambulances, but usually a police officer or fireman trained to the first responder level is the first to arrive on the scene after 911 has been called. First responders are trained to administer CPR and oxygen and to provide basic airway management (i.e., jaw thrust, mouth-to-mask ventilation, bag-valve-mask ventilation, suctioning), as well as basic first aid such as control of hemorrhage, application of splints and bandages, and use of spinal immobilization. In some locations, first responders use automatic external defibrillators (AEDs). The DOT recommends a 40-hour didactic course of instruction. No clinical rotation is included as part of first responder training.[3]

Emergency Medical Technician-Basic (EMT-B)

Formerly known as an EMT-Ambulance (EMT-A), these providers staff basic life support, or the BLS level of ambulance. In addition to the skills of the first responder, EMT-Bs receive additional training in patient assessment skills, triage of multiple victims, emergency childbirth, and transportation skills, including lifting and carrying the patient. Recently added to the BLS curriculum is assistance of patients with their own medications, specifically nitroglycerin, metered-dose inhalers, and oral glucose. BLS providers are trained to use AEDs. The BLS curriculum is approximately 110 hours in length, including didactic training and clinical observation in the hospital. EMT-Bs are required by the National Registry of EMTs to receive 48 hours of continuing medical education and a 24-hour refresher course every 2 years.[4]

BLS or basic ambulances are useful for routine or noncritical patient transports. If the patient requires only oxygen, immobilization, or stretcher transport because of an injury or physical impairment, then a BLS ambulance is appropriate. Although they carry AEDs, BLS units cannot continuously monitor cardiac rhythm and are not suitable for patients with suspected coronary ischemia or cardiac complaints.

Emergency Medical Technician-Intermediate (EMT-I)

The EMT-I curriculum was developed to allow a wider scope of patient care in which paramedic-level care is not available or attainable. EMT-Is usually practice in rural settings or in volunteer EMS systems in which personnel cannot expend the time required for a full paramedic course. The exact skills of the intermediate-level EMT are variable from state to state.

In addition to the BLS skills listed previously, the EMT-I can provide IV therapy, some limited medications (usually some cardiac resuscitation medications), defibrillation, cardiac monitoring, and some adjunctive airway devices (pharyngotracheal lumen airway, esophageal obturator airway, etc.). In some locations, an EMT-I may staff an advanced-level ambulance if it is the most advanced level available in that location. In some places, an advanced-level ambulance may be staffed only if paired with a full paramedic. There is, however, usually not a designation as an "intermediate-level" ambulance. The recommended DOT curriculum for EMT-I is approximately 400 hours in length (in addition to BLS training), which includes didactic, hospital, and field training.[5]

Emergency Medical Technician-Paramedic (EMT-P)

The EMT-P or paramedic is the most advanced prehospital provider and can provide treatment for a wide variety of emergency conditions. In addition to the skill of the EMT-B, the paramedic can provide IV therapy, cardiac monitoring, defibrillation, and transcutaneous cardiac pacing. In many locations, paramedics perform 12-lead electrocardiograms (ECGs) but with only limited or computer-assisted interpretation. They can perform endotracheal intubation orally, nasally, or digitally. They can decompress a tension pneumothorax with a needle, and in some locations, they may perform a needle or surgical cricothyroidotomy. Paramedics administer a variety of medications, including standard cardiac resuscitation drugs, antiarrhythmics, diuretics, β agonists, diazepam, morphine, and others. A list of standard ALS medications used by paramedics is provided in Box 26–1.

Paramedics can operate only under a licensed medical director and can perform patient care by applying medical protocols. Under the approval of their medical director, in some locations they may perform more

---

Box 26–1. *Typical ALS Medications Used by Paramedics*

Activated charcoal	Lidocaine
Adenosine	Magnesium sulfate
Albuterol	Methylprednisolone
Amiodarone	Morphine
Atropine	Naloxone
Bretylium tosylate	Nifedipine
Calcium chloride	Nitroglycerin
Dextrose 50%	Nitrous oxide
Diazepam	Oxygen
Diphenhydramine	Procainamide
Dobutamine	Promethazine
Dopamine	Racemic epinephrine
Epinephrine	Sodium bicarbonate
Furosemide	Syrup of ipecac
Glucagon	Thiamine
Ipratropium bromide	Terbutaline
Labetalol	Verapamil

advanced care such as rapid sequence intubation with paralytic agents. In addition to written protocols, many EMS systems provide on-line medical direction by a physician via radio or cellular phone to assist the paramedic. Paramedics undergo approximately 1500 hours of instruction, in addition to BLS training, including didactic, hospital, and field training.[6] Every 2 years, they must undergo a 48-hour refresher course and 24 additional hours of continuing medical education. Many paramedic training programs are associate degree programs in community colleges.

Any critically ill or potentially critical patient should be transported by an ALS ambulance staffed by paramedics. Patients with cardiac complaints, respiratory problems that potentially need assisted ventilation, seizures, strokes, overdoses, or multiple trauma, and patients who require an IV or an urgent medication need an advanced-level ambulance.

Specialty Transport Services

In addition to standard BLS and ALS ambulances, in many communities there are aeromedical helicopters, "critical care transport," "pediatric life support transport," and other types of transport services available. There are no national standards for these, so the practitioner should contact these services directly to find out exactly the level of service and scope of practice they provide in any particular region. Most are staffed with paramedics who have received additional training and with nurses who have critical care experience. Some may be able to provide physician-level care during transport.

In isolated rural or remote locations, the physician should be familiar with the closest aeromedical helicopter program. How to access care, response time, the need for concurrent activation of the local EMS system, suitable landing zone requirements, payment requirements, and destination options are all items that need to be explored and understood. Typically, helicopters are activated only after the local EMS response to the scene, but in rural locations, it may be prudent to set up potential arrangements in advance. Most aeromedical programs can provide this information ahead of time so that office protocols can be written and easily referred to when an emergency occurs.

For the truly emergent patient, such as one with an acute MI or severe multiple trauma, critically ill children, one with extensive burns, and others, aeromedical transport directly to a specialty or tertiary care facility may be the best option for optimal patient care. If the patient needs urgent airway control or is in active labor, transport to the closest local hospital and subsequent aeromedical evacuation if needed are likely the best courses of action. It may be useful for physician's office personnel to construct a matrix of EMS resources available in their community as a quick reference for services provided, typical response times, means of activation, and other pertinent information. An example is provided in Table 26–1.

"When the Ambulance Arrives, Am I Still in Control of My Patient?"

Paramedics operate under protocols developed by their medical directors; however, there is room for input from the patients' private attending physicians.[7] Most paramedics have predesignated on-line physicians for medical control and advice. If the private attending physician wants to assume medical control of the scene, many jurisdictions have policies that the on-scene physician must then accompany the patient to

Table 26–1. Example Matrix of Emergency Medical Services Resources

Type of Service	Name	How to Call	Typical Response Times	Other
Basic ambulance (oxygen, first aid, stretcher transport)	County Fire and Rescue	911—Present information to dispatcher	4–6 min 15–20 min to community hospital	Will transport only to closest hospital
Advanced ambulance (airway procedures, cardiac monitor and drugs, IV therapy, etc.)	County Fire and Rescue	911—Present information to the dispatcher	8–10 min 15–20 min to community hospital 30 min to university hospital	Paramedics must follow their own medical protocols
Private ambulance BLS and ALS care available	ABC Ambulance Company	202–555–1212	30–90 min	Will take to any destination hospital or nursing facility. Will pick up patient from home. Credit card guarantee of payment required. Minimum $185.00
Helicopter (for critical or specialty care patients)	University Hospital Lifeflight	202–222–2222 Must speak with emergency department physician at university hospital to get approval	20 min 15 min back to university hospital	Must also call 911 to get assistance in setting up landing zone in parking lot. Will only take patient back to university hospital

ALS, Advanced life support; BLS, basic life support.

the hospital if he or she assumes medical control on the scene. Most issues, if they arise, can easily be resolved by having the on-scene physician talk to the designated medical control physician via phone or radio.

Patient Transfers from the Hospital

Although this is not specific to the office setting, when patient transfers are discussed, it is important for the clinician to understand how transfers from the office differ from those from the hospital. Transfers from the office to the hospital are handled at the discretion of the physician and the patient with little regulatory oversight other than statutes regarding EMS systems. Transfers *from* the hospital are very regulated and often scrutinized; thus, an understanding of the correct process is useful for all practitioners.

The situation commonly arises in which hospitalized patients require transfer to another hospital or health care facility. Reasons for transfers include the need for a higher level of care, a specialty procedure not available at the current hospital, patient request, insurance company request, and transfers to extended care facilities. Arrangements for these transfers are often facilitated by nursing staff or social services staff at the hospital, or by HMOs and insurance companies. However, the physician and the hospital have legal and medical responsibility for the patient until he or she arrives at the destination facility—thus an understanding of how to arrange a medically sound transport that also meets federal and state requirements is essential.

All patient transfers (interestingly, a patient discharge is also legally considered a "transfer") are governed by federal regulations found in the Consolidated Omnibus Budget Reconciliation Act (COBRA) of 1985, also known as the "Patient Dumping Law," "Patient Treatment Law," Section 1867 of the Social Security Act, or the Emergency Medical Treatment and Active Labor Act (EMTALA). Further regulations governing transfers are found in COBRA of 1986, specifically under section 9121, which is called "Miscellaneous Provisions."

All hospitals that accept payments from Medicare (which includes essentially all hospitals except military and veterans hospitals) are required to follow EMTALA rules for **all patients**, or risk a fine of up to $50,000 and lose their eligibility to collect Medicare payments. EMTALA is enforced and further interpreted by the Centers for Medicare and Medicaid Services (CMS). No state law that governs health care or patient transfers can supersede the requirements set forth in EMTALA. This is important because some of the newer state-mandated Medicaid managed care plans require transfers that may be in direct conflict with EMTALA.[8]

Transferring Stable Patients

EMTALA regulations regarding transfers do not apply to stable patients. A patient without an "emergency medical condition" is considered stable. An emergency medical condition is defined in EMTALA as "a medical condition manifesting itself by acute symptoms of sufficient severity (including severe pain) such that the absence of immediate medical attention could reasonably be expected to result in placement of the health of the patient or unborn child in serious jeopardy, serious impairment of bodily functions, or serious dysfunction of any bodily organ or part."

Furthermore, a stable patient is defined in EMTALA as one in whom "no material deterioration of the condition is likely, within reasonable medical probability, to result from or during the transfer of the individual." However, if any patient deteriorates en route, retrospectively he or she can be determined to be unstable by CMS or the courts.

Stable patients can be transferred for any reason, including economic ones, and the components for an "appropriate transfer" discussed below are not required under EMTALA. However, for optimum patient care, for uniform compliance when the regulations do apply, and for sound risk management, it is prudent to follow EMTALA rules for *all* patients, stable or unstable.

Transferring Unstable Patients

Unstable patients can be transferred only if they or the legal guardian personally requests in writing that they be transferred after they have been informed of the risks of transfer and of the hospital's obligation to treat or if the transfer is medically necessary. Medically necessary transfers are typically provided for a higher level of care or for special procedures not available at the sending facility. For a medically necessary transfer, the physician must sign a certification that, "based upon information available at the time of the transfer, the medical benefits reasonably expected from the provision of care at another medical facility outweigh the increased risks to the individual and, in the case of labor, to the unborn child from effecting the transfer." Once one of these two conditions is met, the transfer must additionally meet certain other requirements to be deemed "appropriate."

Appropriate Transfers

For a transfer to be appropriate according to EMTALA, the following criteria must be met:
1. The transferring hospital must have provided medical care within its capacity to minimize risks to the individual's or the unborn child's health.

2. The accepting facility must agree to provide the transfer and appropriate medical care. The accepting facility must have available space and qualified personnel to care for the patient.

3. The transferring hospital must send copies of all available medical records, radiographs, and test results regarding the patient's current emergency medical condition. The transferring hospital must also forward the name and address of any on-call physician who failed to appear within a reasonable time to provide necessary stabilizing treatment.

4. The transferring hospital must send a copy of the patient's written consent to transfer or a written certificate signed by a physician that the benefits of transfer outweigh the risks.

5. The transfer is effected through qualified personnel and transportation equipment, including the use of necessary and medically appropriate life support measures during transport.

6. The transfer meets other such requirements as the Secretary (of Health and Human Services) may find necessary in the interest of the health and safety of individuals transferred.

These guidelines are fairly straightforward. The decision to transfer an unstable patient for required treatment that is not available at the current hospital is a clinical judgment, often best made in conjunction with a specialist and the accepting physician. It is important that a physician-to-physician transfer of care be documented. Provision of copies of medical records typically is handled by the nursing or social services staff. Arranging qualified personnel and transportation equipment is often the difficult part of arranging an appropriate transfer.

The sending physician should specify in the transfer order what type of practitioner is required for the transfer—basic EMT, paramedic, nurse, physician, or otherwise. The order should be specific for ground ambulance (basic or advanced) or for helicopter transfer. Any special equipment such as a cardiac monitor or ventilator should be noted. Likewise, orders for any specific drips, medications, and other expected medical interventions en route should be clearly spelled out. Additionally, the transfer order should specifically spell out who will provide on-line medical direction for nonphysician practitioners and by what means during the transfer.[9] Many of these items are worked out by the ambulance company or EMS agency providing the transport, but it is the sending physician's responsibility to see that they are provided for and that they are medically appropriate.

Because the hospital is actually the entity that must be compliant with the law, most hospitals have standing transfer protocols and transfer forms that are well known to the staff. These are usually generated with approval of the hospital's risk management department to ensure compliance with EMTALA. Nevertheless, it is the physician who must sign the certificate of transfer and write the order in the medical record for the transfer. Thus, it is incumbent on all physicians who practice in hospitals to understand the issues and regulations surrounding patient transfers.

References

1. Smith JE: Administration, management, and operations. In Roush WR (ed): Principles of EMS Systems, 2nd ed. Dallas, American College of Emergency Physicians, 1994, p 115.
2. Eisenberg MS, Hallstrom AP, Copass MK, et al: Treatment of ventricular fibrillation: Emergency medical technician defibrillation and paramedic services. JAMA 251:1723–1726, 1984.
3. First responder national standard curriculum. Washington, DC, U.S. Department of Transportation, 1995.
4. Emergency medical technician—basic national standard curriculum. Washington, DC, U.S. Department of Transportation, 1994.
5. Emergency medical technician—intermediate national standard curriculum. Washington, DC, U.S. Department of Transportation, 1999.
6. Emergency medical technician—paramedic national standard curriculum. Washington, DC, U.S. Department of Transportation, 1999.
7. Policy statement: Direction of prehospital care at the scene of medical emergencies. Dallas, American College of Emergency Physicians, 1997.
8. Frew SA: Patient Transfers: How to Comply With the Law, 2nd ed. Dallas, American College of Emergency Physicians, 1995.
9. Policy statement: Medical direction of interfacility patient transfers. Dallas, American College of Emergency Physicians, 1997.

Chapter 27
Bioterrorism
C. Crawford Mechem

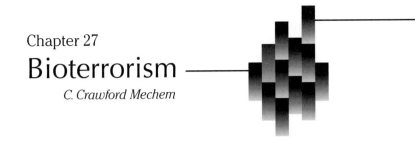

Terrorism has been defined as "premeditated, politically motivated violence perpetrated against noncombatant targets by subnational groups or clandestine agents," usually intended to influence an audience.[1] Bioterrorism refers to the use of biological agents to effect this objective. Until recently, the threat that an individual or terrorist group would use a biological agent against a civilian population seemed to be small. This threat became more real, however, on October 2, 2001, when a 63-year-old photo editor working for a Florida newspaper presented to a local emergency department with fever, vomiting, and confusion.[2] *Bacillus anthracis*, the causative organism for anthrax, was isolated from cultures of both cerebrospinal fluid (CSF) and blood. The patient died on October 5 despite aggressive antibiotic and supportive therapy.[2] Subsequently, a total of 22 confirmed or suspected cases of anthrax resulting from deliberate dissemination through the postal system were identified by the Centers for Disease Control and Prevention (CDC). These included 11 confirmed cases of inhalational anthrax and 11 cases of confirmed or suspected cutaneous anthrax. Five victims died.[11, 12]

The medical response to the 2001 anthrax release involved the close collaboration of federal, state, and local public health and emergency response professionals. Primary care physicians also played a role. Some victims were sick enough to be taken directly to emergency departments. Others first saw their private physicians and were referred to local hospitals. It is anticipated that in the event of a future act of bioterrorism, primary care physicians will play an important role in the response through early recognition of victims, prompt notification of public health officials, and administration of postexposure prophylaxis when indicated. In addition, primary care physicians will be called on to exclude disease diagnosis among those who were never exposed, yet are still concerned— the so-called "worried well."[4]

Classification

Potential bioterrorism weapons include bacteria, viruses, and biological toxins. The CDC has divided these agents into three different categories based on their ease of dissemination or person-to-person transmission, mortality rate, potential to cause panic or social disruption, and requirement for special public health measures to respond to an attack.[5] Category A is the group that is potentially most dangerous. This category consists of the causative agents for anthrax, plague, tularemia, botulism, smallpox, and Ebola and other viral hemorrhagic fevers.[5] Of these, only plague, smallpox, and the viral hemorrhagic fevers are easily transmitted from person to person.[5-7] Category B contains organisms that are moderately easy to disseminate. These organisms are associated with lower mortality rates; they require enhancement of the CDC's diagnostic capacity, as well as enhanced disease surveillance.[5] This group includes the causative organisms for Q fever, glanders, and brucellosis; food safety threats such as *Salmonella* species and *Escherichia coli*; threats to water supplies such as *Vibrio cholerae*; and the toxins ricin and staphylococcal enterotoxin B.[5] Category C includes emerging infectious diseases such as the Hantaviruses, as well as organisms that are genetically engineered or modified to increase their ease of transmission or their potential mortality rates.[5] This chapter discusses agents from Category A.

Clinical Recognition

Acts of bioterrorism will in most cases be covert. Therefore, rapid response requires early recognition of the clues that an incident has occurred. These clues include large numbers of patients seeking care for similar signs and symptoms, many of whom may be critically ill; higher morbidity or mortality from a common disease or failure of the condition to respond to standard therapy; a single case of a very uncommon disease; diagnosis of a disease uncommon for a given geographic area or a given population; multiple clusters of a disease in areas that are not geographically contiguous; a tight cluster of cases with a common point source; and a large number of unexpected deaths among animals.[8, 10] Some of these clues may be recognized by primary care physicians, whereas others are detected through disease surveillance or epidemiologic investigations by public health officials.[9]

Diagnosis of the specific diseases caused by bioterrorism agents is made on clinical grounds combined with laboratory and radiologic testing. Because many of the diagnostic tests are highly specialized and handling of specimens from patients may require elaborate isolation precautions, all diagnostic testing should be conducted in close cooperation with public health officials.

PHONE TRIAGE ◄───────────────────────────

Many of the agents that may be used in acts of bioterrorism initially produce nonspecific symptoms that may be easily confused with benign viral illness.[11] Therefore, making this distinction through telephone interview of patients may be impossible. Once an act of bioterrorism has been identified, however, primary care physicians, working in conjunction with public health officials, can pass specific recommendations on to patients. These can range from seeking immediate medical attention to remaining at home unless specific symptoms develop, thereby minimizing the risk of person-to-person transmission.[9]

Treatment and Disposition

What follows is an overview of the six bioterrorism agents classified in Category A by the CDC. These are agents of highest priority, and their use requires immediate recognition and management.

Anthrax

Anthrax is caused by *Bacillus anthracis*, a large, Gram-positive, spore-forming rod.[12] Under natural conditions, human cases usually occur as a result of occupational exposure to spores on animals or animal hides in the textile or tanning industry.[13] Three distinct forms of anthrax can occur—cutaneous, gastrointestinal, and inhalational. Cutaneous anthrax develops when spores penetrate nonintact skin. The first manifestation is a small, pruritic macule or papule that progresses to a vesicle.[12] After a week, the vesicle ruptures and is replaced by a black eschar.[12] Usually the disease remains localized, but it can disseminate systemically. Gastrointestinal anthrax results when a patient has eaten infected meat. Symptoms include abdominal pain, fever, nausea, vomiting, and diarrhea. Gastrointestinal hemorrhage may be caused by localized intestinal necrosis.

Inhalational anthrax as a result of aerosol release is the form most likely to be encountered in the setting of bioterrorism.[3, 13] Disease results from inhalation of a minimum of 4000 to 8000 spores.[12, 13] After an incubation period of 1 to 6 days, patients develop a prodrome of fever, malaise, headache, adenopathy, dry cough, and chest pressure. Sore throat and rhinorrhea are conspicuously absent, helping to distinguish anthrax from viral upper respiratory tract infections.[12, 13] The patient's condition may briefly improve, but then it abruptly deteriorates, with respiratory distress, hypoxemia, and cyanosis. There may be meningeal involvement in 50% of cases, with meningeal signs and decreased level of consciousness.[12, 13] Without early antimicrobial therapy, bacteremia and death rapidly follow. The mortality rate in untreated cases exceeds 95%.[13]

Diagnosis is made on clinical grounds combined with confirmatory tests, which include Gram stains and cultures of blood and CSF, enzyme-linked immunosorbent assays (ELISAs), and immunohistochemical studies. Health care providers who identify a patient suspected of having been exposed to anthrax should contact their local public health department immediately. Public health officials will arrange for appropriate diagnostic testing and can make recommendations on management.[13]

Treatment of inhalational anthrax involves supportive care combined with antibiotic therapy. The CDC recommends that patients receive a multidrug regimen of either ciprofloxacin or doxycycline administered intravenously combined with one or two additional agents, including a quinolone, rifampin, vancomycin, imipenem, clindamycin, or an aminoglycoside.[13] The mortality rate for fully developed inhalational anthrax approaches 100%.[2] If treatment is initiated during the incubation period, this may be cut to 1%. Because the disease is not spread from person to person, elaborate personal protective equipment for health care providers is not necessary.[14] If the diagnosis is in question, however, use of a high-efficiency particulate air (HEPA) filter mask would be prudent.[14]

Plague

Plague is caused by *Yersinia pestis*. Under natural conditions, the disease is spread by biting fleas that infest rodents such as rats. Plague can manifest in three different clinical forms: bubonic, septicemic, and pneumonic. In the United States, 85% to 90% of cases of naturally acquired disease are of the bubonic form, 10% to 15% are septicemic, and 1% are pneumonic.[5] In the context of bioterrorism, the bacterium would most likely be disseminated as an aerosol.[11] Therefore, the pneumonic form would predominate. Pneumonic plague, the so-called "Black Death" of the Middle Ages, is the most severe form of the disease. Patients present with fever, cough, hemoptysis, and chest pain. Meningitis may also develop. Chest radiography reveals bronchopneumonia that is usually bilateral. Untreated, pneumonic plague has a mortality rate of almost 100%.[5]

Diagnosis may be made by Gram stain of sputum (which demonstrates Gram-negative coccobacilli with a characteristic safety pin morphology) combined with sputum culture. A direct fluorescent antibody stain of capsular antigen is also available.

Treatment of pneumonic plague includes isolation of the patient for up to 96 hours after initiation of antibiotic therapy. Because the disease is readily spread by inhalation of respiratory droplets, gloves, a gown, and respiratory protection such as a HEPA filter mask should be worn by health care providers.[14] Streptomycin is the antibiotic of choice. Chloramphenicol should be added in cases with meningeal involvement. Survival is unlikely if antibiotics are not initiated within 18 hours of symptom onset.

Tularemia

Tularemia is a zoonosis caused by *Francisella tularensis*, a Gram-negative intracellular coccobacillus. In the United States, its principal reservoir is the tick, and it is transmitted by rabbits. The bacterium is readily aerosolized and highly infectious, making it a potent bioterrorism agent.[5] Inhalational tularemia results from inhalation of as few as 10 to 50 organisms; it presents as an acute febrile illness that develops 3 to 5 days after exposure. One of two distinct clinical entities follows—the more common ulceroglandular form and a typhoidal form. The ulceroglandular form is characterized by lesions of the skin or mucous membranes, lymph nodes greater than 1 cm in diameter, or both. The typhoidal form is characterized by lymph nodes less than 1 cm in diameter and no skin lesions. Patients with the ulceroglandular form may develop fever, chills, myalgias, headache, stiff neck, pharyngitis, cough, dyspnea, chest pain, abdominal pain, diarrhea, and back pain. A cutaneous chancre-like lesion up to 3 cm in diameter develops in the majority of cases. Enlarged lymph nodes are frequently seen and may be the only physical finding. Approximately 30% of patients with ulceroglandular tularemia and 80% of patients with the typhoidal form develop pneumonia.

Diagnosis is made by culture or by serologic tests such as an ELISA. Serologic response may be delayed by several weeks after the onset of symptoms, however.

Treatment includes prompt antibiotic administration. Streptomycin is the drug of choice. Gentamicin is an alternative. With appropriate treatment, the mortality rate is 1% to 2%. Patients who are not adequately treated may develop a protracted course of malaise, weakness, and weight loss. Human-to-human transmission is unusual, so respiratory isolation is unnecessary.

Smallpox

Smallpox is caused by the variola virus, an *Orthopoxvirus*. Inhalation of as few as 10 to 100 virus particles is sufficient to cause disease.[7] It is readily transmitted from person to person and is associated with a high mortality rate, making it an important bioterrorism weapon. Historically, the mortality rate among unvaccinated individuals has been 30%.[5, 7] Smallpox is the only infectious disease eradicated as a result of human intervention. Following an aggressive vaccination program, the World

Health Organization declared the disease eradicated in 1980. Currently, there are only two known repositories of smallpox, one at the CDC in Atlanta and one at the Vector Laboratories in Russia. There is strong evidence, however, that the former Soviet Union maintained an active offensive biological warfare program well into the 1990s, which included weaponization of smallpox.[8] The fate of those stocks is a matter of speculation. Therefore, any case of smallpox should be assumed to result from an act of bioterrorism.

After an incubation period of 7 to 17 days, patients develop a prodrome of fever, delirium, myalgias, headache, rigors, vomiting, and backache. The characteristic rash appears 48 to 72 hours after the prodrome. It begins as macules that evolve into papules and then pustules. Lesions begin on the oral mucosa, then spread to the face, forearms, hands, and finally, the lower extremities and trunk. This is in contrast to varicella lesions, which start on the trunk and move peripherally. Also, unlike varicella, the lesions of smallpox develop synchronously.

Definitive diagnosis is made (1) by cultures obtained from swabs of the oropharynx or of freshly opened pustules, (2) by electron microscopy of vesicle fluid, or (3) by polymerase chain reaction (PCR) assays.[7] Isolation of the virus requires a Biosafety Level 4 (BSL-4) laboratory, which is found only at the CDC and the U.S. Army Medical Research Institute of Infectious Diseases (USAMRIID) at Fort Detrick, Maryland.[4] Therefore, local health officials should be notified before any specimens are collected.

Treatment is supportive. The patient should be placed in contact and droplet isolation. The patient and anyone he or she may have contacted within the previous 17 days should remain in isolation until a definitive diagnosis is made, which requires a viral culture performed at the CDC. All individuals exposed to aerosolized smallpox or to clinical cases should be vaccinated immediately. The vaccinia vaccine currently licensed in the United States ameliorates or prevents illness if given within 4 days of exposure. Vaccine is available only from the CDC. Vaccination is not without risk. Approximately 1 of 1 million individuals vaccinated for the first time will die of complications, usually postvaccinial encephalitis or disseminated vaccinia.[15]

Viral Hemorrhagic Fever

Viral hemorrhagic fever (VHF) viruses include the arenavirus, phleboviruses, Nairovirus, Hantaviruses, filoviruses, and flaviviruses.[6] The filoviruses are the most dreaded and include Ebola and Marburg. Ebola virus was first reported in 1976 along the Ebola River in Zaire and Sudan. Two thirds of those infected were health care workers administering to patients. Marburg virus was first reported in 1967 following an outbreak in Marburg, Germany. In the United States, cases of hemorrhagic fever generally involve individuals who have recently arrived from overseas. No human cases of Ebola or Marburg virus disease have been reported in the United States. Any case of viral hemorrhagic fever should raise suspicion for an act of bioterrorism.

Incubation periods range from 2 to 21 days. Initial signs and symptoms may include fever, headache, fatigue, abdominal pain, and myalgias, followed by hematemesis, bloody diarrhea, mucous membrane hemorrhage, diffuse petechiae or ecchymoses, altered mental status, and cardiovascular collapse.[6] Case mortality rates for VHF range from 10% (Dengue hemorrhagic fever) to 90% (Zaire strain of Ebola).

Diagnosis can be made by serologic tests, including ELISA and PCR, or by tissue culture. Any suspected cases should be immediately reported to local public health authorities, who will most likely contact the CDC. Hemorrhagic fevers may be transmitted by body fluids or by respiratory droplet exposure. They may also be spread by aerosol. Thus, patients should be placed in a negative pressure room. Health care providers should use universal precautions combined with a HEPA filter mask. Few specific treatments exist. Intravenous and oral ribavirin have been used successfully for cases of Lassa fever and Hantavirus. Otherwise, management is supportive. Antiplatelet drugs should be avoided. Intravenous line placement should be kept to a minimum because of the risk of uncontrollable bleeding, as well as the risk of needle sticks to health care providers.

Botulism

Botulism results from exposure to toxins produced by *Clostridium botulinum*, a Gram-positive bacillus. Botulinum toxins are the most potent toxins known; they produce their effects by blocking the presynaptic release of acetylcholine. They have a high potential as bioterrorist weapons because of their high lethality, ease of production, and ease of aerosolization. Symptoms develop several hours to days after exposure. Patients may present with a variety of neurologic signs and symptoms, including dysphagia, dysarthria, dysphonia, diplopia, ptosis, blurred vision, mydriasis, descending weakness, and respiratory failure. Sensation remains intact.

Diagnosis is made on clinical grounds. A bioterrorist incident involving botulinum toxin should be suspected if there are multiple victims with descending paralysis and no fever. Laboratory confirmation can be made by ELISA testing of nasal swabs for up to 24 hours after exposure.

Treatment is predominantly supportive. With ventilatory support, the mortality rate should be less than 5%. For confirmed cases, a trivalent equine antitoxin is available.

Pediatrics

Management of pediatric victims of bioterrorism incidents is similar to that of adults. Once disease is suspected or identified, local public health officials should be notified and their recommendations for patient isolation, management, and referral followed. In general, the same antibiotics used for adult victims are used for children. Specific disease information is available from the CDC website at http://www.cdc.gov.

Conclusion

The primary care physician's role in the response to a bioterrorism incident includes early recognition, prompt notification of public health officials, and initiation of treatment or postexposure prophylaxis according to their recommendations. Because any such incident will cause a great deal of anxiety among the general public, primary care physicians will also play an important role in educating their patient population and allaying the concerns of those who have not been exposed.

References

1. Annual country reports on terrorism. U.S. Code, Title 22, Chapter 38, Sec. 2656f. Available at http://www4.law.cornell.edu/uscode/22/2656f.html
2. Bush LM, Abrams BH, Beall AB, Johnson CC: Index case of fatal inhalational anthrax due to bioterrorism in the United States. N Engl J Med 345:1607–1610, 2001.
3. Jernigan JA, Stephens DS, Ashford DA, et al: Bioterrorism-related inhalational anthrax: The first 10 cases reported in the United States. Emerg Infect Dis 7:933–944, 2001.
4. Gerberding JL, Hughes JM, Koplan JP: Bioterrorism preparedness and response: Clinicians and public health agencies as essential partners. JAMA 287:898–900, 2002.
5. Centers for Disease Control and Prevention: Biological diseases/agents listing, 2002. Available at http://www.bt.cdc.gov/Agent/Agentlist.asp
6. Pigott DC, Shope RE, McGovern TW: Viral hemorrhagic fevers. eMed J 3:2002. Available at http://www.emedicine.com/emerg/topic887.html
7. Hogan CJ, Harchelroad F, McGovern TW: Smallpox. eMed J 3:2002. Available at http://www.emedicine.com/emerg/topic885.html
8. Eitzen EM, Office of the Surgeon General: Use of biological weapons. In Sidell FR, Takafuji ET, Franz DR (eds): Medical Aspects of Chemical and Biological Warfare. Washington, DC, TMM Publications, 1997, pp 437-450.
9. Jagminas L, Marcozzi DE, Mothershead JL: Biological warfare mass casualty management. eMed J 2:2001. Available at http://www.emedicine.com/emerg/topic896.html
10. Marcozzi DE, Jagminas L: Evaluation of a biological warfare victim. eMed J 2:2001. Available at http://www.emedicine.com/emerg/topic891.html
11. Dire DJ, McGovern TW: Biological warfare agents. eMed J 3:2002. Available at http://www.emedicine.com/emerg/topic853.html
12. Cranmer H: Anthrax infection. eMed J 3:2002. Available at http://www.emedicine.com/emerg/topic864.html
13. Update: Investigation of bioterrorism-related anthrax and interim guidelines for exposure management and antimicrobial therapy. MMWR Morb Mortal Wkly Rep 50:909–919, 2001.
14. Arnold JL, Lavonas E: Personal protective equipment. eMed J 2:2001. Available at http://www.emedicine.com/emerg/topic894.html
15. Vaccinia (smallpox) vaccine: Recommendations of the Advisory Committee on Immunization Practices (ACIP), 2001. MMWR Morb Mortal Wkly Rep 50(RR-10):1–25, 2001.

BIOTERRORISM

Index